HELPING PARENTS AND TEACHERS UNDERSTAND MEDICATIONS FOR BEHAVIORAL AND EMOTIONAL PROBLEMS

A Resource Book of Medication Information Handouts

FOURTH EDITION

HELPING PARENTS AND TEACHERS UNDERSTAND MEDICATIONS FOR BEHAVIORAL AND EMOTIONAL PROBLEMS

A Resource Book of Medication Information Handouts

FOURTH EDITION

EDITED BY

MINA K. DULCAN, M.D.

RACHEL BALLARD, M.D.

CONTRIBUTORS

Rachel Ballard, M.D.

Thomas Cummins, M.D.

Mina K. Dulcan, M.D.

Nicholas Hatzis, M.D.

Anna Ivanenko, M.D., Ph.D.

Margery Johnson, M.D.

MaryBeth Lake, M.D.

James Mackenzie, D.O.

Rebecca O'Donnell, M.D.

Sigita Plioplys, M.D.

Heide Hullsiek Rollings, M.D.

Alex Timchak, M.D.

Department of Child and Adolescent Psychiatry, Ann & Robert H. Lurie Children's Hospital of Chicago; Division of Child and Adolescent Psychiatry, Northwestern University Feinberg School of Medicine, Chicago, Illinois

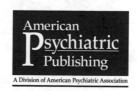

American Psychiatric Publishing
A Division of American Psychiatric Association

Washington, DC
London, England

To buy 25–99 copies of this or any other APPI title, please contact APPI Customer Service at appi@psych.org or 800-368-5777 for a 20% discount. To buy 100 or more copies of the same title, please e-mail bulksales@ psych.org for a price quote.

Manufactured in the United States of America on acid-free paper
18 17 16 15   4 3 2 1
Fourth Edition

Typeset in Adobe's Janson Text, AG Book Rounded, and Frutiger.

American Psychiatric Publishing, Inc.
1000 Wilson Boulevard
Arlington, VA 22209–3901
www.appi.org

Library of Congress Cataloging-in-Publication Data

Helping parents and teachers understand medications for behavioral and emotional problems : a resource book of medication information handouts / edited by Mina K. Dulcan, Rachel Ballard ; contributors, Thomas Cummins [and 11 others]. — Fourth edition.
 p. ; cm.
 Preceded by: Helping parents, youth, and teachers understand medications for behavioral and emotional problems / edited by Mina K. Dulcan ; contributors, Thomas Cummins ... [et al.]. 3rd ed. c2007.
 Includes bibliographical references and index.
 ISBN 978-1-58562-506-2 (pb : alk. paper)
 I. Dulcan, Mina K., editor. II. Ballard, Rachel, 1964– , editor. III. Cummins, Thomas K., contributor. IV. Title.
 [DNLM: 1. Child Behavior Disorders—drug therapy. 2. Adolescent. 3. Child. 4. Patient Education as Topic. 5. Patient Medication Knowledge. 6. Psychotropic Drugs—pharmacology. WS 350.6]
 RJ504.7
 618.92'8918—dc23
                                                                              2014049976

British Library Cataloguing in Publication Data

A CIP record is available from the British Library.

Contents

Contributors

Rachel Ballard, M.D.

Attending Physician, Outpatient Psychiatry, Department of Child and Adolescent Psychiatry, Ann & Robert H. Lurie Children's Hospital of Chicago; Assistant Professor of Psychiatry and Behavioral Sciences, Northwestern University Feinberg School of Medicine, Chicago, Illinois

Thomas Cummins, M.D.

Medical Director, Inpatient Psychiatry, Department of Child and Adolescent Psychiatry, Ann & Robert H. Lurie Children's Hospital of Chicago; Assistant Professor of Psychiatry and Behavioral Sciences, Northwestern University Feinberg School of Medicine, Chicago, Illinois

Mina K. Dulcan, M.D.

Head, Department of Child and Adolescent Psychiatry, Margaret C. Osterman Professor of Child Psychiatry, Ann & Robert H. Lurie Children's Hospital of Chicago; Head, Division of Child and Adolescent Psychiatry, Professor of Psychiatry and Behavioral Sciences and Pediatrics, Northwestern University Feinberg School of Medicine, Chicago, Illinois

Nicholas Hatzis, M.D.

Medical Director, Partial Hospitalization Program, Department of Child and Adolescent Psychiatry, Ann & Robert H. Lurie Children's Hospital of Chicago; Instructor of Psychiatry and Behavioral Sciences, Northwestern University Feinberg School of Medicine, Northwestern University, Chicago, Illinois

Anna Ivanenko, M.D., Ph.D.

Medical Director, Pediatric Sleep Medicine Program, Alexian Brothers Medical Center and Central DuPage Hospital; Associate Professor of Clinical Psychiatry and Behavioral Sciences, Northwestern University Feinberg School of Medicine, Chicago, Illinois

Margery Johnson, M.D.

Medical Director, Outpatient Psychiatry, Department of Child and Adolescent Psychiatry, Ann & Robert H. Lurie Children's Hospital of Chicago; Assistant Professor of Psychiatry and Behavioral Sciences, Northwestern University Feinberg School of Medicine, Chicago, Illinois

MaryBeth Lake, M.D.

Attending Physician, Outpatient Psychiatry, Department of Child and Adolescent Psychiatry, Ann & Robert H. Lurie Children's Hospital of Chicago; Associate Professor of Psychiatry and Behavioral Sciences, Northwestern University Feinberg School of Medicine, Chicago, Illinois

James Mackenzie, D.O.

Medical Director, Consultation/Liaison and Emergency Services, Department of Child and Adolescent Psychiatry, Ann & Robert H. Lurie Children's Hospital of Chicago; Assistant Professor of Psychiatry and Behavioral Sciences, Northwestern University Feinberg School of Medicine, Chicago, Illinois

Rebecca O'Donnell, M.D.

Attending Physician, Outpatient Psychiatry, Department of Child and Adolescent Psychiatry, Ann & Robert H. Lurie Children's Hospital of Chicago; Instructor of Psychiatry and Behavioral Sciences, Northwestern University Feinberg School of Medicine, Chicago, Illinois

Sigita Plioplys, M.D.

Attending Physician, Outpatient Psychiatry, Department of Child and Adolescent Psychiatry, Ann & Robert H. Lurie Children's Hospital of Chicago; Assistant Professor of Psychiatry and Behavioral Sciences, Northwestern University Feinberg School of Medicine, Chicago, Illinois

Heide Hullsiek Rollings, M.D.

Fellow, Department of Child and Adolescent Psychiatry, Ann & Robert H. Lurie Children's Hospital of Chicago, Chicago, Illinois

Alex Timchak, M.D.
Attending Physician, Outpatient Psychiatry and Partial Hospitalization Program, Department of Child, Adolescent, and Adult Psychiatry, Compass Health Center, Northbrook, Illinois

The following contributor to this book has indicated a financial interest in or other affiliation with a commercial supporter, manufacturer of a commercial product, and/or provider of a commercial service as listed below:

Mina K. Dulcan, M.D.—*Consultant:* Care Management Technologies, Inc. (a company that develops medication guidelines for managed care and Medicaid)

Introduction for Clinicians to the Fourth Edition

The medication information handouts in this book are intended for use in the context of clinical psychiatric evaluation and treatment of children and adolescents. The purpose of these handouts is to share basic information about medications with parents and teachers. The information sheets do not cover all possible side effects and are not intended for use as informed consent forms. They do not include educational information about psychiatric disorders. Suggested resources are provided in the pages following this introduction, preceding the medication information sheets. The medication information sheets should be used by prescribing physicians, advanced practice nurses, and physician assistants with patients and families to supplement an ongoing dialogue regarding the indications for medications, medication effects, and side effects. The sheets are not meant to be guides for prescribing medicine but rather to be used once the decision is made to prescribe a particular medication for a particular patient or for parents to learn more about a medication before agreeing to its prescription for their child. The sheets are valuable for teachers (and school nurses) in helping understand the medications used by students. In our clinical practice at Ann & Robert H. Lurie Children's Hospital of Chicago, nonphysician mental health professionals have found these sheets to be useful when proposing to patients and families an evaluation for possible medication.

This edition welcomes a new coeditor, Rachel Ballard, M.D., who is both a child and adolescent psychiatrist and a pediatrician, with clinical experience in both specialties.

Information on each medication in this fourth edition has been completely updated from the third edition (published in 2007). New medications and new formulations of older medications have been added, along with several supplements that are often used for mental health problems and that have some empirical support. The medications used for sleep have been reorganized, to group similar drugs. New concerns about potential side effects and U.S. Food and Drug Administration (FDA) black box warnings have been addressed. The medications are placed alphabetically by their generic names. The various formulations of stimulant medications are placed in two information sheets according to the active ingredient, methylphenidate/dexmethylphenidate or amphetamine. It is always a dilemma whether to focus on generic names or brand names. In this edition, we have chosen to use the generic names more often, because more medications are going off-patent and more formulations are available and to minimize the commercial focus. As before, we use only U.S. brand names. For some drugs (e.g., amitriptyline and chlorpromazine) the brand name drugs are no longer available, but the brand names are so commonly used that we continue to list them along with the generic names.

Appendices list medications typically used for certain indications, in case the clinician wishes to discuss options with the family or to check off which medications have been tried as he or she reviews the patient's medication history with the family. The information on additional mental health resources—books, journals, newsletters, and Internet sites—has been updated.

We have not included some medications (like monoamine oxidase inhibitors or cognitive enhancers) that are virtually never used for youth because of unacceptable side-effect profiles and/or lack of evidence for efficacy. Some medications have been included although they are rarely, if ever, prescribed in our practice because we have observed those drugs being used in the community, and we feel that patients should have the opportunity for information. For medications not included in this book, or for more sophisticated and detailed information targeted at highly educated "consumers," an excellent resource is *What Your Patients Need to Know About Psychiatric Medications*, by Hales, Yudofsky, and Chew (American Psychiatric Publishing 2005). The format and intended use are the same as this book, but the target audience is psychiatrists caring for adult patients.

All of the contributors to this book are experienced child and adolescent psychiatrist clinicians who use psychopharmacology as one component of comprehensive mental health treatment of children and adolescents. In the years since the publication of the third edition, we have found that many families have become more sophisticated about psychotropic medications due to increasingly available helpful information from patient–professional advocacy groups and more dramatic but less helpful attention from the media. The decision with regard to the complexity of the information sheets must always be weighed against the reality of the variability in reading levels in order for the information sheets to be accessible to the largest possible audience of families. We hope that we have found the right balance. For brevity and readability, many details and much explanation have been omitted, as well as very rare or poorly documented side effects. Each clinician is likely to disagree with some aspect of what we have written. The handouts are offered as a resource to those who find them useful, not as a standard for psychopharmacology practice. Only the most common indications are included. If a specific indication has been omitted, that does not necessarily mean that it is inappropriate.

The information provided in these sheets is based on the available scientific literature and the clinical experience of the authors and their colleagues. Many of the clinical indications for medication have not received FDA approval and therefore are not listed in the *Physicians' Desk Reference* (PDR). However, once a drug is approved for any indication, the FDA regulates only the company's advertising of the drug, not what physicians may prescribe. Nearly all psychopharmacological agents and indications (and the majority of the drugs used in pediatrics, as well) lack pediatric labeling and are "unapproved" or "off-label" for use in children, at least for certain age groups and indications. Off-label use may be accepted practice, appropriate, and rational. It is important to note that the FDA guidelines as published in the PDR cannot be relied on for appropriate indications, age ranges, or dosages for children. Sources such as the PDR are increasingly available to lay consumers, making the information in this book even more necessary. Lack of FDA approval for an age group or a disorder does not imply improper or illegal use. As a result of pressure from the FDA and financial incentives (via extending the patent on drugs), pharmaceutical companies have increased their attention to research in children. The Best Pharmaceuticals for Children Act mandates that for any drug that receives pediatric exclusivity (i.e., 6-month extension of patent exclusivity) the manufacturer must submit data to the FDA on all pediatric adverse event reports for 1 year following the granting of extended exclusivity. This requirement, in addition to applications for new indications, has increased the opportunities for discussion of potential side effects. However, while knowledge of potential risks is clearly beneficial, the resulting FDA hearings and advisory committee meetings have given antipsychiatry groups, such as the Citizens Commission on Human Rights and the Alliance for Human Research Protection, highly visible opportunities for testimony opposing psychiatric medications and even questioning the validity of diagnoses. Unfortunately, this attention to supposed side effects, fueled by attention from the media and plaintiff attorneys, has frightened parents and some physicians and is also likely to dampen industry enthusiasm to pursue needed research in pediatric psychopharmacology. The National Institute of Mental Health budget is unlikely to allow for the large, long-term studies needed to assess efficacy and safety. In the meantime, practitioners must do the best they can to help children and families struggling with mental illness, using the available evidence, good clinical judgment, and appropriate caution.

Selected Additional Reading for Health and Mental Health Professionals

Books

Barkley RA: *Attention-Deficit Hyperactivity Disorder: A Handbook for Diagnosis and Treatment*, 4th Edition. New York, Guilford, 2014

Dulcan MK, Lake MB: *Concise Guide to Child and Adolescent Psychiatry*, 4th Edition. Washington, DC, American Psychiatric Publishing, 2012

Elbe D, Bezchlibnyk-Butler KZ, Virani AS, et al. (eds): *Clinical Handbook of Psychotropic Drugs for Children and Adolescents.* Boston, MA, Hogrefe Publishing, 2015

Klykylo WM, Bowers R, et al.: *Green's Child and Adolescent Clinical Psychopharmacology*, 5th Edition. Philadelphia, PA, Lippincott Williams & Wilkins, 2014

McVoy M, Findling RL: *Clinical Manual of Child and Adolescent Psychopharmacology*, 2nd Edition. Washington, DC, American Psychiatric Publishing, 2013

Journals

Journal of the American Academy of Child and Adolescent Psychiatry, Elsevier; www.jaacap.com

Journal of Child and Adolescent Psychopharmacology, Mary Ann Liebert; www.liebertpub.com

Newsletters

The Brown University Child and Adolescent Psychopharmacology Update, John Wiley & Sons, http://onlinelibrary.wiley.com/journal/10.1002/(ISSN)1556-7567

Child and Adolescent Psychopharmacology News, Guilford Press, http://www.guilford.com/journals/Child-and-Adolescent-Psychopharmacology-News/Robert-Findling/10850295

Internet

American Academy of Child and Adolescent Psychiatry; www.aacap.org/

Published Resources for Parents and Teachers

Books

American Academy of Child and Adolescent Psychiatry: *Your Child: What Every Parent Needs to Know*. New York, HarperCollins, 1998

American Academy of Child and Adolescent Psychiatry: *Your Adolescent: Emotional, Behavioral and Cognitive Development From Early Adolescence Through the Teen Years*. New York, HarperCollins, 1999

American Academy of Pediatrics: *ADHD: A Complete and Authoritative Guide*. Elk Grove Village, IL, American Academy of Pediatrics, 2004

Attwood T: *The Complete Guide to Asperger's Syndrome*. Philadelphia, PA, Jessica Kingsley Publishers, 2007

Barkley RA: *Taking Charge of ADHD: The Complete, Authoritative Guide for Parents*, 3rd Edition. New York, Guilford, 20013

Barkley RA, Benton CM: *Your Defiant Child*, 2nd Edition. New York, Guilford, 2013

Birmaher B: *New Hope for Children and Teens With Bipolar Disorder*. New York, Three Rivers Press, 2004

Braaten E, Felopulos G: *Straight Talk About Psychological Testing for Kids*. New York, Guilford, 2004

Braaten E, Willoughby B: *Bright Kids Who Can't Keep Up*. New York, Guilford, 2014

Clark L: *SOS! Help for Parents: A Practical Guide for Handling Common Everyday Behavior Problems*, 2nd Edition. Berkeley, CA, Parents Press, 1996

Evans DL, Wasmer Andrews L: *If Your Adolescent Has Depression or Bipolar Disorder: An Essential Resource for Parents*. New York, Oxford University Press, 2005

Foa EB, Andrews LW: *If Your Adolescent Has an Anxiety Disorder: An Essential Resource for Parents*. New York, Oxford University Press, 2006

Fristad MA, Arnold JSG: *Raising a Moody Child: How to Cope With Depression and Bipolar Disorder*. New York, Guilford, 2004

Green RW: *The Explosive Child*, 3rd Edition. New York, Harper, 2014

Gur RE, Johnson AB: *If Your Adolescent Has Schizophrenia: An Essential Resource for Parents*. New York, Oxford University Press, 2006

Jensen P: *Making the System Work for Your Child with ADHD*. New York, Guilford, 2004

Kazdin AE: *The Kazdin Method for Parenting the Defiant Child*. New York, Mariner Books, 2009

Last CG: *Help for Worried Kids: How Your Child Can Conquer Anxiety and Fear*. New York, Guilford, 2006

Lederman J, Fink C: *The Ups and Downs of Raising a Bipolar Child: A Survival Guide for Parents*. New York, Simon & Schuster, 2003

Lock J, LeGrange D: *Help Your Teenager Beat an Eating Disorder*. New York, Guilford, 2005

Manassis K: *Keys to Parenting Your Anxious Child*. Hauppage, NY, Barron's Educational Books, 1996

Manassis K, Levac AM: *Helping Your Teenager Beat Depression: A Problem-Solving Approach for Families*. Bethesda, MD, Woodbine House, 2004

March JS: *Talking Back to OCD*. New York, Guilford, 2007

Miklowitz DJ, George EL: *The Bipolar Teen: What You Can Do to Help Your Child and Your Family*. New York, Guilford, 2008

Ozonoff S, Dawson G, McPartland J: *A Parent's Guide to Asperger Syndrome and High-Functioning Autism*. New York, Guilford, 2002

Phelan TW: *1-2-3 Magic: Effective Discipline for Children 2-12*, 3rd Edition. Glen Ellyn, IL, ParentMagic, 2003

Rapee RM, Spence S, Cobham V, et al: *Helping Your Anxious Child: A Step-by-Step Guide for Parents*. Oakland, CA, New Harbinger Publications, 2000

Sederer LI: *The Family Guide to Mental Health Care*. New York, WW Norton, 2013

Siegel B: *Getting the Best for Your Child with Autism: An Expert's Guide to Treatment*. New York, Guilford, 2008

Szatmari P: *A Mind Apart: Understanding Children With Autism and Asperger Syndrome*. New York, Guilford, 2004

Walsh BT, Cameron VL: *If Your Adolescent Has an Eating Disorder*. New York, Oxford University Press, 2005

Wilens TE: *Straight Talk About Psychiatric Medications for Kids*, 3rd Edition. New York, Guilford, 2009

Zeigler Dendy CA: *Teenagers With ADD and ADHD: A Guide for Parents and Professionals*. Bethesda, MD, Woodbine House, 2006

Information on the Internet

ADHD Parents Medication Guide
www.parentsmedguide.org/parentguide_english.pdf

American Academy of Child and Adolescent Psychiatry (AACAP)
3615 Wisconsin Avenue, NW
Washington, DC 20016-3007
1-202-966-7300
www.aacap.org

American Academy of Pediatrics
www.aap.org

American Psychiatric Association
www.healthyminds.org

American Psychiatric Association and American Academy of Child and Adolescent Psychiatry
Information on ADHD (English and Spanish), bipolar disorder, and child and adolescent depression
parentsmedguide.org

Autism Society of America
4340 East-West Highway, Suite 350
Bethesda, MD 20814
1-800-3-AUTISM
www.autism-society.org

Beyond OCD
http://beyondocd.org

Bright Futures
http://brightfutures.org

Canadian Alliance for Monitoring Effectiveness and Safety of Antipsychotics in Children (CAMESA)
http://camesaguideline.org
www.childmind.org

Center for Mental Health Services (CMHS)
Information on child and adolescent mental health and on family mental health resources
www.mentalhealth.gov

Child and Adolescent Bipolar Foundation
1000 Skokie Boulevard, Suite 425
Wilmette, IL 60091
1-847-256-8525
www.bpkids.org

Child Mind Institute
Council of Educators for Students with Disabilities
13091 Pond Springs Road, Suite 300
Austin, TX 78729
1-512-219-5043
www.504idea.org

Children and Adults with Attention-Deficit/Hyperactivity Disorder (CHADD)
8181 Professional Place, Suite 150
Landover, MD 20785
1-301-306-7070 (business)
1-800-233-4050 (National Resource Center)
www.chadd.org

Depression and Bipolar Support Alliance
730 North Franklin Street, Suite 501
Chicago, IL 60610
1-800-826-3632 or 1-312-642-0049
www.dbsalliance.org

National Alliance on Mental Illness (NAMI)
3803 North Fairfax Drive, Suite 100
Arlington, VA 22203
1-703-524-7600
1-800-950-NAMI (Information Helpline)
www.nami.org

National Child Traumatic Stress Network
www.nctsnet.org

National Institute of Mental Health
Public Information and Communications Branch
6001 Executive Boulevard
Room 8184, MSC 9663
Bethesda, MD 20892-9663
1-866-615-6464 or 1-301-443-4513
www.nimh.nih.gov

National Resource Center on AD/HD
A cooperative venture of CHADD and the Centers
for Disease Control and Prevention
www.help4adhd.org/library.cfm

NYU Child Study Center
Wide variety of information on mental health and
treatment, including tutorials on teaching a child to
swallow pills.
www.aboutourkids.org

**Online Asperger Syndrome Information and
Support (OASIS)**
www.aspergersyndrome.org

**The Annenberg Foundation Trust at
Sunnylands Adolescent Mental Health Initiative**
MindZone—a mental health site for teens
www.CopeCareDeal.org

Tourette Syndrome Association
42-40 Bell Boulevard
Bayside, NY 11361
1-718-224-2999
www.tsa-usa.org

Online Access

Accessing the Medication Handouts Online

Purchasers of this book may download the medication information handouts, resource lists, and appendices from http://www.appi.org/Dulcan in Adobe's Portable Document Format (PDF). The PDF files are essentially pictures of the book pages, and these files will allow you to view, print, and e-mail the handouts exactly as they appear in the book. You will need Adobe's Acrobat Reader to view and print the PDF files. Please note that you can only view and print the PDF files with the Acrobat Reader; you cannot modify them.

Minimum System Requirements for Installing Adobe's Acrobat Reader

Windows

- 1.3GHz or faster processor
- Microsoft® Windows® XP with Service Pack 3 for 32 bit or Service Pack 2 for 64 bit; Windows Server® 2003 R2 (32 bit and 64 bit); Windows Server 2008 or 2008 R2 (32 bit and 64 bit); Windows 7 (32 bit and 64 bit); Windows 8 or 8.1 (32 bit and 64 bit)
- 256MB of RAM (512MB recommended)
- 320MB of available hard-disk space

Macintosh

- Intel® processor
- Mac OS X v10.6.4, v10.7.2, or v10.8
- 1GB of RAM
- 350MB of available hard-disk space

Medication Information for Parents and Teachers

Alprazolam—Xanax

General Information About Medication

Each child and adolescent is different. No one has exactly the same combination of medical and psychological problems. It is a good idea to talk with the doctor or nurse about the reasons a medicine is being used. It is very important to keep all appointments and to be in touch by telephone if you have concerns. It is important to communicate with the doctor, nurse, or therapist. An *advanced practice nurse* (APN) has additional education and training after becoming a registered nurse (RN). Your child's medication may be prescribed by a medical doctor (MD or DO) or an APN. In addition, a *physician assistant* (PA) working with a physician may prescribe certain medications. In this information sheet, "doctor" includes medical doctors as well as APNs and PAs who prescribe medication. Often a nurse (RN) will be part of the team and answer questions and give information.

It is very important that the medicine be taken exactly as the doctor instructs. However, once in a while, everyone forgets to give a medicine on time. It is a good idea to ask the doctor or nurse what to do if this happens. Do not stop or change a medicine without asking the doctor or nurse first.

If the medicine seems to stop working, it may be because it is not being taken regularly. The youth may be "cheeking" or hiding the medicine or forgetting to take it (especially at school). The doses may be too far apart or a different dose or medicine may be needed. Something at school, at home, or in the neighborhood may be upsetting the youth, or he or she may need special help for learning disabilities or tutoring. Please discuss your concerns with the doctor. **Do not just increase the dose.** It is also very important not to decrease the dose or stop the medicine without talking to the doctor first. The problem being treated may come back, or there could be uncomfortable or even dangerous results.

All medicines should be kept in a safe place, out of the reach of children, and should be supervised by an adult. If someone takes too much of a medicine, call the doctor, the poison control center, or a hospital emergency room.

Each medicine has a "generic" or chemical name. Just like laundry detergents or paper towels, some medicines are sold by more than one company under different brand names. The same medicine may be available under a generic name and several brand names. The generic medications are usually less expensive than the brand name ones. The generic medications have the same chemical formula, but they may or may not be exactly the same strength as the brand-name medications. Also, some brands of pills contain dye or other things that can cause allergic reactions. It is a good idea to talk to the doctor and the pharmacist about whether it is important to use a specific brand of medicine.

Any medicine can cause an allergic reaction. Examples are hives, itching, rashes, swelling, and trouble breathing. Even a tiny amount of a medicine can cause a reaction in patients who are allergic to that medicine. Be *sure* to talk to the doctor before restarting a medicine that has caused an allergic reaction and tell the doctor about any reactions to medicine that your child has had before.

Taking more than one medicine at the same time may cause more side effects or cause one of the medicines to not work as well. Always ask the doctor, nurse, or pharmacist before adding another

1

medicine, either prescription or bought without a prescription in a store or on the Internet. **Be sure that each doctor knows about *all* of the medicines your child is taking. Also tell the doctor about any vitamins, herbal medicines, or supplements your child may be taking.** Some of these may have side effects alone or when taken with this medication. It is a very good idea to keep a list with you of the names and doses of all medicines that your child is taking.

Everyone taking medicine should have a physical examination at least once a year.

If you think that your child may be using drugs or alcohol, please tell the doctor right away.

Pregnancy requires special care in the use of medicine. Some medicines can cause birth defects if taken by a pregnant mother. **Please tell the doctor immediately if you suspect the teenager is at risk of becoming pregnant.** The doctor may wish to discuss sexual behavior and/or birth control with your daughter.

Printed information like this applies to children and adolescents in general. If you have questions about the medicine, or if you notice changes or anything unusual, please ask the doctor or nurse. As scientific research advances, knowledge increases and advice changes. Even experts do not always agree. Many medicines have not been "approved" by the U.S. Food and Drug Administration (FDA) for use in children or use for particular problems. For this reason, use of the medicine for a problem or age group often is not listed in the *Physicians' Desk Reference*. This does not necessarily mean that the medicine is dangerous or does not work, only that the company that makes the medicine has not received permission to advertise the medicine for use in children. Companies often do not apply for this permission because it is expensive to do the tests needed to apply for approval for use in children. Once a medication is approved by the FDA for any purpose, a doctor is allowed to prescribe it according to research and clinical experience.

Note to Teachers

It is a good idea to talk with the parent(s) about the reason(s) that a medication is being used. If the parent(s) sign consent to release information, it is often helpful for you to talk with the doctor. If the parent(s) give permission, the doctor may ask you to fill out rating forms about your experience with the student's behavior, feelings, academic performance, and medication side effects. This information is very useful in selecting and monitoring medication treatment. If you have observations that you think are important, do not hesitate to share these with the student's parent(s) and treating clinicians (with parental consent).

It is very important that the medicine be taken exactly as the doctor instructs. However, everyone forgets to give a medicine on time once in a while. It is a good idea to ask the parent(s) in advance what to do if this happens. Do not stop or change the time you are giving a medicine at school without parental permission. If a medication is to be taken with food, but lunchtime or snack time changes, be sure to notify the parent(s) so appropriate adjustments can be made.

All medicines should be kept in a secure place and should be supervised by an adult. If someone takes too much of a medicine, follow your school procedure for an urgent medical problem.

Taking medicine is a private matter and is best managed discreetly and confidentially. It is important to be sensitive to the student's feelings about taking medicine.

If you suspect that the student is using drugs or alcohol, please tell the parent(s) or a school counselor right away.

Please tell the parent(s) or school nurse if you suspect medication side effects.

Modifications of the classroom environment or assignments may be useful in addition to medication. The student may need to be evaluated for additional help or a 504 plan or an Individualized Education Plan for learning problems or emotional or behavioral issues.

Any expression of suicidal thoughts or feelings or self-harm by a child or adolescent is a signal of distress and should be taken seriously. These behaviors should not be dismissed as "attention seeking." School procedures for safety issues should be followed.

What Is Alprazolam (Xanax)?

Alprazolam is a *benzodiazepine* or *antianxiety* medicine. It used to be called a *minor tranquilizer*. It is sometimes called an *anxiolytic* or *sedative*. It comes in Xanax brand name and generic immediate-release tablets, Xanax XR and generic extended-release tablets, Intensol concentrated liquid, and generic orally disintegrating tablets.

How Can This Medicine Help?

Alprazolam can decrease anxiety, nervousness, fears, and excessive worrying. It can help anxious people to be calm enough to learn—with therapy and practice (exposure to feared things or situations)—to understand and tolerate their worries or fears and even to overcome them. People with generalized anxiety disorder, social phobia, posttraumatic stress disorder (PTSD), or panic disorder can be helped by alprazolam. Most often, it is used for a short time when symptoms are very uncomfortable or frightening or when they make it hard to do important things such as going to school. Alprazolam can decrease the severe physical symptoms (rapid heartbeat, trouble breathing, dizziness, sweating) of panic attacks and phobias.

Alprazolam also can be used for sleep problems, such as night terrors (sudden waking up from sleep with great fear) or sleepwalking, when these problems put the youth at risk of an accident or make it impossible for other family members to get enough sleep. Alprazolam can help with insomnia (difficulty falling asleep) when used for a short time along with a behavioral program.

Sometimes alprazolam is used for a few days to treat agitation in mania or psychosis until other medicines start to work.

Occasionally the benzodiazepines are used to reduce the side effects of other medicines.

How Does This Medicine Work?

Alprazolam works by calming the parts of the brain that are too excitable in anxious people. The medicine does this by working on *receptors* (special places on brain cells) in certain parts of the brain to change the action of *GABA*—a *neurotransmitter*—a chemical that the brain makes for brain cells to communicate with each other.

How Long Does This Medicine Last?

Alprazolam usually needs to be taken three times a day. The extended-release tablets may be taken only once a day. For acute symptoms of anxiety or agitation, it can be taken occasionally, as needed. When used for sleep, it is taken at bedtime. There may still be some effects in the morning.

How Will the Doctor Monitor This Medicine?

The doctor will review your child's medical history and physical examination before starting alprazolam. The doctor may order some blood or urine tests or an ECG (electrocardiogram or heart rhythm test) to be sure your child does not have a hidden medical condition. The doctor or nurse may measure your child's height, weight, pulse, and blood pressure before starting alprazolam.

After the medicine is started, the doctor will want to have regular appointments with you and your child to see how the medicine is working, to see if a dose change is needed, to watch for side effects, to see if alprazolam is still needed, and to see if any other treatment is needed. The doctor or nurse may check your child's height, weight, pulse, and blood pressure.

What Side Effects Can This Medicine Have?

Any medicine can have side effects, including an allergy to the medicine. Because each patient is different, the doctor will monitor the youth closely, especially when the medicine is started. The doctor will work with you to increase the positive effects and decrease the negative effects of the medicine. Please tell the doctor if any of the listed side effects appear or if you think that the medicine is causing any other problems. Not all of the rare or unusual side effects are listed.

Side effects are most common after starting the medicine or after a dose increase. Many side effects can be avoided or lessened by starting with a very low dose and increasing it slowly—ask the doctor.

Allergic Reaction

Tell the doctor in a day or two (if possible, before the next dose of medicine):

- Hives
- Itching
- Rash

Stop the medicine and get *immediate* medical care:

- Trouble breathing or chest tightness
- Swelling of lips, tongue, or throat

Alprazolam is usually very safe when used for short periods as the doctor prescribes.

The most common side effect is daytime sleepiness. Alprazolam can also cause dizziness, feeling "spacey," or decreased coordination. If the medicine is causing any of these problems it is very important not to drive a car, ride a bicycle or motorcycle, or operate machinery.

Alprazolam can cause decreased concentration and memory. These problems, along with daytime sleepiness, may decrease learning and performance in school.

People who take alprazolam must not drink alcohol. Severe sleepiness or even loss of consciousness may result.

It is possible to become psychologically and physically dependent on alprazolam, but that is not a common problem for patients who see their doctors regularly. Because some people abuse benzodiazepines, it is illegal to give or sell these medicines to someone other than the patient for whom they were prescribed.

Very rarely, alprazolam causes excitement, irritability, anger, aggression, trouble sleeping, nightmares, uncontrollable behavior, or memory loss. This is called *disinhibition* or a *paradoxical effect*. Stop the medicine and call the doctor if this happens.

Some Interactions With Other Medicines or Food

Please note that the following are only the most likely interactions with other medicines or food.

Alprazolam may be taken with or without food.

Grapefruit juice can increase the levels of alprazolam and increase side effects.

Antibiotics such as erythromycin, oral antifungal agents such as ketoconazole, oral contraceptives (birth control pills), fluoxetine (Prozac), fluvoxamine (Luvox), propranolol (Inderal), valproate (Depakote), and other medicines may increase the levels of alprazolam and increase side effects, especially sedation.

Antacids, carbamazepine (Tegretol), theophylline, and St. John's wort can decrease the positive effects of alprazolam.

It is important not to use other sedatives, tranquilizers, sleeping pills, or antihistamines (such as Benadryl) when taking alprazolam because of greatly increased side effects.

It is better to limit drinks with caffeine (coffee, tea, soft drinks) because caffeine works in the opposite way from this medicine, and the positive effects might be decreased.

What Could Happen if This Medicine Is Stopped Suddenly?

Many medicines cause problems if stopped suddenly. Alprazolam must be decreased slowly (tapered) rather than stopped suddenly. When alprazolam is stopped suddenly, there are withdrawal symptoms that are uncomfortable and may even be dangerous. Problems are more likely in patients taking high doses of alprazolam for 2 months or longer, but even after taking alprazolam for just a few weeks it is important to stop it slowly. Withdrawal symptoms may include anxiety, irritability, shaking, sweating, aches and pains, muscle cramps, vomiting, confusion, and trouble sleeping. If large doses taken for a long time are stopped suddenly, seizures (fits, convulsions), hallucinations (hearing voices or seeing things that are not there), or out-of-control behavior may result.

How Long Will This Medicine Be Needed?

Alprazolam is usually prescribed for only a few weeks to allow the patient to be calm enough to learn new ways to cope with anxiety and to allow the nervous system to become less excitable. Sometimes antianxiety medicines are used for longer periods to treat panic attacks or anxiety that remains after therapy is completed. Each person is unique, and some people may need these medicines for months or years.

What Else Should I Know About This Medicine?

Because benzodiazepines can be abused (especially by people who abuse alcohol or drugs) and can cause psychological dependence or physical dependence (addiction), they are regulated by special state and federal laws as *controlled substances*. These laws place limitations on telephone prescriptions and refills.

Sometimes alprazolam (Xanax) and lorazepam (Ativan) get mixed up; be sure to check the prescription.

People with sleep apnea (breathing stops while they are asleep) should not take alprazolam. Tell the doctor if your child snores very loudly.

Alprazolam should be avoided during pregnancy, especially in the first 3 months, because it may cause birth defects in the baby. If taken regularly at the end of pregnancy, alprazolam may cause withdrawal symptoms in the baby.

Notes

Use this space to take notes or to write down questions you want to ask the doctor.

_____

_____

_____

_____

_____

_____

_____

_____

_____

_____

_____

_____

From Dulcan MK, Ballard R (editors): _Helping Parents and Teachers Understand Medications for Behavioral and Emotional Problems: A Resource Book of Medication Information Handouts_, Fourth Edition. Washington, DC, American Psychiatric Publishing, 2015

Amitriptyline

General Information About Medication

Each child and adolescent is different. No one has exactly the same combination of medical and psychological problems. It is a good idea to talk with the doctor or nurse about the reasons a medicine is being used. It is very important to keep all appointments and to be in touch by telephone if you have concerns. It is important to communicate with the doctor, nurse, or therapist. An *advanced practice nurse* (APN) has additional education and training after becoming a registered nurse (RN). Your child's medication may be prescribed by a medical doctor (MD or DO) or an APN. In addition, a *physician assistant* (PA) working with a physician may prescribe certain medications. In this information sheet, "doctor" includes medical doctors as well as APNs and PAs who prescribe medication. Often a nurse (RN) will be part of the team and answer questions and give information.

It is very important that the medicine be taken exactly as the doctor instructs. However, once in a while, everyone forgets to give a medicine on time. It is a good idea to ask the doctor or nurse what to do if this happens. Do not stop or change a medicine without asking the doctor or nurse first.

If the medicine seems to stop working, it may be because it is not being taken regularly. The youth may be "cheeking" or hiding the medicine or forgetting to take it (especially at school). The doses may be too far apart or a different dose or medicine may be needed. Something at school, at home, or in the neighborhood may be upsetting the youth, or he or she may need special help for learning disabilities or tutoring. Please discuss your concerns with the doctor. **Do not just increase the dose.** It is also very important not to decrease the dose or stop the medicine without talking to the doctor first. The problem being treated may come back, or there could be uncomfortable or even dangerous results.

All medicines should be kept in a safe place, out of the reach of children, and should be supervised by an adult. If someone takes too much of a medicine, call the doctor, the poison control center, or a hospital emergency room.

Each medicine has a "generic" or chemical name. Just like laundry detergents or paper towels, some medicines are sold by more than one company under different brand names. The same medicine may be available under a generic name and several brand names. The generic medications are usually less expensive than the brand name ones. The generic medications have the same chemical formula, but they may or may not be exactly the same strength as the brand-name medications. Also, some brands of pills contain dye or other things that can cause allergic reactions. It is a good idea to talk to the doctor and the pharmacist about whether it is important to use a specific brand of medicine.

Any medicine can cause an allergic reaction. Examples are hives, itching, rashes, swelling, and trouble breathing. Even a tiny amount of a medicine can cause a reaction in patients who are allergic to that medicine. Be *sure* to talk to the doctor before restarting a medicine that has caused an allergic reaction and tell the doctor about any reactions to medicine that your child has had before.

Taking more than one medicine at the same time may cause more side effects or cause one of the medicines to not work as well. Always ask the doctor, nurse, or pharmacist before adding another

medicine, either prescription or bought without a prescription in a store or on the Internet. Be sure that each doctor knows about *all* of the medicines your child is taking. Also tell the doctor about any vitamins, herbal medicines, or supplements your child may be taking. Some of these may have side effects alone or when taken with this medication. It is a very good idea to keep a list with you of the names and doses of all medicines that your child is taking.

Everyone taking medicine should have a physical examination at least once a year.

If you think that your child may be using drugs or alcohol, please tell the doctor right away.

Pregnancy requires special care in the use of medicine. Some medicines can cause birth defects if taken by a pregnant mother. **Please tell the doctor immediately if you suspect the teenager is at risk of becoming pregnant.** The doctor may wish to discuss sexual behavior and/or birth control with your daughter.

Printed information like this applies to children and adolescents in general. If you have questions about the medicine, or if you notice changes or anything unusual, please ask the doctor or nurse. As scientific research advances, knowledge increases and advice changes. Even experts do not always agree. Many medicines have not been "approved" by the U.S. Food and Drug Administration (FDA) for use in children or use for particular problems. For this reason, use of the medicine for a problem or age group often is not listed in the *Physicians' Desk Reference*. This does not necessarily mean that the medicine is dangerous or does not work, only that the company that makes the medicine has not received permission to advertise the medicine for use in children. Companies often do not apply for this permission because it is expensive to do the tests needed to apply for approval for use in children. Once a medication is approved by the FDA for any purpose, a doctor is allowed to prescribe it according to research and clinical experience.

Note to Teachers

It is a good idea to talk with the parent(s) about the reason(s) that a medication is being used. If the parent(s) sign consent to release information, it is often helpful for you to talk with the doctor. If the parent(s) give permission, the doctor may ask you to fill out rating forms about your experience with the student's behavior, feelings, academic performance, and medication side effects. This information is very useful in selecting and monitoring medication treatment. If you have observations that you think are important, do not hesitate to share these with the student's parent(s) and treating clinicians (with parental consent).

It is very important that the medicine be taken exactly as the doctor instructs. However, everyone forgets to give a medicine on time once in a while. It is a good idea to ask the parent(s) in advance what to do if this happens. Do not stop or change the time you are giving a medicine at school without parental permission. If a medication is to be taken with food, but lunchtime or snack time changes, be sure to notify the parent(s) so appropriate adjustments can be made.

All medicines should be kept in a secure place and should be supervised by an adult. If someone takes too much of a medicine, follow your school procedure for an urgent medical problem.

Taking medicine is a private matter and is best managed discreetly and confidentially. It is important to be sensitive to the student's feelings about taking medicine.

If you suspect that the student is using drugs or alcohol, please tell the parent(s) or a school counselor right away.

Please tell the parent(s) or school nurse if you suspect medication side effects.

Modifications of the classroom environment or assignments may be useful in addition to medication. The student may need to be evaluated for additional help or a 504 plan or an Individualized Education Plan for learning problems or emotional or behavioral issues.

Any expression of suicidal thoughts or feelings or self-harm by a child or adolescent is a signal of distress and should be taken seriously. These behaviors should not be dismissed as "attention seeking." School procedures for safety issues should be followed.

You may notice the following side effects at school:

Common Side Effects

- Dry mouth—Allow the student to chew sugar-free gum, carry a water bottle, or make extra trips to the water fountain.
- Constipation—Allow the student to drink more fluids or to use the bathroom more often.
- Daytime sleepiness—The student should not drive, ride a bicycle or motorcycle, or operate machinery.
- Dizziness (especially when standing up quickly)—This may happen in the classroom or during physical education. Suggest that the student stand up more slowly.
- Irritability

Occasional Side Effects

- Stuttering
- Increased risk of sunburn (this may be a problem if recess or physical education is outdoors in warm weather)—The student should wear sunscreen or protective clothing or stay out of the sun.

Less Common Side Effects

- Nausea—The student may need to take the medicine after a meal or snack.
- Trouble urinating—The student may need more time in the bathroom.
- Blurred vision—The student may have trouble seeing the blackboard.
- Motor tics (fast, repeated movements) or muscle twitches (jerking movements) of parts of the body
- Increased activity, rapid speech, feeling "speeded up," being very excited or irritable (cranky)
- Skin rash

Rare, but Potentially Serious, Side Effects

Call the parent(s) or follow your school's emergency procedures *immediately:*

- Seizure (fit, convulsion) **(This is a medical emergency.)**
- Very fast or irregular heartbeat **(This is a medical emergency.)**
- Fainting
- Hallucinations (hearing voices or seeing things that are not there)
- Inability to urinate
- Confusion
- Severe change in behavior

What Is Amitriptyline?

Amitriptyline is called a *tricyclic antidepressant.* It was first used to treat depression but is now used to treat abdominal pain, chronic or severe migraine headaches, fibromyalgia, or other kinds of chronic pain. There are no brand name tablets of amitriptyline sold in the United States, but in other countries it is sometimes called Elavil or Endep.

How Can This Medicine Help?

When taken regularly, amitriptyline can reduce chronic pain, including in fibromyalgia. The side effect of sleepiness may help people with chronic pain to fall asleep and stay asleep.

How Does This Medicine Work?

Tricyclic antidepressants affect *neurotransmitters*—the natural substances that work in the brain and the nerves throughout the body.

How Long Does This Medicine Last?

Although a dose lasts for a whole day in adults and older teenagers, in younger children several doses a day may be needed.

How Will the Doctor Monitor This Medicine?

The doctor will review your child's medical history and physical examination, paying special attention to pulse rate, blood pressure, weight, and height, before starting amitriptyline. These measurements will be taken when the dose is increased and occasionally as long as the medicine is continued. The doctor may order some blood or urine tests to be sure your child does not have a hidden medical condition that would make it unsafe to use this medicine.

Tricyclic antidepressants can slow the speed at which signals move through the heart. This effect is not dangerous if the heart is normal, which is why an ECG (electrocardiogram or heart rhythm test) is done before starting the medicine. The ECG may be repeated as the dose is increased and occasionally while the medicine is being taken. Changes in the heart from the medicine usually can be seen on the ECG before they become a problem, so your child's doctor will order an ECG every so often.

To find possible hidden heart risks, it is especially important to tell the doctor if your child or anyone in the family has a history of fainting, palpitations, or irregular heartbeat or if anyone in the family died suddenly.

Be sure to tell the doctor if your child or anyone in the family has bipolar disorder or has tried to kill himself or herself.

Because amitriptyline may increase the risk of seizures (fits, convulsions), the doctor will want to know whether your child has ever had a seizure or a head injury and if there is any family history of epilepsy. Your child's doctor may want to order an EEG (electroencephalogram or brain wave test) before starting the medicine.

After the medicine is started, the doctor will want to have regular appointments with you and your child to see how the medicine is working, to see if a dose change is needed, to watch for side effects, to see if amitriptyline is still needed, and to see if any other treatment is needed. The doctor or nurse may check your child's height, weight, pulse, and blood pressure or order tests, such as an ECG.

Before using this medicine and at times afterward, the doctor may ask your child to fill out a rating scale about pain, to help see how your child is doing.

10

What Side Effects Can This Medicine Have?

Any medicine can have side effects, including an allergy to the medicine. Because each patient is different, the doctor will monitor the youth closely, especially when the medicine is started. The doctor will work with you to increase the positive effects and decrease the negative effects of the medicine. Please tell the doctor if any of the listed side effects appear or if you think that the medicine is causing any other problems. Not all of the rare or unusual side effects are listed.

Side effects are most common after starting the medicine or after a dose increase. Many side effects can be avoided or lessened by starting with a very low dose and increasing it slowly—ask the doctor.

Allergic Reaction

Tell the doctor in a day or two (if possible, before the next dose of medicine):

- Hives
- Itching
- Rash (may be caused by an allergy to the medicine or to a dye in the specific brand of pill)

Stop medicine and get *immediate* medical care:

- Trouble breathing or chest tightness
- Swelling of lips, tongue, or throat

Common Side Effects

Tell the doctor within a week or two:

- Dry mouth—Have your child try using sugar-free gum or candy.
- Constipation—Encourage your child to drink more fluids and eat high-fiber foods; if necessary, the doctor may recommend a fiber medicine such as Benefiber or a stool softener such as Colace or mineral oil.
- Daytime sleepiness—Do not allow your child to drive, ride a bicycle or motorcycle, or operate machinery if this happens.
- Dizziness—This side effect is worse when the child stands up quickly, especially when getting out of bed in the morning; try having the child stand up slowly.
- Weight gain
- Loss of appetite and weight loss
- Irritability
- Acne

Occasional Side Effects

Tell the doctor within a week or two:

- Nightmares
- Stuttering
- Blurred vision

11

- Increase in breast size, nipple discharge, or both (in girls)
- Increase in breast size (in boys)

Less Common, but More Serious, Side Effects

Call the doctor within a day or two:

- High or low blood pressure
- Nausea
- Trouble urinating
- Motor tics (fast, repeated movements) or muscle twitches (jerking movements)
- Increased activity, rapid speech, feeling "speeded up," decreased need for sleep, being very excited or irritable (cranky)

Rare, but Potentially Serious, Side Effects

Call the doctor *immediately*:

- Seizure (fit, convulsion)—**Go to an emergency room.**
- Very fast or irregular heartbeat—**Go to an emergency room.**
- Fainting
- Hallucinations (hearing voices or seeing things that are not there)
- Inability to urinate
- Confusion
- Severe change in behavior
- Yellowing of skin or eyes, dark urine, pale bowel movements, abdominal pain or fullness, unexplained flu-like symptoms, itchy skin—These side effects are extremely rare but could be signs of liver damage.

Some Interactions With Other Medicines or Food

Please note that the following are only the most likely interactions with other medicines or food.

Check with your child's doctor before giving your child decongestants or over-the-counter cold medicine.

Taking another antidepressant or valproate (Depakote) with amitriptyline may increase the level of amitriptyline and increase side effects.

Taking carbamazepine (Tegretol) with amitriptyline may decrease the positive effects of amitriptyline and increase the side effects of carbamazepine.

It can be *very dangerous* to take amitriptyline at the same time as or even within a month of taking another type of medicine called a *monoamine oxidase inhibitor* (MAOI), such as selegiline (Eldepryl), phenelzine (Nardil), tranylcypromine (Parnate), or isocarboxazid (Marplan).

Do not give linezolid or pimozide with amitriptyline.

Caffeine may worsen side effects on the heart or symptoms of anxiety. It is best not to drink coffee, tea, or soft drinks with caffeine while taking this medicine.

What Could Happen if This Medicine Is Stopped Suddenly?

Stopping the medicine suddenly or skipping a dose is not dangerous but can be very uncomfortable. Your child may feel like he or she has the flu—with a headache, muscle aches, stomachache, and upset stomach. Behavioral problems, sadness, nervousness, or trouble sleeping also may occur. If these feelings appear every day, the medicine may need to be given more often during each day.

How Long Will This Medicine Be Needed?

There is no way to know how long a person will need to take this medicine. Parents work together with the doctor to determine what is right for each child.

What Else Should I Know About This Medicine?

In youth who have bipolar disorder or who might be at risk for bipolar disorder, any antidepressant medicine may increase the risk of hypomania or mania (excitement, agitation, increased activity, decreased sleep).

An overdose by accident or on purpose with this medicine is *very dangerous*! You must closely supervise the medicine. You may have to lock up the medicine if your child or teenager is suicidal or if young children live in or visit your home.

Tricyclic antidepressants may cause dry mouth, which could increase the chance of tooth decay. Regular brushing of teeth and checkups with the dentist are especially important.

This medicine causes increased risk of sunburn. Be sure that your child wears sunscreen or protective clothing or stays out of the sun.

People who take tricyclic antidepressants must not drink alcohol or use tranquilizers. Severe sleepiness, loss of consciousness, or even death may result.

Black Box Antidepressant Warning

In 2004, an advisory committee to the FDA decided that there might be an increased risk of suicidal behavior for some youth taking medicines called *antidepressants*. In the research studies that the committee reviewed, about 3%–4% of youth with depression who took an antidepressant medicine—and 1%–2% of youth with depression who took a placebo (pill without active medicine)—talked about suicidal thoughts (thinking about killing themselves or wishing they were dead) or did something to harm themselves. This means that almost twice as many youth who were taking an antidepressant to treat their depression talked about suicide or had suicidal behavior compared with youth with depression who were taking inactive medicine. There were *no* completed suicides in any of these research studies, which included more than 4,000 children and adolescents. For youth being treated for anxiety, there was no difference in suicidal talking or behavior between those taking antidepressant medication and those taking placebo.

The FDA told drug companies to add a *black box warning* label to all antidepressant medicines. Because of this label, a doctor (or advanced practice nurse) prescribing one of these medicines has to warn youth and their families that there might be more suicidal thoughts and actions in youth taking these medicines.

On the other hand, in places where more youth are taking the newer antidepressant medicines, the number of adolescents who commit suicide has gotten smaller. Also, thinking about or attempting suicide is more common in surveys of teenagers in the community than it is in depressed youth treated in research studies with antidepressant medicine.

If a youth is being treated with this medicine and is doing well, then no changes are needed as a result of this warning. Increased suicidal talk or action is most likely to happen in the first few months of treatment with a medicine. If your child has recently started this medicine or is about to start, then you and your doctor (or advanced practice nurse) should watch for any changes in behavior. People who are depressed often have suicidal thoughts or actions. It is hard to know whether suicidal thoughts or actions in depressed people are caused by the depression itself or by the medicine. Also, as their depression is getting better, some people talk more about the suicidal thoughts that they had before but did not talk about. As young people get better from depression, they might be at higher risk of doing something about suicidal thoughts that they have had for some time, because they have more energy.

What Should a Parent Do?

1. Be honest with your child about possible risks and benefits of medicine.

2. Talk to your child about whether he or she is having any suicidal thoughts, and tell your child to come to you if he or she is having such thoughts.

3. You, your child, and your child's doctor or nurse should develop a safety plan. Pick adults whom your child can tell if he or she is thinking about suicide.

4. Be sure to tell your child's doctor, nurse, or therapist if you suspect that your child is using alcohol or drugs or if something has happened that might make your child feel worse, such as a family separation, breaking up with a boyfriend or girlfriend, someone close dying or attempting suicide, physical or sexual abuse, or failure in school.

5. Be sure that there are no guns in the home and that all medicines (including over-the-counter medicines like Tylenol) are closely supervised by an adult and kept in a safe place.

6. Watch for new or worse thoughts of suicide, self-harm, depression, anxiety (nerves), feeling very agitated or restless, being angry or aggressive, having more trouble sleeping, or anything else that you see for the first time, seems worse, or worries your child or you. If these appear, contact a mental health professional **right away.** Do not just stop or change the dose of the medicine on your own. If the problems are serious, and you cannot reach one of your clinicians, call a 24-hour psychiatry emergency telephone number or take your child to an emergency room.

Youth taking antidepressant medicine should be watched carefully by their parent(s), clinician(s) (doctor, advanced practice nurse, nurse, therapist), and other concerned adults for the first weeks of treatment. It is a good idea to have regular contact with the doctor, APN, nurse, or therapist for the first months to check for feelings of depression or sadness, thoughts of killing or harming himself or herself, and any problems with the medication. If you have questions, be sure to ask the doctor, APN, nurse, or therapist.

For more information, see http://www.parentsmedguide.org/.

Notes

Use this space to take notes or to write down questions you want to ask the doctor.

_____

_____

_____

_____

_____

_____

_____

Medication Information for Parents and Teachers

Amphetamine—Dexedrine, ProCentra, Zenzedi, Adderall, Vyvanse

General Information About Medication

Each child and adolescent is different. No one has exactly the same combination of medical and psychological problems. It is a good idea to talk with the doctor or nurse about the reasons a medicine is being used. It is very important to keep all appointments and to be in touch by telephone if you have concerns. It is important to communicate with the doctor, nurse, or therapist. An *advanced practice nurse* (APN) has additional education and training after becoming a registered nurse (RN). Your child's medication may be prescribed by a medical doctor (MD or DO) or an APN. In addition, a *physician assistant* (PA) working with a physician may prescribe certain medications. In this information sheet, "doctor" includes medical doctors as well as APNs and PAs who prescribe medication. Often a nurse (RN) will be part of the team and answer questions and give information.

It is very important that the medicine be taken exactly as the doctor instructs. However, once in a while, everyone forgets to give a medicine on time. It is a good idea to ask the doctor or nurse what to do if this happens. Do not stop or change a medicine without asking the doctor or nurse first.

If the medicine seems to stop working, it may be because it is not being taken regularly. The youth may be "cheeking" or hiding the medicine or forgetting to take it (especially at school). The doses may be too far apart or a different dose or medicine may be needed. Something at school, at home, or in the neighborhood may be upsetting the youth, or he or she may need special help for learning disabilities or tutoring. Please discuss your concerns with the doctor. **Do not just increase the dose.** It is also very important not to decrease the dose or stop the medicine without talking to the doctor first. The problem being treated may come back, or there could be uncomfortable or even dangerous results.

All medicines should be kept in a safe place, out of the reach of children, and should be supervised by an adult. If someone takes too much of a medicine, call the doctor, the poison control center, or a hospital emergency room.

Each medicine has a "generic" or chemical name. Just like laundry detergents or paper towels, some medicines are sold by more than one company under different brand names. The same medicine may be available under a generic name and several brand names. The generic medications are usually less expensive than the brand name ones. The generic medications have the same chemical formula, but they may or may not be exactly the same strength as the brand-name medications. Also, some brands of pills contain dye or other things that can cause allergic reactions. It is a good idea to talk to the doctor and the pharmacist about whether it is important to use a specific brand of medicine.

Any medicine can cause an allergic reaction. Examples are hives, itching, rashes, swelling, and trouble breathing. Even a tiny amount of a medicine can cause a reaction in patients who are allergic to that medicine. Be *sure* to talk to the doctor before restarting a medicine that has caused an allergic reaction and tell the doctor about any reactions to medicine that your child has had before.

Taking more than one medicine at the same time may cause more side effects or cause one of the medicines to not work as well. Always ask the doctor, nurse, or pharmacist before adding another

medicine, either prescription or bought without a prescription in a store or on the Internet. Be sure that each doctor knows about *all* of the medicines your child is taking. Also tell the doctor about any vitamins, herbal medicines, or supplements your child may be taking. Some of these may have side effects alone or when taken with this medication. It is a very good idea to keep a list with you of the names and doses of all medicines that your child is taking.

Everyone taking medicine should have a physical examination at least once a year.

If you think that your child may be using drugs or alcohol, please tell the doctor right away.

Pregnancy requires special care in the use of medicine. Some medicines can cause birth defects if taken by a pregnant mother. **Please tell the doctor immediately if you suspect the teenager is at risk of becoming pregnant.** The doctor may wish to discuss sexual behavior and/or birth control with your daughter.

Printed information like this applies to children and adolescents in general. If you have questions about the medicine, or if you notice changes or anything unusual, please ask the doctor or nurse. As scientific research advances, knowledge increases and advice changes. Even experts do not always agree. Many medicines have not been "approved" by the U.S. Food and Drug Administration (FDA) for use in children or use for particular problems. For this reason, use of the medicine for a problem or age group often is not listed in the *Physicians' Desk Reference*. This does not necessarily mean that the medicine is dangerous or does not work, only that the company that makes the medicine has not received permission to advertise the medicine for use in children. Companies often do not apply for this permission because it is expensive to do the tests needed to apply for approval for use in children. Once a medication is approved by the FDA for any purpose, a doctor is allowed to prescribe it according to research and clinical experience.

Note to Teachers

It is a good idea to talk with the parent(s) about the reason(s) that a medication is being used. If the parent(s) sign consent to release information, it is often helpful for you to talk with the doctor. If the parent(s) give permission, the doctor may ask you to fill out rating forms about your experience with the student's behavior, feelings, academic performance, and medication side effects. This information is very useful in selecting and monitoring medication treatment. If you have observations that you think are important, do not hesitate to share these with the student's parent(s) and treating clinicians (with parental consent).

It is very important that the medicine be taken exactly as the doctor instructs. However, everyone forgets to give a medicine on time once in a while. It is a good idea to ask the parent(s) in advance what to do if this happens. Do not stop or change the time you are giving a medicine at school without parental permission. If a medication is to be taken with food, but lunchtime or snack time changes, be sure to notify the parent(s) so appropriate adjustments can be made.

All medicines should be kept in a secure place and should be supervised by an adult. If someone takes too much of a medicine, follow your school procedure for an urgent medical problem.

Taking medicine is a private matter and is best managed discreetly and confidentially. It is important to be sensitive to the student's feelings about taking medicine.

If you suspect that the student is using drugs or alcohol, please tell the parent(s) or a school counselor right away.

Please tell the parent(s) or school nurse if you suspect medication side effects.

Modifications of the classroom environment or assignments may be useful in addition to medication. The student may need to be evaluated for additional help or a 504 plan or an Individualized Education Plan for learning problems or emotional or behavioral issues.

Any expression of suicidal thoughts or feelings or self-harm by a child or adolescent is a signal of distress and should be taken seriously. These behaviors should not be dismissed as "attention seeking." School procedures for safety issues should be followed.

What Is Amphetamine (Dexedrine, ProCentra, Zenzedi, Adderall, Vyvanse)?

Amphetamine is called a *stimulant*. It is used to treat attention-deficit/hyperactivity disorder (ADHD), whether the person has hyperactivity (increased moving around) or not. It comes in a generic form and several brand name formulations (see table below). Although all of these medicines have amphetamine as the active ingredient, they are made differently, so that there are many different ways to take amphetamine. This helps the doctor to find just the right form of the medicine for each person.

Generic and brand name formulations
Short-acting, or immediate-release dextroamphetamine (3–5 hours)
Generic dextroamphetamine
Dexedrine
Zenzedi
ProCentra (liquid)
Long-acting dextroamphetamine (6–8 hours)
Dexedrine Spansule (capsule with particles)
Dextroamphetamine ER (extended release)
Very long-acting lisdexamfetamine dimesylate: dextroamphetamine prodrug (turns into dextroamphetamine when digested) (12–14 hours)
Vyvanse (capsule may be opened and dissolved in water or mixed with yogurt or orange juice and taken right away)
Mixed amphetamine salts
Generic mixed amphetamine salts (immediate release) (3–5 hours)
Adderall (immediate release, short acting) (3–5 hours)
Adderall XR (extended release, very long acting; capsule with beads—may be sprinkled on food) (10–12 hours)
Generic mixed amphetamine salts extended release (10–12 hours)

How Can This Medicine Help?

Amphetamine can increase attention and the ability to follow instructions. It can improve attention span, decrease distractibility, increase the ability to finish things, decrease hyperactivity, and improve the ability to think before acting (decrease impulsivity). Handwriting and completion of schoolwork and homework can improve. Amphetamine can improve willingness to follow directions and decrease stubbornness in youngsters with both ADHD and oppositional defiant disorder (ODD).

Many people with Tourette's disorder (chronic motor and vocal tics) also have symptoms of ADHD. Amphetamine may be used cautiously to reduce these symptoms of hyperactivity, impulsivity, and trouble paying attention and usually does not make the tics worse. If the tics get worse, talk with your child's doctor. Lowering the dose or stopping the amphetamine will usually lead to the tics decreasing again. Tics also increase and decrease for a lot of reasons that are not related to medicine.

Medicine may not resolve all symptoms in children with ADHD. These children may also need special help in school and behavior modification at home and at school. Some youngsters and families are helped by family therapy or group social skills therapy.

Stimulant medicines last for different amounts of time. ADHD symptoms may come back when the medicine wears off. This does not mean the medicine is not working but means that longer coverage may be needed.

Amphetamine is also used to help people with narcolepsy (sudden and uncontrollable episodes of deep sleep) to stay awake.

How Does This Medicine Work?

In people who have ADHD, parts of the brain are not working as well as they should. An example would be the part that controls impulsive actions ("the brakes"). Amphetamine helps these parts of the brain work better by acting as a stimulant, increasing the activity of neurotransmitters—mostly *dopamine* but also *norepinephrine*. *Neurotransmitters* are the chemicals that the brain makes for the nerve cells to communicate with each other.

Amphetamine is not a tranquilizer or sedative. It works in the same way in children and adults and in people with or without ADHD.

Methylphenidate and amphetamine are both stimulant medicines, but they work in different ways on the neurotransmitters. A person with ADHD might be helped by one stimulant but not the other, so if one is not working, the doctor may try the other one.

How Long Does This Medicine Last?

All types of amphetamine start working in 30–60 minutes after taking them. Different forms last for different lengths of time. The immediate-release or short-acting forms last for 3–5 hours. The long-acting forms of dextroamphetamine last for 6–8 hours. Adderall XR lasts for 10–12 hours. Vyvanse can take up to an hour to start working, but it lasts for 12–14 hours. The length of time is different for different people, and the medicine may work longer for some symptoms than for others. An advantage of the longer-acting forms is that they do not have to be given during the school day.

How Will the Doctor Monitor This Medicine?

The doctor will review your child's medical history and physical examination before starting amphetamine. The doctor may order some blood or urine tests to be sure your child does not have a hidden medical condition. Be sure to tell the doctor if your child or anyone in the family was born with or has had heart problems, seizures, irregular heartbeat (pulse), high blood pressure (hypertension), dizziness, fainting, shortness of breath, glaucoma, hyperthyroidism, or severe tiredness. Tell the doctor if anyone in the family has died suddenly. People who have a history of heart problems generally should not take amphetamine. Talk to your doctor if your child has a history of seizures, as amphetamines may lower the seizure threshold in some children with a history of seizure disorders. Also tell the doctor if your child or anyone in the family has had motor or vocal tics (hard-to-control repeated movements or sounds) or Tourette's disorder (also called Tourette's syndrome). The doctor or nurse will measure your child's height, weight, pulse, and blood pressure before starting the medicine. The doctor will usually ask parents and teachers to fill out behavior rating scales (checklists).

After the medicine is started, the doctor will want to have regular appointments with you and your child to see how the medicine is working, to see if a dose change is needed, to watch for side effects, to see if amphetamine is still needed, and to see if any other treatment is needed. The doctor or nurse may check your child's height, weight, pulse, and blood pressure. With parental permission, the doctor will usually ask for reports (rating scale, checklist, testing results, comments) from the teacher(s) to keep track of progress in learning and behavior. Some young people take the medicine three or four times a day, every day. Others need to take it only once or twice a day or only on school days. You and your child's doctor will work out the doses and timing and type of medicine that is best for your child and his or her symptoms and schedule.

What Side Effects Can This Medicine Have?

Any medicine can have side effects, including an allergy to the medicine. Because each patient is different, the doctor will monitor the youth closely, especially when the medicine is started. The doctor will work with you to increase the positive effects and decrease the negative effects of the medicine. Please tell the doctor if any of the listed side effects appear or if you think that the medicine is causing any other problems. Not all of the rare or unusual side effects are listed.

Side effects are most common after starting the medicine or after a dose increase. Many side effects can be avoided or lessened by starting with a very low dose and increasing it slowly—ask the doctor.

Allergic Reaction

Tell the doctor in a day or two (if possible, before the next dose of medicine):

- Hives
- Itching
- Rash

Stop the medicine and get *immediate* medical care:

- Trouble breathing or chest tightness
- Swelling of lips, tongue, or throat

Common Side Effects

If the following side effects do not go away after about 2 weeks, ask the doctor about lowering your child's dose:

- Lack of appetite and weight loss—Encourage your child to eat a good breakfast and afternoon and evening snacks; give medicine during or after meals.
- Insomnia (trouble falling asleep)—This may be the ADHD coming back and not a side effect. Talk with your child's doctor. Changing the time or dose of medicine, starting a bedtime routine, or adding another medicine may help.
- Headaches
- Stomachaches
- Irritability, crankiness, crying, emotional sensitivity
- Loss of interest in friends
- Staring into space
- Rapid pulse rate (heartbeat) or increased blood pressure

Less Common Side Effects

Tell the doctor within a week or two if you notice

- Rebound—As the medicine wears off, hyperactivity or bad mood may get worse than before the medicine was taken. The doctor can make adjustments to help this problem.
- Slowing of growth—This is why your child's height and weight are checked regularly; if this is a problem, growth usually catches up if the medicine is stopped or the dose is decreased.
- Nervous habits—Examples are picking at skin or biting nails (although these habits are also common in children with ADHD who do not take medicine).
- Stuttering

Rare, but Serious, Side Effects

If any of the following occur, call the doctor or go to an emergency room *right away:*

- Chest pain that does not go away after a few minutes
- Very fast or irregular heartbeat not related to exercise or exertion
- Shortness of breath not related to exercise or exertion
- Fainting
- Seizures (fits, convulsions)

Call the doctor within a day or two:

- Motor or vocal tics (fast, repeated movements or sounds) or muscle twitches (jerking movements) of parts of the body
- Pain, numbness, or changes in skin color or temperature sensitivity in fingers and/or toes
- Sadness that lasts more than a few days
- Auditory, visual, or tactile hallucinations (hearing, seeing, or feeling things that are not there)
- Any behavior that is very unusual for your child

Some Interactions With Other Medicines or Food

Please note that the following are only the most likely interactions with other medicines or food.

Caffeine may increase side effects.

Amphetamine may be taken with or without food. Very acid juices (like grapefruit or tomato) or vitamin C may decrease levels of amphetamine so that it does not work as well.

It is not a good idea to combine stimulants with nasal decongestants or cough and cold medicines that contain ingredients such as pseudoephedrine or phenylpropanolamine, because rapid pulse rate (heartbeat) or high blood pressure may develop. If a stuffy nose is really troublesome, it is better to use a nasal spray. Check with the pharmacist before giving an over-the-counter medicine. Also, many children with ADHD become cranky or more hyperactive while taking antihistamines (such as Benadryl). If medicine for allergies is needed, ask your child's doctor.

Using amphetamine together with imipramine (Tofranil), nortriptyline (Pamelor), or amitriptyline (Elavil) may be dangerous because these combinations can increase the risk of serious heart problems.

Amphetamine should not be taken at the same time as or even within a month of taking another type of medicine called a *monoamine oxidase inhibitor* (MAOI), such as selegiline (Eldepryl), phenelzine (Nardil), tranylcypromine (Parnate), or isocarboxazid (Marplan). The combination could cause dangerous high blood pressure.

What Could Happen if This Medicine Is Stopped Suddenly?

No medical withdrawal effects occur if prescribed amphetamine is stopped suddenly. The ADHD symptoms will come back as soon as the medicine wears off. Some people may have irritability, trouble sleeping, or increased hyperactivity for a day or two if they have been taking the medicine every day for a long time, especially at high doses. It may be better to decrease the medicine slowly (taper) over a week or so.

How Long Will This Medicine Be Needed?

There is no way to know how long a person will need to take amphetamine. The parent(s), the doctor, and the school will work together to determine what is right for each patient. Sometimes the medicine is needed for a few years, but many people need to take medicine for ADHD even as adults.

What Else Should I Know About This Medicine?

Many people have incorrect information about stimulants. If you hear anything that worries you, please check with your doctor.

Unlike methylphenidate, amphetamines are FDA approved for children younger than 6 years old. This is a historical accident that happened as rules changed for approval of medicines. There is actually less research on using amphetamines for ADHD in young children than there is for methylphenidate.

Stimulants do not *cause* drug use or addiction. However, because the patient or other people (especially if they have a history of drug abuse) may abuse these medicines, adult supervision is especially important. Some teenagers may try to sell or share their medicine, so it should be kept in a secure place and given by an adult. Amphetamine will not help people who do not have ADHD to get better grades or do better on tests, but some people think that it will, so they try to take someone else's medicine. It is important to talk to your teenager about why he or she should never give away or sell medication. This is called *diversion* and can be considered a federal crime.

The government considers amphetamine to be a *controlled substance*. There are special rules for how much of this medicine may be prescribed at one time and how soon prescriptions must be filled after they are written. Prescriptions may not have refills and may not be telephoned to the pharmacy. The doctor must write a new prescription for stimulants each time. Prescriptions may be mailed or picked up at the doctor's office.

It is important for the child *not* to chew the long-acting tablets because doing so releases too much medicine all at once.

For children who cannot swallow pills, the capsule forms may be opened and the tiny beads inside sprinkled onto a spoonful of applesauce. The mixture of applesauce and medicine should be swallowed right away without chewing. The beads should not be mixed in liquid. The medicine should not be mixed into food and then stored. Do not divide the dose.

Some of these medicines have similar names but have different strengths or last different amounts of time (for example, Adderall and Adderall XR). Be sure to check your prescription to be sure you have the correct medicine from the pharmacy.

Questions have been raised after a very small number of people died suddenly while taking amphetamine. Clearly, amphetamine in very high doses can be dangerous. However, the chance of sudden death when taking amphetamine as prescribed by a doctor is not higher than without medication. In most of the deaths, problems in the shape, size, or rhythm of the heart were found that were not related to the amphetamine use. Be sure to tell the doctor if your child or anyone in the family has had heart problems or if a family member died suddenly.

Notes

Use this space to take notes or to write down questions you want to ask the doctor.

_____

_____

_____

_____

_____

_____

_____

_____

_____

_____

_____

_____

_____

all the possible uses, precautions, side effects, or interactions of this drug. For a complete listing of side effects, see the manufacturer's package insert, which can be obtained from your physician or pharmacist. As medical research and practice advance, therapeutic standards may change. For this reason and because human and mechanical errors sometimes occur, we recommend that readers follow the advice of a physician who is directly involved in their care or the care of a member of their family.

From Dulcan MK, Ballard R (editors): *Helping Parents and Teachers Understand Medications for Behavioral and Emotional Problems: A Resource Book of Medication Information Handouts*, Fourth Edition. Washington, DC, American Psychiatric Publishing, 2015

Medication Information for Parents and Teachers

Aripiprazole—Abilify

General Information About Medication

Each child and adolescent is different. No one has exactly the same combination of medical and psychological problems. It is a good idea to talk with the doctor or nurse about the reasons a medicine is being used. It is very important to keep all appointments and to be in touch by telephone if you have concerns. It is important to communicate with the doctor, nurse, or therapist. An *advanced practice nurse* (APN) has additional education and training after becoming a registered nurse (RN). Your child's medication may be prescribed by a medical doctor (MD or DO) or an APN. In addition, a *physician assistant* (PA) working with a physician may prescribe certain medications. In this information sheet, "doctor" includes medical doctors as well as APNs and PAs who prescribe medication. Often a nurse (RN) will be part of the team and answer questions and give information.

It is very important that the medicine be taken exactly as the doctor instructs. However, once in a while, everyone forgets to give a medicine on time. It is a good idea to ask the doctor or nurse what to do if this happens. Do not stop or change a medicine without asking the doctor or nurse first.

If the medicine seems to stop working, it may be because it is not being taken regularly. The youth may be "cheeking" or hiding the medicine or forgetting to take it (especially at school). The doses may be too far apart or a different dose or medicine may be needed. Something at school, at home, or in the neighborhood may be upsetting the youth, or he or she may need special help for learning disabilities or tutoring. Please discuss your concerns with the doctor. **Do not just increase the dose.** It is also very important not to decrease the dose or stop the medicine without talking to the doctor first. The problem being treated may come back, or there could be uncomfortable or even dangerous results.

All medicines should be kept in a safe place, out of the reach of children, and should be supervised by an adult. If someone takes too much of a medicine, call the doctor, the poison control center, or a hospital emergency room.

Each medicine has a "generic" or chemical name. Just like laundry detergents or paper towels, some medicines are sold by more than one company under different brand names. The same medicine may be available under a generic name and several brand names. The generic medications are usually less expensive than the brand name ones. The generic medications have the same chemical formula, but they may or may not be exactly the same strength as the brand-name medications. Also, some brands of pills contain dye or other things that can cause allergic reactions. It is a good idea to talk to the doctor and the pharmacist about whether it is important to use a specific brand of medicine.

Any medicine can cause an allergic reaction. Examples are hives, itching, rashes, swelling, and trouble breathing. Even a tiny amount of a medicine can cause a reaction in patients who are allergic to that medicine. Be *sure* to talk to the doctor before restarting a medicine that has caused an allergic reaction and tell the doctor about any reactions to medicine that your child has had before.

Taking more than one medicine at the same time may cause more side effects or cause one of the medicines to not work as well. Always ask the doctor, nurse, or pharmacist before adding another medicine, either prescription or bought without a prescription in a store or on the Internet. Be sure

that each doctor knows about *all* of the medicines your child is taking. Also tell the doctor about any vitamins, herbal medicines, or supplements your child may be taking. Some of these may have side effects alone or when taken with this medication. It is a very good idea to keep a list with you of the names and doses of all medicines that your child is taking.

Everyone taking medicine should have a physical examination at least once a year.

If you think that your child may be using drugs or alcohol, please tell the doctor right away.

Pregnancy requires special care in the use of medicine. Some medicines can cause birth defects if taken by a pregnant mother. **Please tell the doctor immediately if you suspect the teenager is at risk of becoming pregnant.** The doctor may wish to discuss sexual behavior and/or birth control with your daughter.

Printed information like this applies to children and adolescents in general. If you have questions about the medicine, or if you notice changes or anything unusual, please ask the doctor or nurse. As scientific research advances, knowledge increases and advice changes. Even experts do not always agree. Many medicines have not been "approved" by the U.S. Food and Drug Administration (FDA) for use in children or use for particular problems. For this reason, use of the medicine for a problem or age group often is not listed in the *Physicians' Desk Reference.* This does not necessarily mean that the medicine is dangerous or does not work, only that the company that makes the medicine has not received permission to advertise the medicine for use in children. Companies often do not apply for this permission because it is expensive to do the tests needed to apply for approval for use in children. Once a medication is approved by the FDA for any purpose, a doctor is allowed to prescribe it according to research and clinical experience.

Note to Teachers

It is a good idea to talk with the parent(s) about the reason(s) that a medication is being used. If the parent(s) sign consent to release information, it is often helpful for you to talk with the doctor. If the parent(s) give permission, the doctor may ask you to fill out rating forms about your experience with the student's behavior, feelings, academic performance, and medication side effects. This information is very useful in selecting and monitoring medication treatment. If you have observations that you think are important, do not hesitate to share these with the student's parent(s) and treating clinicians (with parental consent).

It is very important that the medicine be taken exactly as the doctor instructs. However, everyone forgets to give a medicine on time once in a while. It is a good idea to ask the parent(s) in advance what to do if this happens. Do not stop or change the time you are giving a medicine at school without parental permission. If a medication is to be taken with food, but lunchtime or snack time changes, be sure to notify the parent(s) so appropriate adjustments can be made.

All medicines should be kept in a secure place and should be supervised by an adult. If someone takes too much of a medicine, follow your school procedure for an urgent medical problem.

Taking medicine is a private matter and is best managed discreetly and confidentially. It is important to be sensitive to the student's feelings about taking medicine.

If you suspect that the student is using drugs or alcohol, please tell the parent(s) or a school counselor right away.

Please tell the parent(s) or school nurse if you suspect medication side effects.

Modifications of the classroom environment or assignments may be useful in addition to medication. The student may need to be evaluated for additional help or a 504 plan or an Individualized Education Plan for learning problems or emotional or behavioral issues.

Any expression of suicidal thoughts or feelings or self-harm by a child or adolescent is a signal of distress and should be taken seriously. These behaviors should not be dismissed as "attention seeking." School procedures for safety issues should be followed.

What Is Aripiprazole (Abilify)?

This medicine is called an *atypical* or *second-generation antipsychotic*. It is sometimes called an *atypical psychotropic agent*, or simply an *atypical*. It comes in brand name Abilify tablets, disks that dissolve under the tongue, and liquid. Abilify Maintena long-acting injection is given in a shot once a month.

How Can This Medicine Help?

Aripiprazole is used to treat psychosis, such as in schizophrenia, mania, or very severe depression. It can reduce *positive symptoms* such as hallucinations (hearing voices or seeing things that are not there); delusions (troubling beliefs that other people do not share); agitation; and very unusual thinking, speech, and behavior. It is also used to lessen the *negative symptoms* of schizophrenia, such as lack of interest in doing things (apathy), lack of motivation, social withdrawal, and lack of energy.

Aripiprazole may be used as a *mood stabilizer* in patients with bipolar disorder or severe mood swings. It can reduce mania and may be able to help maintain a stable mood.

Aripiprazole may be used to treat irritability and associated problem behaviors in young people with autism spectrum disorders.

Sometimes aripiprazole is used to reduce severe aggression or very serious behavioral problems in young people with conduct disorder or intellectual disability.

Aripiprazole may be used for behavior problems after a head injury.

This medicine is very powerful and is used to treat very serious problems or symptoms that other medicines do not help. Be patient; the positive effects of this medicine may not appear for 2–3 weeks.

How Does This Medicine Work?

Cells in the brain communicate using chemicals called *neurotransmitters*. Too much or too little of these substances in parts of the brain can cause problems. Aripiprazole works by changing the effects of two of these neurotransmitters—*dopamine and serotonin*—in certain areas of the brain.

How Long Does This Medicine Last?

Aripiprazole can usually be taken only once a day.

How Will the Doctor Monitor This Medicine?

The doctor will review your child's medical history and physical examination before starting aripiprazole. The doctor may order some blood or urine tests to be sure your child does not have a hidden medical condition that would make it unsafe to use this medicine. The doctor or nurse may measure your child's pulse and blood pressure before starting aripiprazole. The doctor may order other tests, such as baseline tests for blood sugar and cholesterol.

Be sure to tell the doctor if anyone in the family has diabetes, high blood pressure, high cholesterol, or heart disease.

Before your child starts taking aripiprazole and every so often afterward, the doctor or nurse may use a test such as the Abnormal Involuntary Movement Scale (AIMS) to check your child's tongue, legs, and arms for unusual movements that could be caused by the medicine.

After the medicine is started, the doctor will want to have regular appointments with you and your child to see how the medicine is working, to see if a dose change is needed, to watch for side effects, to see if aripiprazole is still needed, and to see if any other treatment is needed. The doctor or nurse may check your child's height, weight, pulse, and blood pressure and watch for abnormal movements. Sometimes blood tests are needed to watch for diabetes or increased cholesterol.

What Side Effects Can This Medicine Have?

Any medicine can have side effects, including an allergy to the medicine. Because each patient is different, the doctor will monitor the youth closely, especially when the medicine is started. The doctor will work with you to increase the positive effects and decrease the negative effects of the medicine. Please tell the doctor if any of the listed side effects appear or if you think that the medicine is causing any other problems. Not all of the rare or unusual side effects are listed.

Side effects are most common after starting the medicine or after a dose increase. Many side effects can be avoided or lessened by starting with a very low dose and increasing it slowly—ask the doctor.

Allergic Reaction

Tell the doctor in a day or two (if possible, before the next dose of medicine):

- Hives
- Itching
- Rash

Stop the medicine and get *immediate* medical care:

- Trouble breathing or chest tightness
- Swelling of lips, tongue, or throat

Common, but Not Usually Serious, Side Effects

Discuss the following side effects with your child's doctor when convenient. These side effects often can be helped by lowering the dose of medicine, changing the times medicine is taken, or adding another medicine.

- Daytime sleepiness or tiredness—Do not allow your child to drive, ride a bicycle or motorcycle, or operate machinery if this happens. This problem may be lessened by taking the medicine at bedtime.
- Insomnia (trouble sleeping)
- Headache
- Nausea
- Vomiting
- Increased appetite

- Weight gain—Seek nutritional counseling; provide your child with low-calorie snacks and encourage regular exercise.

Rare, but Not Usually Serious, Side Effects

Discuss the following side effects with your child's doctor when convenient. These side effects often can be helped by lowering the dose of medicine, changing the times medicine is taken, or adding another medicine.

- Dry mouth—Have your child try using sugar-free gum or candy.
- Dizziness—This side effect is worse when the child stands up quickly, especially when getting out of bed in the morning; try having the child stand up slowly.
- Increased restlessness or inability to sit still
- Shaking of hands and fingers
- Decreased or slowed movement and decreased facial expressions

Very Rare, but Serious, Side Effects

Call the doctor immediately:

- Stiffness of the tongue, jaw, neck, back, or legs
- Seizure (fit, convulsion)—This is more common in people with a history of seizures or head injury.
- Increased thirst, frequent urination (having to go to the bathroom often), lethargy, tiredness, dizziness, and blurred vision—These could be signs of diabetes, especially if your child is overweight or there is a family history of diabetes. **Talk to a doctor within a day.**
- Extreme stiffness or lack of movement, very high fever, mental confusion, irregular pulse rate, or eye pain—**This is a medical emergency. Go to an emergency room right away.**
- Sudden stiffness and inability to breathe or swallow—**Go to an emergency room or call 911. Tell the paramedics, nurses, and doctors that the patient is taking aripiprazole. Other medicines can be used to treat this problem quickly.**

What Else Should I Know About Side Effects?

Most side effects lessen over time. If they are troublesome, talk with your child's doctor. Some side effects can be decreased by taking a smaller dose of medicine, by stopping the medicine, by changing to another medicine, or by adding another medicine.

Sometimes people who take aripiprazole gain weight, although this is less a problem with aripiprazole than with some other atypicals. Children seem to have more problems with weight gain than adults. The weight gain may be from increased appetite and also from ways that the medicine changes how the body processes food. Aripiprazole may also change the way that the body handles glucose (sugar) and cause high levels of blood sugar (*hyperglycemia*). People who take aripiprazole, especially those who gain a lot of weight, might be at increased risk of developing *diabetes* and of having increased fats (*lipids—cholesterol and triglycerides*) in their blood. Over time, both diabetes and increased fats in the blood may lead to heart disease, stroke, and other complications. The FDA has put warnings on all atypical agents about the increased risks of hyperglycemia, diabetes, and increased blood cholesterol and triglycerides when taking one of these medicines. It is much easier to prevent weight gain than to lose weight later. When your child first starts taking aripiprazole, it is a good idea to be sure that he or she eats a well-balanced diet without "junk food" and with healthy snacks like fruits and vegetables, not sweets or fried foods. He or she should drink water or skim milk, not pop, sodas, soft drinks, or sugary juices. Regular exercise is important for maintaining a healthy weight (and may also help with sleep).

One very rare side effect that may not go away is *tardive dyskinesia* (or TD). Patients with tardive dyskinesia have involuntary movements (movements that they cannot help making) of the body, especially the mouth and tongue. The patient may look as though he or she is making faces over and over again. Jerky movements of the arms, legs, or body may occur. There may be fine, wormlike, or sudden repeated movements of the tongue, or the person may appear to be chewing something or smacking or puckering his or her lips. The fingers may look as though they are rolling something. If you notice any unusual movements, be sure to tell the doctor. The doctor may use the AIMS test to look for these movements.

Neuroleptic malignant syndrome is a very rare side effect that can lead to death. The symptoms are severe muscle stiffness, high fever, increased heart rate and blood pressure, irregular heartbeat (pulse), and sweating. It may lead to unconsciousness. If you suspect this, **call 911 or go to an emergency room right away.**

Sometimes this medicine can cause a *dystonic reaction*. This is a sudden stiffening of the muscles, most often in the jaw, neck, tongue, face, or shoulders. If this happens, and your child is not having trouble breathing, you may give a dose of diphenhydramine (Benadryl). Follow the dose instructions on the package for your child's age. This should relax the muscles in a few minutes. Then call your doctor to tell him or her what happened. If the muscles do not relax, take your child to the emergency department.

Some Interactions With Other Medicines or Food

Please note that the following are only the most likely interactions with other medicines or food.

Aripiprazole can be taken with or without food.

Taking aripiprazole together with fluoxetine (Prozac), cimetidine (Tagamet), or paroxetine (Paxil) can increase levels of aripiprazole and increase the risk of side effects.

Taking aripiprazole together with carbamazepine (Tegretol) can decrease the levels of aripiprazole so that it does not work as well.

It is better to limit drinks with caffeine (coffee, tea, soft drinks) because caffeine works in the opposite way from this medicine, and the positive effects might be decreased.

What Could Happen if This Medicine Is Stopped Suddenly?

Involuntary movements, or *withdrawal dyskinesias*, may appear within 1–4 weeks of lowering the dose or stopping the medicine. Usually these go away, but they can last for days to months. If aripiprazole is stopped suddenly, emotional disturbance (such as irritability, nervousness, moodiness, or oppositional behavior) or physical problems (such as stomachache, loss of appetite, nausea, vomiting, diarrhea, sweating, indigestion, trouble sleeping, trembling, or shaking) may appear. These problems usually last only a few days to a few weeks. If they happen, you should tell your child's doctor. The medicine dose may need to be lowered more slowly (tapered). Always check with the doctor before stopping a medicine.

How Long Will This Medicine Be Needed?

How long your child will need to take this medicine depends partly on the reason that it was prescribed. Some problems last for only a few months, whereas others last much longer. It is important to ask the doctor whether medicine is still needed, especially with medicines as powerful as this one. Every few months, you should discuss with your child's doctor the reasons for using the medicine and whether the medicine may be stopped or the dose lowered.

What Else Should I Know About This Medicine?

There are other medicines that are used for the same kinds of problems. If your child is having bad side effects or the medicine does not seem to be working, ask the doctor if another medicine might work as well or better and have fewer side effects for your child. Each person reacts differently to medicines.

Taking this medicine could make overheating or heatstroke more likely. Have your child decrease activity in hot weather, stay out of the sun, and drink water to prevent this.

Notes

Use this space to take notes or to write down questions you want to ask the doctor.

_____

_____

_____

_____

_____

_____

_____

_____

_____

_____

_____

_____

community and accepted child psychiatric practice. The information on this medication sheet does not cover all the possible uses, precautions, side effects, or interactions of this drug. For a complete listing of side effects, see the manufacturer's package insert, which can be obtained from your physician or pharmacist. As medical research and practice advance, therapeutic standards may change. For this reason and because human and mechanical errors sometimes occur, we recommend that readers follow the advice of a physician who is directly involved in their care or the care of a member of their family.

From Dulcan MK, Ballard R (editors): *Helping Parents and Teachers Understand Medications for Behavioral and Emotional Problems: A Resource Book of Medication Information Handouts*, Fourth Edition. Washington, DC, American Psychiatric Publishing, 2015

Medication Information for Parents and Teachers

Asenapine—Saphris

General Information About Medication

Each child and adolescent is different. No one has exactly the same combination of medical and psychological problems. It is a good idea to talk with the doctor or nurse about the reasons a medicine is being used. It is very important to keep all appointments and to be in touch by telephone if you have concerns. It is important to communicate with the doctor, nurse, or therapist. An *advanced practice nurse* (APN) has additional education and training after becoming a registered nurse (RN). Your child's medication may be prescribed by a medical doctor (MD or DO) or an APN. In addition, a *physician assistant* (PA) working with a physician may prescribe certain medications. In this information sheet, "doctor" includes medical doctors as well as APNs and PAs who prescribe medication. Often a nurse (RN) will be part of the team and answer questions and give information.

It is very important that the medicine be taken exactly as the doctor teaches. However, once in a while, everyone forgets to give a medicine on time. It is a good idea to ask the doctor or nurse what to do if this happens. Do not stop or change a medicine without asking the doctor or nurse first.

If the medicine seems to stop working, it may be because it is not being taken regularly. The youth may be "cheeking" or hiding the medicine or forgetting to take it (especially at school). The doses may be too far apart or a different dose or medicine may be needed. Something at school, at home, or in the neighborhood may be upsetting the youth, or he or she may need special help for learning disabilities or tutoring. Please discuss your concerns with the doctor. **Do not just increase the dose.** It is also very important not to decrease the dose or stop the medicine without talking to the doctor first. The problem being treated may come back, or there could be uncomfortable or even dangerous results.

All medicines should be kept in a safe place, out of the reach of children, and should be supervised by an adult. If someone takes too much of a medicine, call the doctor, the poison control center, or a hospital emergency room.

Each medicine has a "generic" or chemical name. Just like laundry detergents or paper towels, some medicines are sold by more than one company under different brand names. The same medicine may be available under a generic name and several brand names. The generic medications are usually less expensive than the brand name ones. The generic medications have the same chemical formula, but they may or may not be exactly the same strength as the brand-name medications. Also, some brands of pills contain dye or other things that can cause allergic reactions. It is a good idea to talk to the doctor and the pharmacist about whether it is important to use a specific brand of medicine.

Any medicine can cause an allergic reaction. Examples are hives, itching, rashes, swelling, and trouble breathing. Even a tiny amount of a medicine can cause a reaction in patients who are allergic to that medicine. Be *sure* to talk to the doctor before restarting a medicine that has caused an allergic reaction and tell the doctor about any reactions to medicine that your child has had before.

Taking more than one medicine at the same time may cause more side effects or cause one of the medicines to not work as well. Always ask the doctor, nurse, or pharmacist before adding another medicine, either prescription or bought without a prescription in a store or on the Internet. Be sure

35

that each doctor knows about *all* of the medicines your child is taking. Also tell the doctor about any vitamins, herbal medicines, or supplements your child may be taking. Some of these may have side effects alone or when taken with this medication. It is a very good idea to keep a list with you of the names and doses of all medicines that your child is taking.

Everyone taking medicine should have a physical examination at least once a year.

If you think that your child may be using drugs or alcohol, please tell the doctor right away.

Pregnancy requires special care in the use of medicine. Some medicines can cause birth defects if taken by a pregnant mother. **Please tell the doctor immediately if you suspect the teenager is at risk of becoming pregnant.** The doctor may wish to discuss sexual behavior and/or birth control with your daughter.

Printed information like this applies to children and adolescents in general. If you have questions about the medicine, or if you notice changes or anything unusual, please ask the doctor or nurse. As scientific research advances, knowledge increases and advice changes. Even experts do not always agree. Many medicines have not been "approved" by the U.S. Food and Drug Administration (FDA) for use in children or use for particular problems. For this reason, use of the medicine for a problem or age group often is not listed in the *Physicians' Desk Reference*. This does not necessarily mean that the medicine is dangerous or does not work, only that the company that makes the medicine has not received permission to advertise the medicine for use in children. Companies often do not apply for this permission because it is expensive to do the tests needed to apply for approval for use in children. Once a medication is approved by the FDA for any purpose, a doctor is allowed to prescribe it according to research and clinical experience.

Note to Teachers

It is a good idea to talk with the parent(s) about the reason(s) that a medication is being used. If the parent(s) sign consent to release information, it is often helpful for you to talk with the doctor. If the parent(s) give permission, the doctor may ask you to fill out rating forms about your experience with the student's behavior, feelings, academic performance, and medication side effects. This information is very useful in selecting and monitoring medication treatment. If you have observations that you think are important, do not hesitate to share these with the student's parent(s) and treating clinicians (with parental consent).

It is very important that the medicine be taken exactly as the doctor instructs. However, everyone forgets to give a medicine on time once in a while. It is a good idea to ask the parent(s) in advance what to do if this happens. Do not stop or change the time you are giving a medicine at school without parental permission. If a medication is to be taken with food, but lunchtime or snack time changes, be sure to notify the parent(s) so appropriate adjustments can be made.

All medicines should be kept in a secure place and should be supervised by an adult. If someone takes too much of a medicine, follow your school procedure for an urgent medical problem.

Taking medicine is a private matter and is best managed discreetly and confidentially. It is important to be sensitive to the student's feelings about taking medicine.

If you suspect that the student is using drugs or alcohol, please tell the parent(s) or a school counselor right away.

Please tell the parent(s) or school nurse if you suspect medication side effects.

Modifications of the classroom environment or assignments may be useful in addition to medication. The student may need to be evaluated for additional help or a 504 plan or an Individualized Education Plan for learning problems or emotional or behavioral issues.

Any expression of suicidal thoughts or feelings or self-harm by a child or adolescent is a signal of distress and should be taken seriously. These behaviors should not be dismissed as "attention seeking." School procedures for safety issues should be followed.

What Is Asenapine (Saphris)?

This medicine is called an *atypical* or *second-generation antipsychotic*. It is sometimes called an *atypical psychotropic agent*, or simply an *atypical*. It comes in brand name Saphris sublingual tablets that are placed under the tongue and allowed to dissolve there.

How Can This Medicine Help?

Asenapine is used to treat psychosis, such as in schizophrenia, mania, or very severe depression. It can reduce *positive symptoms* such as hallucinations (hearing voices or seeing things that are not there); delusions (troubling beliefs that other people do not share); agitation; and very unusual thinking, speech, and behavior. It is also used to lessen the *negative symptoms* of schizophrenia, such as lack of interest in doing things (apathy), lack of motivation, social withdrawal, and lack of energy.

Asenapine may be used as a *mood stabilizer* in patients with bipolar disorder or severe mood swings. It can reduce mania and may be able to help maintain a stable mood.

Sometimes asenapine is used to reduce severe aggression or very serious behavioral problems in young people with conduct disorder, intellectual disability, or autism spectrum disorder. This medicine is very powerful and is used to treat very serious problems or symptoms that other medicines do not help. Be patient; the positive effects of this medicine may not appear for 2–3 weeks.

How Does This Medicine Work?

Cells in the brain communicate using chemicals called *neurotransmitters*. Too much or too little of these substances in parts of the brain can cause problems. Asenapine works by blocking the action of two of these neurotransmitters—*dopamine and serotonin*—in certain areas of the brain.

How Long Does This Medicine Last?

Asenapine is usually taken twice a day.

How Will the Doctor Monitor This Medicine?

The doctor will review your child's medical history and physical examination before starting asenapine. The doctor may order some blood or urine tests to be sure your child does not have a hidden medical condition that would make it unsafe to use this medicine. The doctor or nurse may measure your child's pulse and blood pressure before starting asenapine. The doctor may order other tests, such as baseline tests for blood sugar and cholesterol or an ECG (electrocardiogram or heart rhythm test).

Be sure to tell the doctor if anyone in the family has diabetes, high blood pressure, high cholesterol, or heart disease.

Before your child starts taking asenapine and every so often afterward, a test such as the Abnormal Involuntary Movement Scale (AIMS) may be used to check your child's tongue, legs, and arms for unusual movements that could be caused by the medicine.

After the medicine is started, the doctor will want to have regular appointments with you and your child to see how the medicine is working, to see if a dose change is needed, to watch for side effects, to see if asenapine is still needed, and to see if any other treatment is needed. The doctor or nurse will check your child's height, weight, pulse, and blood pressure and watch for abnormal movements. Sometimes blood tests are needed to watch for diabetes or increased cholesterol.

What Side Effects Can This Medicine Have?

Any medicine can have side effects, including an allergy to the medicine. Because each patient is different, the doctor will monitor the youth closely, especially when the medicine is started. The doctor will work with you to increase the positive effects and decrease the negative effects of the medicine. Please tell the doctor if any of the listed side effects appear or if you think that the medicine is causing any other problems. Not all of the rare or unusual side effects are listed.

Side effects are most common after starting the medicine or after a dose increase. Many side effects can be avoided or lessened by starting with a very low dose and increasing it slowly—ask the doctor.

Allergic Reaction

Tell the doctor in a day or two (if possible, before the next dose of medicine):

- Hives
- Itching
- Rash

Stop the medicine and get *immediate* medical care:

- Trouble breathing or chest tightness
- Swelling of lips, tongue, or throat
- Feeling faint or dizzy (low blood pressure) and very fast heartbeat

Common, but Not Usually Serious, Side Effects

Discuss the following side effects with your child's doctor when convenient. These side effects often can be helped by lowering the dose of medicine, changing the times medicine is taken, or adding another medicine.

- Daytime sleepiness or tiredness—Do not allow your child to drive, ride a bicycle or motorcycle, or operate machinery if this happens. This problem may be lessened by taking the medicine at bedtime.
- Dry mouth—Have your child try using sugar-free gum or candy.
- Constipation—Encourage your child to drink more fluids and eat high-fiber foods; if necessary, the doctor may recommend a fiber medicine such as Benefiber or a stool softener such as Colace or mineral oil.
- Dizziness—This side effect is worse when the child stands up quickly, especially when getting out of bed in the morning; try having the child stand up slowly.
- Increased appetite

- Weight gain—Seek nutritional counseling; provide your child with low-calorie snacks and encourage regular exercise.
- Increased risk of sunburn—Have your child wear sunscreen or protective clothing or stay out of the sun.
- Nausea
- Vomiting
- Insomnia (trouble sleeping)

Less Common, but Not Usually Serious, Side Effects

Discuss the following side effects with your child's doctor when convenient. These side effects often can be helped by lowering the dose of medicine, changing the times medicine is taken, or adding another medicine.

- Drooling
- Increased restlessness or inability to sit still
- Shaking of hands and fingers
- Decreased or slowed movement and decreased facial expressions
- Decreased sexual interest or ability
- Changes in menstrual cycle
- Increase in breast size or discharge from the breasts (in both boys and girls)—This may go away with time.

Less Common, but Potentially Serious, Side Effects

Call the doctor *immediately*:

- Stiffness of the tongue, jaw, neck, back, or legs
- Seizure (fit, convulsion)—This is more common in people with a history of seizures or head injury.
- Increased thirst, frequent urination (having to go to the bathroom often), lethargy, tiredness, dizziness, and blurred vision—These could be signs of diabetes, especially if your child is overweight or there is a family history of diabetes. **Talk to a doctor within a day.**

Very Rare, but Serious, Side Effects

- Extreme stiffness or lack of movement, very high fever, mental confusion, irregular pulse rate, or eye pain—**This is a medical emergency. Go to an emergency room right away.**
- Sudden stiffness and inability to breathe or swallow—**Go to an emergency room or call 911.** Tell the paramedics, nurses, and doctors that the patient is taking asenapine. Other medicines can be used to treat this problem quickly.

What Else Should I Know About Side Effects?

Most side effects lessen over time. If they are troublesome, talk with your child's doctor. Some side effects can be decreased by taking a smaller dose of medicine, by stopping the medicine, by changing to another medicine, or by adding another medicine.

Many young people who take asenapine gain weight. The weight gain may be from increased appetite and also from ways that the medicine changes how the body processes food. Asenapine may also change the way that the body handles glucose (sugar) and cause high levels of blood sugar (*hyperglycemia*). People who take asenapine, especially those who gain a lot of weight, might be at increased risk of developing *diabetes* and of having increased fats (*lipids—cholesterol and triglycerides*) in their blood. Over time, both diabetes and increased fats in the blood may lead to heart disease, stroke, and other complications. The FDA has put warnings on all atypical agents about the increased risks of hyperglycemia, diabetes, and increased blood cholesterol and triglycerides when taking one of these medicines. It is much easier to prevent weight gain than to lose weight later. When your child first starts taking asenapine, it is a good idea to be sure that he or she eats a well-balanced diet without "junk food" and with healthy snacks like fruits and vegetables, not sweets or fried foods. He or she should drink water or skim milk, not pop, sodas, soft drinks, or sugary juices. Regular exercise is important for maintaining a healthy weight (and may also help with sleep).

The medicine may increase the level of *prolactin*, a natural hormone made in the part of the brain called the *pituitary*. This may cause side effects such as breast tenderness or swelling or production of milk in both boys and girls. It also may interfere with sexual functioning in teenage boys and with regular menstrual cycles (periods) in teenage girls. A blood test can measure the level of prolactin. If these side effects do not go away and are troublesome, talk with your child's doctor about substituting another medicine for asenapine.

One very rare side effect that may not go away is *tardive dyskinesia* (or TD). Patients with tardive dyskinesia have involuntary movements (movements that they cannot help making) of the body, especially the mouth and tongue. The patient may look as though he or she is making faces over and over again. Jerky movements of the arms, legs, or body may occur. There may be fine, wormlike, or sudden repeated movements of the tongue, or the person may appear to be chewing something or smacking or puckering his or her lips. The fingers may look as though they are rolling something. If you notice any unusual movements, be sure to tell the doctor. The doctor may use the AIMS test to look for these movements.

Neuroleptic malignant syndrome is a very rare side effect that can lead to death. The symptoms are severe muscle stiffness, high fever, increased heart rate and blood pressure, irregular heartbeat (pulse), and sweating. It may lead to unconsciousness. If you suspect this, **call 911 or go to an emergency room right away.**

Sometimes this medicine can cause a *dystonic reaction*. This is a sudden stiffening of the muscles, most often in the jaw, neck, tongue, face, or shoulders. If this happens, and your child is not having trouble breathing, you may give a dose of diphenhydramine (Benadryl). Follow the dose instructions on the package for your child's age. This should relax the muscles in a few minutes. Then call your doctor to tell him or her what happened. If the muscles do not relax, take your child to the emergency department.

Some Interactions With Other Medicines or Food

Please note that the following are only the most likely interactions with other medicines or food.

Asenapine should be taken without food and one should not eat or drink for at least 10 minutes after taking this medicine. The tablet should be allowed to dissolve and should not be chewed or swallowed.

Fluoxetine (Prozac), fluvoxamine (Luvox), and other selective serotonin reuptake inhibitor (SSRI) antidepressants can increase the levels of asenapine and increase the risk of side effects.

Heart problems are more common if other medicines that affect the heart are being taken as well. Be sure to tell all your child's doctors and your pharmacist about all medications your child is taking.

It is better to limit drinks with caffeine (coffee, tea, soft drinks) because caffeine works in the opposite way from this medicine, and the positive effects might be decreased.

What Could Happen if This Medicine Is Stopped Suddenly?

Involuntary movements, or *withdrawal dyskinesias*, may appear within 1–4 weeks of lowering the dose or stopping the medicine. Usually these go away, but they can last for days to months. If asenapine is stopped suddenly, emotional disturbance (such as irritability, nervousness, moodiness, or oppositional behavior) or physical problems (such as stomachache, loss of appetite, nausea, vomiting, diarrhea, sweating, indigestion, trouble sleeping, trembling, or shaking) may appear. These problems usually last only a few days to a few weeks. If they happen, you should tell your child's doctor. The medicine dose may need to be lowered more slowly (tapered). Always check with the doctor before stopping a medicine.

How Long Will This Medicine Be Needed?

How long your child will need to take this medicine depends partly on the reason that it was prescribed. Some problems last for only a few months, whereas others last much longer. It is important to ask the doctor whether medicine is still needed, especially with medicines as powerful as this one. Every few months, you should discuss with your child's doctor the reasons for using the medicine and whether the medicine may be stopped or the dose lowered.

What Else Should I Know About This Medicine?

There are other medicines that are used for the same kinds of problems. If your child is having bad side effects or the medicine does not seem to be working, ask the doctor if another medicine might work as well or better and have fewer side effects for your child. Each person reacts differently to medicines.

Taking this medicine could make overheating or heatstroke more likely. Have your child decrease activity in hot weather, stay out of the sun, and drink water to prevent this.

Notes

Use this space to take notes or to write down questions you want to ask the doctor.

_____

_____

_____

_____

_____

_____

_____

_____

_____

_____

_____

From Dulcan MK, Ballard R (editors): _Helping Parents and Teachers Understand Medications for Behavioral and Emotional Problems: A Resource Book of Medication Information Handouts_, Fourth Edition. Washington, DC, American Psychiatric Publishing, 2015

Medication Information for Parents and Teachers

Atenolol—Tenormin

General Information About Medication

Each child and adolescent is different. No one has exactly the same combination of medical and psychological problems. It is a good idea to talk with the doctor or nurse about the reasons a medicine is being used. It is very important to keep all appointments and to be in touch by telephone if you have concerns. It is important to communicate with the doctor, nurse, or therapist. An *advanced practice nurse* (APN) has additional education and training after becoming a registered nurse (RN). Your child's medication may be prescribed by a medical doctor (MD or DO) or an APN. In addition, a *physician assistant* (PA) working with a physician may prescribe certain medications. In this information sheet, "doctor" includes medical doctors as well as APNs and PAs who prescribe medication. Often a nurse (RN) will be part of the team and answer questions and give information.

It is very important that the medicine be taken exactly as the doctor instructs. However, once in a while, everyone forgets to give a medicine on time. It is a good idea to ask the doctor or nurse what to do if this happens. Do not stop or change a medicine without asking the doctor or nurse first.

If the medicine seems to stop working, it may be because it is not being taken regularly. The youth may be "cheeking" or hiding the medicine or forgetting to take it (especially at school). The doses may be too far apart or a different dose or medicine may be needed. Something at school, at home, or in the neighborhood may be upsetting the youth, or he or she may need special help for learning disabilities or tutoring. Please discuss your concerns with the doctor. **Do not just increase the dose.** It is also very important not to decrease the dose or stop the medicine without talking to the doctor first. The problem being treated may come back, or there could be uncomfortable or even dangerous results.

All medicines should be kept in a safe place, out of the reach of children, and should be supervised by an adult. If someone takes too much of a medicine, call the doctor, the poison control center, or a hospital emergency room.

Each medicine has a "generic" or chemical name. Just like laundry detergents or paper towels, some medicines are sold by more than one company under different brand names. The same medicine may be available under a generic name and several brand names. The generic medications are usually less expensive than the brand name ones. The generic medications have the same chemical formula, but they may or may not be exactly the same strength as the brand-name medications. Also, some brands of pills contain dye or other things that can cause allergic reactions. It is a good idea to talk to the doctor and the pharmacist about whether it is important to use a specific brand of medicine.

Any medicine can cause an allergic reaction. Examples are hives, itching, rashes, swelling, and trouble breathing. Even a tiny amount of a medicine can cause a reaction in patients who are allergic to that medicine. Be *sure* to talk to the doctor before restarting a medicine that has caused an allergic reaction and tell the doctor about any reactions to medicine that your child has had before.

Taking more than one medicine at the same time may cause more side effects or cause one of the medicines to not work as well. Always ask the doctor, nurse, or pharmacist before adding another medicine, either prescription or bought without a prescription in a store or on the Internet. Be sure

43

that each doctor knows about *all* of the medicines your child is taking. **Also tell the doctor about any vitamins, herbal medicines, or supplements your child may be taking.** Some of these may have side effects alone or when taken with this medication. It is a very good idea to keep a list with you of the names and doses of all medicines that your child is taking.

Everyone taking medicine should have a physical examination at least once a year.

If you think that your child may be using drugs or alcohol, please tell the doctor right away.

Pregnancy requires special care in the use of medicine. Some medicines can cause birth defects if taken by a pregnant mother. **Please tell the doctor immediately if you suspect the teenager is at risk of becoming pregnant.** The doctor may wish to discuss sexual behavior and/or birth control with your daughter.

Printed information like this applies to children and adolescents in general. If you have questions about the medicine, or if you notice changes or anything unusual, please ask the doctor or nurse. As scientific research advances, knowledge increases and advice changes. Even experts do not always agree. Many medicines have not been "approved" by the U.S. Food and Drug Administration (FDA) for use in children or use for particular problems. For this reason, use of the medicine for a problem or age group often is not listed in the *Physicians' Desk Reference.* This does not necessarily mean that the medicine is dangerous or does not work, only that the company that makes the medicine has not received permission to advertise the medicine for use in children. Companies often do not apply for this permission because it is expensive to do the tests needed to apply for approval for use in children. Once a medication is approved by the FDA for any purpose, a doctor is allowed to prescribe it according to research and clinical experience.

Note to Teachers

It is a good idea to talk with the parent(s) about the reason(s) that a medication is being used. If the parent(s) sign consent to release information, it is often helpful for you to talk with the doctor. If the parent(s) give permission, the doctor may ask you to fill out rating forms about your experience with the student's behavior, feelings, academic performance, and medication side effects. This information is very useful in selecting and monitoring medication treatment. If you have observations that you think are important, do not hesitate to share these with the student's parent(s) and treating clinicians (with parental consent).

It is very important that the medicine be taken exactly as the doctor instructs. However, everyone forgets to give a medicine on time once in a while. It is a good idea to ask the parent(s) in advance what to do if this happens. Do not stop or change the time you are giving a medicine at school without parental permission. If a medication is to be taken with food, but lunchtime or snack time changes, be sure to notify the parent(s) so appropriate adjustments can be made.

All medicines should be kept in a secure place and should be supervised by an adult. If someone takes too much of a medicine, follow your school procedure for an urgent medical problem.

Taking medicine is a private matter and is best managed discreetly and confidentially. It is important to be sensitive to the student's feelings about taking medicine.

If you suspect that the student is using drugs or alcohol, please tell the parent(s) or a school counselor right away.

Please tell the parent(s) or school nurse if you suspect medication side effects.

Modifications of the classroom environment or assignments may be useful in addition to medication. The student may need to be evaluated for additional help or a 504 plan or an Individualized Education Plan for learning problems or emotional or behavioral issues.

Any expression of suicidal thoughts or feelings or self-harm by a child or adolescent is a signal of distress and should be taken seriously. These behaviors should not be dismissed as "attention seeking." School procedures for safety issues should be followed.

What Is Atenolol (Tenormin)?

Atenolol is called a *beta-blocker*. It was first used to treat high blood pressure and irregular heartbeat. A newer use is the treatment of emotional and behavioral problems. It is also sometimes used to treat *akathisia*, which is a side effect of some antipsychotic medications. It is used for migraine headaches and a number of other medical conditions. It comes in generic and brand name Tenormin tablets.

How Can This Medicine Help?

Atenolol can decrease aggressive or violent behavior in children and adolescents. It may be particularly useful for patients who have developmental delays or autism spectrum disorder. In addition, atenolol may reduce the aggression and anger that sometimes follow brain injuries. It may reduce some symptoms of anxiety (nervousness) and help children and adolescents who have experienced very frightening events and have posttraumatic stress disorder (PTSD). Atenolol may reduce the severe restlessness resulting from other medicines.

Your child may need to continue taking atenolol for at least 4 weeks before the doctor is able to decide whether the medicine is working.

How Does This Medicine Work?

When atenolol is prescribed for patients with anxiety, aggression, or other behavioral problems, this medicine stops the effect of certain chemicals on nerves that are causing the symptoms. For example, atenolol can decrease the physical anxiety symptoms of shaking, sweating, and fast heartbeat.

How Long Does This Medicine Last?

Atenolol is usually taken twice a day.

How Will the Doctor Monitor This Medicine?

The doctor will review your child's medical history and physical examination before starting atenolol. Extreme caution is needed for children and adolescents with asthma, heart disease, diabetes, kidney disease, or thyroid disease. Please be sure to tell the doctor if your child or anyone in the family has one of these problems. The doctor may order some blood or urine tests to be sure your child does not have a hidden medical condition that would make it unsafe to use this medicine. The doctor or nurse will measure your child's height, weight, pulse, and blood pressure before starting atenolol. The doctor may order an ECG (electrocardiogram or heart rhythm test) before starting atenolol.

After the medicine is started, the doctor will want to have regular appointments with you and your child to see how the medicine is working, to see if a dose change is needed, to watch for side effects, to see if atenolol is still needed, and to see if any other treatment is needed. The doctor or nurse will measure pulse rate and blood pressure at each visit, particularly as the dose is increased. Sometimes these measurements are taken

45

while the patient is both sitting or lying down and standing up. If either pulse rate or blood pressure drops too low, a pill may not be given at that time or the regular dose may be decreased.

What Side Effects Can This Medicine Have?

Any medicine can have side effects, including an allergy to the medicine. Because each patient is different, the doctor will monitor the youth closely, especially when the medicine is started. The doctor will work with you to increase the positive effects and decrease the negative effects of the medicine. Please tell the doctor if any of the listed side effects appear or if you think that the medicine is causing any other problems. Not all of the rare or unusual side effects are listed.

Side effects are most common after starting the medicine or after a dose increase. Many side effects can be avoided or lessened by starting with a very low dose and increasing it slowly—ask the doctor.

Allergic Reaction

Tell the doctor in a day or two (if possible, before the next dose of medicine):

- Hives
- Itching
- Rash

Stop the medicine and get *immediate* medical care:

- Trouble breathing or chest tightness
- Swelling of lips, tongue, or throat

Occasional Side Effects

Tell the doctor within a week or two:

- Tingling, numbness, cold, or pain in the fingers or toes (Raynaud's phenomenon)
- Tiredness or weakness, especially with exercise
- Slow heartbeat
- Low blood pressure
- Dizziness or light-headedness—When standing up quickly, especially when getting out of bed in the morning; try having the child stand up slowly.
- Cough

Uncommon Side Effects

Call the doctor within a day or two:

- Sadness or irritability lasting more than a few days
- Nausea
- Trouble sleeping or nightmares
- Diarrhea

- Muscle cramps
- Swelling of the face, fingers, or feet

Serious Side Effects

Call the doctor *immediately*:

- Wheezing or shortness of breath
- Chest pain or discomfort
- Fast heartbeat
- Fainting
- Hallucinations (hearing voices or seeing things that are not there)

Some Interactions With Other Medicines or Food

Please note that the following are only the most likely interactions with other medicines or food.

Giving atenolol with food will decrease side effects.

Atenolol interacts with many other medicines. Be sure to tell the doctor about all medicines being taken. A doctor may use atenolol in combination with other medicines to treat a behavioral problem. Talk with your doctor and pharmacist about possible medicine interactions.

What Could Happen if This Medicine Is Stopped Suddenly?

Stopping atenolol suddenly may cause a fast or irregular heartbeat, high blood pressure, or severe emotional problems. Atenolol should be decreased slowly over at least 2 weeks under a doctor's supervision. It is especially important not to miss doses of this medicine, because withdrawal problems may occur. **Be sure not to let the prescription run out!**

How Long Will This Medicine Be Needed?

The length of time atenolol will be needed depends on how well the medicine works for your child, whether any side effects occur, and what condition is being treated. Sometimes medicine is needed for a short time to treat a particular problem. Occasionally a person may require treatment lasting for several months or may need to start the medicine again if symptoms return.

What Else Should I Know About This Medicine?

Atenolol may be confused with albuterol or Tylenol. Tenormin may be confused with Norpramin or thiamine. Be sure to check the medicine when you get it from the pharmacy.

People with diabetes should be very careful if taking atenolol because it can hide symptoms of low blood sugar.

Notes

Use this space to take notes or to write down questions you want to ask the doctor.

_____

_____

_____

_____

_____

_____

_____

_____

_____

_____

_____

_____

_____

From Dulcan MK, Ballard R (editors): _Helping Parents and Teachers Understand Medications for Behavioral and Emotional Problems: A Resource Book of Medication Information Handouts_, Fourth Edition. Washington, DC, American Psychiatric Publishing, 2015

Medication Information for Parents and Teachers

Atomoxetine—Strattera

General Information About Medication

Each child and adolescent is different. No one has exactly the same combination of medical and psychological problems. It is a good idea to talk with the doctor or nurse about the reasons a medicine is being used. It is very important to keep all appointments and to be in touch by telephone if you have concerns. It is important to communicate with the doctor, nurse, or therapist. An *advanced practice nurse* (APN) has additional education and training after becoming a registered nurse (RN). Your child's medication may be prescribed by a medical doctor (MD or DO) or an APN. In addition, a *physician assistant* (PA) working with a physician may prescribe certain medications. In this information sheet, "doctor" includes medical doctors as well as APNs and PAs who prescribe medication. Often a nurse (RN) will be part of the team and answer questions and give information.

It is very important that the medicine be taken exactly as the doctor instructs. However, once in a while, everyone forgets to give a medicine on time. It is a good idea to ask the doctor or nurse what to do if this happens. Do not stop or change a medicine without asking the doctor or nurse first.

If the medicine seems to stop working, it may be because it is not being taken regularly. The youth may be "cheeking" or hiding the medicine or forgetting to take it (especially at school). The doses may be too far apart or a different dose or medicine may be needed. Something at school, at home, or in the neighborhood may be upsetting the youth, or he or she may need special help for learning disabilities or tutoring. Please discuss your concerns with the doctor. **Do not just increase the dose.** It is also very important not to decrease the dose or stop the medicine without talking to the doctor first. The problem being treated may come back, or there could be uncomfortable or even dangerous results.

All medicines should be kept in a safe place, out of the reach of children, and should be supervised by an adult. If someone takes too much of a medicine, call the doctor, the poison control center, or a hospital emergency room.

Each medicine has a "generic" or chemical name. Just like laundry detergents or paper towels, some medicines are sold by more than one company under different brand names. The same medicine may be available under a generic name and several brand names. The generic medications are usually less expensive than the brand name ones. The generic medications have the same chemical formula, but they may or may not be exactly the same strength as the brand-name medications. Also, some brands of pills contain dye or other things that can cause allergic reactions. It is a good idea to talk to the doctor and the pharmacist about whether it is important to use a specific brand of medicine.

Any medicine can cause an allergic reaction. Examples are hives, itching, rashes, swelling, and trouble breathing. Even a tiny amount of a medicine can cause a reaction in patients who are allergic to that medicine. Be *sure* to talk to the doctor before restarting a medicine that has caused an allergic reaction and tell the doctor about any reactions to medicine that your child has had before.

Taking more than one medicine at the same time may cause more side effects or cause one of the medicines to not work as well. Always ask the doctor, nurse, or pharmacist before adding another medicine, either prescription or bought without a prescription in a store or on the Internet. Be sure

that each doctor knows about *all* of the medicines your child is taking. Also tell the doctor about any vitamins, herbal medicines, or supplements your child may be taking. Some of these may have side effects alone or when taken with this medication. It is a very good idea to keep a list with you of the names and doses of all medicines that your child is taking.

Everyone taking medicine should have a physical examination at least once a year.

If you think that your child may be using drugs or alcohol, please tell the doctor right away.

Pregnancy requires special care in the use of medicine. Some medicines can cause birth defects if taken by a pregnant mother. **Please tell the doctor immediately if you suspect the teenager is at risk of becoming pregnant.** The doctor may wish to discuss sexual behavior and/or birth control with your daughter.

Printed information like this applies to children and adolescents in general. If you have questions about the medicine, or if you notice changes or anything unusual, please ask the doctor or nurse. As scientific research advances, knowledge increases and advice changes. Even experts do not always agree. Many medicines have not been "approved" by the U.S. Food and Drug Administration (FDA) for use in children or use for particular problems. For this reason, use of the medicine for a problem or age group often is not listed in the *Physicians' Desk Reference.* This does not necessarily mean that the medicine is dangerous or does not work, only that the company that makes the medicine has not received permission to advertise the medicine for use in children. Companies often do not apply for this permission because it is expensive to do the tests needed to apply for approval for use in children. Once a medication is approved by the FDA for any purpose, a doctor is allowed to prescribe it according to research and clinical experience.

Note to Teachers

It is a good idea to talk with the parent(s) about the reason(s) that a medication is being used. If the parent(s) sign consent to release information, it is often helpful for you to talk with the doctor. If the parent(s) give permission, the doctor may ask you to fill out rating forms about your experience with the student's behavior, feelings, academic performance, and medication side effects. This information is very useful in selecting and monitoring medication treatment. If you have observations that you think are important, do not hesitate to share these with the student's parent(s) and treating clinicians (with parental consent).

It is very important that the medicine be taken exactly as the doctor instructs. However, everyone forgets to give a medicine on time once in a while. It is a good idea to ask the parent(s) in advance what to do if this happens. Do not stop or change the time you are giving a medicine at school without parental permission. If a medication is to be taken with food, but lunchtime or snack time changes, be sure to notify the parent(s) so appropriate adjustments can be made.

All medicines should be kept in a secure place and should be supervised by an adult. If someone takes too much of a medicine, follow your school procedure for an urgent medical problem.

Taking medicine is a private matter and is best managed discreetly and confidentially. It is important to be sensitive to the student's feelings about taking medicine.

If you suspect that the student is using drugs or alcohol, please tell the parent(s) or a school counselor right away.

Please tell the parent(s) or school nurse if you suspect medication side effects.

Modifications of the classroom environment or assignments may be useful in addition to medication. The student may need to be evaluated for additional help or a 504 plan or an Individualized Education Plan for learning problems or emotional or behavioral issues.

Any expression of suicidal thoughts or feelings or self-harm by a child or adolescent is a signal of distress and should be taken seriously. These behaviors should not be dismissed as "attention seeking." School procedures for safety issues should be followed.

What Is Atomoxetine (Strattera)?

Atomoxetine is a medicine developed to treat attention-deficit/hyperactivity disorder (ADHD) in children, adolescents, and adults. Atomoxetine is not a stimulant (like methylphenidate or amphetamine), and it works in a different way than the stimulant medicines. It is sometimes called a *selective norepinephrine reuptake inhibitor.*

How Can This Medicine Help?

Atomoxetine can increase attention and the ability to follow instructions. It can improve attention span, decrease distractibility, increase the ability to finish things, decrease hyperactivity, and improve the ability to think before acting (decrease impulsivity). Handwriting and completion of schoolwork and homework can improve. Atomoxetine can improve willingness to follow directions and decrease stubbornness in youngsters who have both ADHD and oppositional defiant disorder (ODD). Atomoxetine can decrease depression (sadness) and anxiety (nervousness, worrying) in children with ADHD who have these emotional symptoms.

Medicine may not remove all symptoms in people with ADHD. Children may also need special help in school and behavior modification at home and at school. Some youngsters and families are helped by family therapy or group social skills therapy.

How Does This Medicine Work?

Atomoxetine helps certain parts of the brain that control impulsive actions ("the brakes") work better by increasing the activity of the neurotransmitter *norepinephrine. Neurotransmitters* are the chemicals that the brain makes for the nerve cells to communicate with each other.

How Long Does This Medicine Last?

When given once or twice a day, atomoxetine works around the clock. It must be taken every day.

How Will the Doctor Monitor This Medicine?

The doctor will review your child's medical history and physical examination before starting atomoxetine. The doctor or nurse may measure your child's height, weight, pulse (heart rate), and blood pressure before starting atomoxetine. The doctor will usually ask parents and teachers to fill out behavior rating scales (checklists).

Unlike most medicines used for behavioral and emotional problems, the correct dose of atomoxetine depends on the youth's weight. The doctor will start with a low dose and increase the dose over several weeks to a "target dose." Often, atomoxetine is started in two divided doses—with breakfast and dinner—to decrease uncomfortable side effects. Once a person is used to the medicine, it can be given once a day, either with breakfast or with dinner. If daytime sleepiness is a problem, it can be given just before or at bedtime.

After the medicine is started, the doctor will want to have regular appointments with you and your child to see how the medicine is working, to see if a dose change is needed, to watch for side effects, to see if atomoxetine is still needed, and to see if any other treatment is needed. The doctor or nurse may check your child's height, weight, pulse, and blood pressure. With parental permission, the doctor will usually ask for reports (rating scale, checklist, testing results, comments) from the teacher(s) to keep track of progress in learning and behavior.

What Side Effects Can This Medicine Have?

Any medicine can have side effects, including an allergy to the medicine. Because each patient is different, the doctor will monitor the youth closely, especially when the medicine is started. The doctor will work with you to increase the positive effects and decrease the negative effects of the medicine. Please tell the doctor if any of the listed side effects appear or if you think that the medicine is causing any other problems. Not all of the rare or unusual side effects are listed.

Side effects are most common after starting the medicine or after a dose increase. Many side effects can be avoided or lessened by starting with a very low dose and increasing it slowly—ask the doctor.

Allergic Reaction

Tell the doctor in a day or two (if possible, before the next dose of medicine):

- Hives
- Itching
- Rash

Stop the medicine and get *immediate* medical care:

- Trouble breathing or chest tightness
- Swelling of lips, tongue, or throat

Common Side Effects

If the following side effects do not go away after a week or two, ask the doctor about lowering your child's dose:

- Sedation, fatigue, sleepiness—These side effects can be helped by giving more of the medicine with dinner. Do not allow your child to drive, ride a bicycle or motorcycle, or operate machinery if this happens.
- Nausea, upset stomach, stomachache—These side effects can be helped by giving the medicine in two doses a day, with meals.
- Decreased appetite, mild weight loss
- Dizziness
- Headache

Less Common Side Effects

Tell the doctor within a week or two:

- Rapid pulse rate (heartbeat)
- Increased blood pressure

- Motor tics (fast, repeated movements) or muscle twitches (jerking movements)
- Vomiting
- Irritability, jitteriness, nervousness
- Insomnia (trouble sleeping)
- Constipation—Encourage your child to drink more fluids and eat high-fiber foods; if necessary, the doctor may recommend a fiber medicine such as Benefiber or a stool softener such as Colace or mineral oil.
- Dry mouth

Less Common, but More Serious, Side Effects

Call the doctor within a day or two:

- Increased aggression or hostility
- Increased moodiness
- Problems urinating (passing urine)

Rare, but Serious, Side Effects

Call the doctor within a day:

- Any unusual change in behavior
- Thoughts of suicide or hurting himself or herself (very rare)
- Hurting himself or herself on purpose (very rare)
- Increased activity, agitation, rapid speech, feeling "speeded up," decreased need for sleep, being very excited or irritable (cranky)—This is likely to be manic activation. It has been seen only in people who have bipolar disorder together with ADHD.
- Yellowing of skin or eyes, dark urine, pale bowel movements, abdominal pain or fullness, unexplained flu-like symptoms, itchy skin—These side effects are extremely rare but could be signs of liver damage.

Boys only

Go to an emergency room *right away*:

- Erection of the penis lasting more than 1 hour (also called *priapism*)—This may be painful and could cause permanent damage.

Some Interactions With Other Medicines or Food

Please note that the following are only the most likely interactions with other medicines or food.

Atomoxetine may be taken with food.

Caffeine may increase side effects.

Atomoxetine is safe to use together with a stimulant medication (methylphenidate or amphetamine) if neither type of medicine alone works well enough for your child.

Atomoxetine may increase the side effects of albuterol (Ventolin) inhalers; these side effects include palpitations, fast heart rate (pulse), and increased blood pressure.

When atomoxetine is taken together with fluoxetine (Prozac), paroxetine (Paxil), cimetidine (Tagamet), or bupropion (Wellbutrin), the dose of atomoxetine may need to be lowered.

Atomoxetine should not be taken at the same time as or even within a month of taking another type of medicine called a _monoamine oxidase inhibitor_ (MAOI), such as selegiline (Eldepryl), phenelzine (Nardil), tranylcypromine (Parnate), or isocarboxazid (Marplan). The combination could cause severe high blood pressure.

What Could Happen if This Medicine Is Stopped Suddenly?

There are no known medical side effects from stopping atomoxetine suddenly. The symptoms of ADHD will gradually come back.

How Long Will This Medicine Be Needed?

There is no way to know how long a person will need to take atomoxetine. The parent(s), the doctor, and the school will work together to determine what is right for each patient. Sometimes the medicine is needed for a few years, but many people need to take medicine for ADHD even as adults.

What Else Should I Know About This Medicine?

Unlike stimulant medicines (methylphenidate or amphetamine), atomoxetine takes several weeks to work (although side effects may show up right away). The full positive effects of a certain dose of atomoxetine may not show for several months, so it helps to be patient.

It is important that the child swallow the capsule whole and not chew it or open it, because the liquid inside can burn the eyes or mouth.

The FDA has required that the label for atomoxetine include a warning regarding possible increased risk of suicidal thinking in children and adolescents being treated with this medicine. The risk of this is very low, but it is important to be careful.

What Should a Parent Do?

1. Be honest with your child about possible risks and benefits of medicine.
2. Talk to your child about whether he or she is having any suicidal thoughts, and tell your child to come to you if he or she is having such thoughts.
3. You, your child, and your child's doctor or nurse should develop a safety plan. Pick adults whom your child can tell if he or she is thinking about suicide.
4. Be sure to tell your child's doctor, nurse, or therapist if you suspect that your child is using alcohol or drugs or if something has happened that might make your child feel worse, such as a family separation, breaking up with a boyfriend or girlfriend, someone close dying or attempting suicide, physical or sexual abuse, or failure in school.
5. Be sure that there are no guns in the home and that all medicines (including over-the-counter medicines like Tylenol) are closely supervised by an adult and kept in a safe place.
6. Watch for new or worse thoughts of suicide, self-harm, depression, anxiety (nerves), feeling very agitated

or restless, being angry or aggressive, having more trouble sleeping, or anything else that you see for the first time, seems worse, or worries your child or you. If these appear, contact a mental health professional **right away.** Do not just stop or change the dose of the medicine on your own. If the problems are serious, and you cannot reach one of your clinicians, call a 24-hour psychiatry emergency telephone number or take your child to an emergency room.

The FDA has also required a warning about possible severe liver injury in patients taking atomoxetine. This problem happened only a few times in a very large number of children and adolescents taking this medicine, but if your child develops itchy skin, yellow skin or eyes, dark urine, abdominal pain or fullness, or unexplained flu-like symptoms, stop the medicine and see the doctor right away.

Notes

Use this space to take notes or to write down questions you want to ask the doctor.

_____

_____

_____

_____

_____

_____

_____

_____

_____

_____

_____

_____

concerning drug dosages, schedules, routes of administration, and side effects is accurate as of the time of publication and consistent with standards set by the U.S. Food and Drug Administration and the general medical community and accepted child psychiatric practice. The information on this medication sheet does not cover all the possible uses, precautions, side effects, or interactions of this drug. For a complete listing of side effects, see the manufacturer's package insert, which can be obtained from your physician or pharmacist. As medical research and practice advance, therapeutic standards may change. For this reason and because human and mechanical errors sometimes occur, we recommend that readers follow the advice of a physician who is directly involved in their care or the care of a member of their family.

From Dulcan MK, Ballard R (editors): *Helping Parents and Teachers Understand Medications for Behavioral and Emotional Problems: A Resource Book of Medication Information Handouts*, Fourth Edition. Washington, DC, American Psychiatric Publishing, 2015

Medication Information for Parents and Teachers

Benzodiazepines Used for Sleep:
Estazolam—ProSom
Flurazepam
Temazepam—Restoril
Triazolam—Halcion

General Information About Medication

Each child and adolescent is different. No one has exactly the same combination of medical and psychological problems. It is a good idea to talk with the doctor or nurse about the reasons a medicine is being used. It is very important to keep all appointments and to be in touch by telephone if you have concerns. It is important to communicate with the doctor, nurse, or therapist. An *advanced practice nurse* (APN) has additional education and training after becoming a registered nurse (RN). Your child's medication may be prescribed by a medical doctor (MD or DO) or an APN. In addition, a *physician assistant* (PA) working with a physician may prescribe certain medications. In this information sheet, "doctor" includes medical doctors as well as APNs and PAs who prescribe medication. Often a nurse (RN) will be part of the team and answer questions and give information.

It is very important that the medicine be taken exactly as the doctor instructs. However, once in a while, everyone forgets to give a medicine on time. It is a good idea to ask the doctor or nurse what to do if this happens. Do not stop or change a medicine without asking the doctor or nurse first.

If the medicine seems to stop working, it may be because it is not being taken regularly. The youth may be "cheeking" or hiding the medicine or forgetting to take it (especially at school). The doses may be too far apart or a different dose or medicine may be needed. Something at school, at home, or in the neighborhood may be upsetting the youth, or he or she may need special help for learning disabilities or tutoring. Please discuss your concerns with the doctor. **Do not just increase the dose.** It is also very important not to decrease the dose or stop the medicine without talking to the doctor first. The problem being treated may come back, or there could be uncomfortable or even dangerous results.

All medicines should be kept in a safe place, out of the reach of children, and should be supervised by an adult. If someone takes too much of a medicine, call the doctor, the poison control center, or a hospital emergency room.

Each medicine has a "generic" or chemical name. Just like laundry detergents or paper towels, some medicines are sold by more than one company under different brand names. The same medicine may be available under a generic name and several brand names. The generic medications are usually less expensive than the brand name ones. The generic medications have the same chemical formula, but they may or may not be exactly the same strength as the brand-name medications. Also, some brands of pills contain dye or other things that can cause allergic reactions. It is a good idea to talk to the doctor and the pharmacist about whether it is important to use a specific brand of medicine.

Any medicine can cause an allergic reaction. Examples are hives, itching, rashes, swelling, and trouble breathing. Even a tiny amount of a medicine can cause a reaction in patients who are allergic to that medicine. Be *sure* to talk to the doctor before restarting a medicine that has caused an allergic reaction and tell the doctor about any reactions to medicine that your child has had before.

Taking more than one medicine at the same time may cause more side effects or cause one of the medicines to not work as well. Always ask the doctor, nurse, or pharmacist before adding another medicine, either prescription or bought without a prescription in a store or on the Internet. Be sure that each doctor knows about *all* of the medicines your child is taking. Also tell the doctor about any vitamins, herbal medicines, or supplements your child may be taking. Some of these may have side effects alone or when taken with this medication. It is a very good idea to keep a list with you of the names and doses of all medicines that your child is taking.

Everyone taking medicine should have a physical examination at least once a year.

If you think that your child may be using drugs or alcohol, please tell the doctor right away.

Pregnancy requires special care in the use of medicine. Some medicines can cause birth defects if taken by a pregnant mother. **Please tell the doctor immediately if you suspect the teenager is at risk of becoming pregnant.** The doctor may wish to discuss sexual behavior and/or birth control with your daughter.

Printed information like this applies to children and adolescents in general. If you have questions about the medicine, or if you notice changes or anything unusual, please ask the doctor or nurse. As scientific research advances, knowledge increases and advice changes. Even experts do not always agree. Many medicines have not been "approved" by the U.S. Food and Drug Administration (FDA) for use in children or use for particular problems. For this reason, use of the medicine for a problem or age group often is not listed in the *Physicians' Desk Reference*. This does not necessarily mean that the medicine is dangerous or does not work, only that the company that makes the medicine has not received permission to advertise the medicine for use in children. Companies often do not apply for this permission because it is expensive to do the tests needed to apply for approval for use in children. Once a medication is approved by the FDA for any purpose, a doctor is allowed to prescribe it according to research and clinical experience.

Note to Teachers

It is a good idea to talk with the parent(s) about the reason(s) that a medication is being used. If the parent(s) sign consent to release information, it is often helpful for you to talk with the doctor. If the parent(s) give permission, the doctor may ask you to fill out rating forms about your experience with the student's behavior, feelings, academic performance, and medication side effects. This information is very useful in selecting and monitoring medication treatment. If you have observations that you think are important, do not hesitate to share these with the student's parent(s) and treating clinicians (with parental consent).

It is very important that the medicine be taken exactly as the doctor instructs. However, everyone forgets to give a medicine on time once in a while. It is a good idea to ask the parent(s) in advance what to do if this happens. Do not stop or change the time you are giving a medicine at school without parental permission. If a medication is to be taken with food, but lunchtime or snack time changes, be sure to notify the parent(s) so appropriate adjustments can be made.

All medicines should be kept in a secure place and should be supervised by an adult. If someone takes too much of a medicine, follow your school procedure for an urgent medical problem.

Taking medicine is a private matter and is best managed discreetly and confidentially. It is important to be sensitive to the student's feelings about taking medicine.

If you suspect that the student is using drugs or alcohol, please tell the parent(s) or a school counselor right away.

Please tell the parent(s) or school nurse if you suspect medication side effects.

Modifications of the classroom environment or assignments may be useful in addition to medication. The student may need to be evaluated for additional help or a 504 plan or an Individualized Education Plan for learning problems or emotional or behavioral issues.

Any expression of suicidal thoughts or feelings or self-harm by a child or adolescent is a signal of distress and should be taken seriously. These behaviors should not be dismissed as "attention seeking." School procedures for safety issues should be followed.

What Are Benzodiazepines Used for Sleep?

Benzodiazepines used for sleep are a family of sedative-hypnotics that include the following:

- Estazolam—comes in brand name ProSom and generic tablets
- Flurazepam—comes in generic capsules
- Temazepam—comes in brand name Restoril and generic capsules
- Triazolam—comes in brand name Halcion and generic tablets

These medications are classified as *benzodiazepine receptor agonist hypnotics*.

How Can These Medicines Help?

Some benzodiazepines are used to treat insomnia—problems falling asleep or staying asleep—when used for a short time along with a behavioral program. They can also be used for problem sleep behaviors, called *parasomnias*, such as night terrors (sudden waking up from sleep with great fear), sleepwalking, or sleeptalking, when these put the youth at risk of an accident or make it impossible for other family members to get enough sleep.

How Do These Medicines Work?

Benzodiazepines work on *receptors* (special places on brain cells) in certain parts of the brain to change the action of *GABA*, a *neurotransmitter*—a chemical that the brain makes for brain cells to communicate with each other.

How Long Do These Medicines Last?

Benzodiazepines are taken before bedtime and start working within 15 minutes to 1 hour depending on the individual drug's properties. Triazolam starts working within 15–30 minutes. It is a short-acting benzodiazepine, so it is less likely to cause sleepiness and memory problems the next day or to build up in the body if taken every day.

Temazepam, flurazepam, and estazolam start working within 30 minutes and are long-acting benzodiazepines, so they are more likely to cause sleepiness and memory problems the next day. If taken every night, these medicines can make daytime drowsiness even worse.

How Will the Doctor Monitor These Medicines?

The doctor will review your child's medical history and physical examination before starting a benzodiazepine.

After the medicine is started, the doctor will want to have regular appointments with you and your child to see how the medicine is working, to see if a dose change is needed, to watch for side effects, to see if medicine is still needed, and to see if any other treatment is needed. Usually these medicines are used for only a short time, along with setting a regular bedtime and other behavioral and environmental changes to promote a healthy sleep pattern.

What Side Effects Can These Medicines Have?

Any medicine can have side effects, including an allergy to the medicine. Because each patient is different, the doctor will monitor the youth closely, especially when the medicine is started. The doctor will work with you to increase the positive effects and decrease the negative effects of the medicine. Please tell the doctor if any of the listed side effects appear or if you think that the medicine is causing any other problems. Not all of the rare or unusual side effects are listed.

Side effects are most common after starting the medicine or after a dose increase. Many side effects can be avoided or lessened by starting with a very low dose and increasing it slowly—ask the doctor.

Allergic Reaction

Tell the doctor in a day or two (if possible, before the next dose of medicine):

- Hives
- Itching
- Rash

Stop the medicine and get *immediate* medical care:

- Trouble breathing or chest tightness
- Swelling of lips, tongue, or throat

Benzodiazepines are usually very safe when used for short periods as the doctor prescribes.

The most common side effect is daytime sleepiness. Benzodiazepines can also cause dizziness, feeling "spacey," or decreased coordination. If the medicine is causing any of these problems it is very important not to drive a car, ride a bicycle or motorcycle, or operate machinery.

Benzodiazepines can cause decreased concentration and memory. These problems, along with daytime sleepiness, may decrease learning and performance in school.

People who take benzodiazepines must not drink alcohol. Severe sleepiness or even loss of consciousness may result.

It is possible to become psychologically and physically dependent on benzodiazepines, but that is not a common problem for patients who see their doctors regularly. Because some people abuse benzodiazepines, it is illegal to give or sell these medicines to someone other than the patient for whom they were prescribed.

Very rarely, benzodiazepines cause excitement, irritability, anger, aggression, agitation, trouble sleeping, nightmares, uncontrollable behavior, or memory loss. This is called *disinhibition* or a *paradoxical effect*. This may be more common in younger children. Stop the medicine and call the doctor if this happens.

Some Interactions With Other Medicines or Food

Please note that the following are only the most likely interactions with other medicines or food.

Caffeine may cause trouble sleeping and make benzodiazepines less effective. If caffeine is eliminated, a lower dose of benzodiazepine may be needed, or medicine may not be needed at all.

Oral contraceptives (birth control pills) may increase the levels of benzodiazepines and increase side effects.

It is important not to use other sedatives, tranquilizers, or sleeping pills or antihistamines (such as Benadryl) when taking benzodiazepines because of greatly increased side effects that could be dangerous.

Some antibiotics may increase levels of triazolam (Halcion) and increase side effects—ask the doctor.

What Could Happen if These Medicines Are Stopped Suddenly?

Many medicines cause problems if stopped suddenly. Benzodiazepines must be decreased slowly (tapered) rather than stopped suddenly. When a benzodiazepine medicine is stopped suddenly, there are withdrawal symptoms that are uncomfortable and may even be dangerous. Problems are more likely in patients taking high doses of benzodiazepines for 2 months or longer, but even after taking benzodiazepines for just a few weeks, it is important to stop these medications slowly. Withdrawal symptoms may include anxiety, irritability, shaking, sweating, aches and pains, muscle cramps, vomiting, confusion, and trouble sleeping. If large doses taken for a long time are stopped suddenly, seizures (fits, convulsions), hallucinations (hearing voices or seeing things that are not there), or out-of-control behavior may result.

How Long Will These Medicines Be Needed?

The length of time depends on why the benzodiazepine is being used. When used for sleep, it is usually prescribed for only a week or so. A behavioral program, such as regular soothing routines at bedtime and increased exercise in the daytime, should be used along with the medicine to improve sleep. This program can be continued after the medicine is tapered (stopped slowly) or when the medicine is used only occasionally.

When used for night terrors or other parasomnias, the medicine may be needed for months or years.

What Else Should I Know About These Medicines?

Because benzodiazepines can be abused (especially by people who abuse alcohol or drugs) and can cause psychological dependence or physical dependence (addiction), they are regulated by special state and federal laws as *controlled substances*. These laws place limitations on telephone prescriptions and refills, and prescriptions expire if they are not filled promptly.

People with sleep apnea (breathing stops while they are asleep) should not take benzodiazepines. Be sure to tell the doctor if your child snores very loudly.

Benzodiazepines should be avoided during pregnancy, especially in the first 3 months, because they may cause birth defects in the baby. Your doctor may consider ordering a pregnancy test before your daughter starts this medication. If your daughter decides to start sexual activity while taking this medication, she should plan to talk with her doctor about birth control and other health issues related to sex. If taken regularly at the end of pregnancy, benzodiazepines may cause withdrawal symptoms in the baby.

Notes

Use this space to take notes or to write down questions you want to ask the doctor.

_____

_____

_____

_____

_____

_____

_____

_____

_____

_____

_____

_____

From Dulcan MK, Ballard R (editors): *Helping Parents and Teachers Understand Medications for Behavioral and Emotional Problems: A Resource Book of Medication Information Handouts*, Fourth Edition. Washington, DC, American Psychiatric Publishing, 2015

Medication Information for Parents and Teachers

Benztropine—Cogentin

General Information About Medication

Each child and adolescent is different. No one has exactly the same combination of medical and psychological problems. It is a good idea to talk with the doctor or nurse about the reasons a medicine is being used. It is very important to keep all appointments and to be in touch by telephone if you have concerns. It is important to communicate with the doctor, nurse, or therapist. An *advanced practice nurse* (APN) has additional education and training after becoming a registered nurse (RN). Your child's medication may be prescribed by a medical doctor (MD or DO) or an APN. In addition, a *physician assistant* (PA) working with a physician may prescribe certain medications. In this information sheet, "doctor" includes medical doctors as well as APNs and PAs who prescribe medication. Often a nurse (RN) will be part of the team and answer questions and give information.

It is very important that the medicine be taken exactly as the doctor instructs. However, once in a while, everyone forgets to give a medicine on time. It is a good idea to ask the doctor or nurse what to do if this happens. Do not stop or change a medicine without asking the doctor or nurse first.

If the medicine seems to stop working, it may be because it is not being taken regularly. The youth may be "cheeking" or hiding the medicine or forgetting to take it (especially at school). The doses may be too far apart or a different dose or medicine may be needed. Something at school, at home, or in the neighborhood may be upsetting the youth, or he or she may need special help for learning disabilities or tutoring. Please discuss your concerns with the doctor. **Do not just increase the dose.** It is also very important not to decrease the dose or stop the medicine without talking to the doctor first. The problem being treated may come back, or there could be uncomfortable or even dangerous results.

All medicines should be kept in a safe place, out of the reach of children, and should be supervised by an adult. If someone takes too much of a medicine, call the doctor, the poison control center, or a hospital emergency room.

Each medicine has a "generic" or chemical name. Just like laundry detergents or paper towels, some medicines are sold by more than one company under different brand names. The same medicine may be available under a generic name and several brand names. The generic medications are usually less expensive than the brand name ones. The generic medications have the same chemical formula, but they may or may not be exactly the same strength as the brand-name medications. Also, some brands of pills contain dye or other things that can cause allergic reactions. It is a good idea to talk to the doctor and the pharmacist about whether it is important to use a specific brand of medicine.

Any medicine can cause an allergic reaction. Examples are hives, itching, rashes, swelling, and trouble breathing. Even a tiny amount of a medicine can cause a reaction in patients who are allergic to that medicine. Be *sure* to talk to the doctor before restarting a medicine that has caused an allergic reaction and tell the doctor about any reactions to medicine that your child has had before.

Taking more than one medicine at the same time may cause more side effects or cause one of the medicines to not work as well. Always ask the doctor, nurse, or pharmacist before adding another

medicine, either prescription or bought without a prescription in a store or on the Internet. **Be sure that each doctor knows about *all* of the medicines your child is taking. Also tell the doctor about any vitamins, herbal medicines, or supplements your child may be taking.** Some of these may have side effects alone or when taken with this medication. It is a very good idea to keep a list with you of the names and doses of all medicines that your child is taking.

Everyone taking medicine should have a physical examination at least once a year.

If you think that your child may be using drugs or alcohol, please tell the doctor right away.

Pregnancy requires special care in the use of medicine. Some medicines can cause birth defects if taken by a pregnant mother. **Please tell the doctor immediately if you suspect the teenager is at risk of becoming pregnant.** The doctor may wish to discuss sexual behavior and/or birth control with your daughter.

Printed information like this applies to children and adolescents in general. If you have questions about the medicine, or if you notice changes or anything unusual, please ask the doctor or nurse. As scientific research advances, knowledge increases and advice changes. Even experts do not always agree. Many medicines have not been "approved" by the U.S. Food and Drug Administration (FDA) for use in children or use for particular problems. For this reason, use of the medicine for a problem or age group often is not listed in the *Physicians' Desk Reference.* This does not necessarily mean that the medicine is dangerous or does not work, only that the company that makes the medicine has not received permission to advertise the medicine for use in children. Companies often do not apply for this permission because it is expensive to do the tests needed to apply for approval for use in children. Once a medication is approved by the FDA for any purpose, a doctor is allowed to prescribe it according to research and clinical experience.

Note to Teachers

It is a good idea to talk with the parent(s) about the reason(s) that a medication is being used. If the parent(s) sign consent to release information, it is often helpful for you to talk with the doctor. If the parent(s) give permission, the doctor may ask you to fill out rating forms about your experience with the student's behavior, feelings, academic performance, and medication side effects. This information is very useful in selecting and monitoring medication treatment. If you have observations that you think are important, do not hesitate to share these with the student's parent(s) and treating clinicians (with parental consent).

It is very important that the medicine be taken exactly as the doctor instructs. However, everyone forgets to give a medicine on time once in a while. It is a good idea to ask the parent(s) in advance what to do if this happens. Do not stop or change the time you are giving a medicine at school without parental permission. If a medication is to be taken with food, but lunchtime or snack time changes, be sure to notify the parent(s) so appropriate adjustments can be made.

All medicines should be kept in a secure place and should be supervised by an adult. If someone takes too much of a medicine, follow your school procedure for an urgent medical problem.

Taking medicine is a private matter and is best managed discreetly and confidentially. It is important to be sensitive to the student's feelings about taking medicine.

If you suspect that the student is using drugs or alcohol, please tell the parent(s) or a school counselor right away.

Please tell the parent(s) or school nurse if you suspect medication side effects.

Modifications of the classroom environment or assignments may be useful in addition to medication. The student may need to be evaluated for additional help or a 504 plan or an Individualized Education Plan for learning problems or emotional or behavioral issues.

Any expression of suicidal thoughts or feelings or self-harm by a child or adolescent is a signal of distress and should be taken seriously. These behaviors should not be dismissed as "attention seeking." School procedures for safety issues should be followed.

What Is Benztropine (Cogentin)?

Benztropine is called an *anticholinergic* or *antiparkinson* medicine. It is not used alone, but together with some antipsychotic medicines, such as haloperidol, fluphenazine, risperidone, and trifluoperazine. Benztropine comes in generic tablets and brand name Cogentin and generic injections (shots).

How Can This Medicine Help?

Benztropine can reduce some of the movement side effects of the antipsychotic medicines, such as severe restlessness, agitation, and pacing *(akathisia)*; muscle spasms *(dystonia)*; muscle stiffness *(cogwheeling rigidity)*; or trembling. Sometimes these are called *parkinsonian* or *extrapyramidal* symptoms. Benztropine can be given regularly as a pill to prevent or treat these problems. If there is a sudden, severe muscle spasm, benztropine may be given as a shot so that it works within 15 minutes.

How Does This Medicine Work?

Benztropine counteracts the effects of the antipsychotic medicines in parts of the brain that control muscle action, but without decreasing the effects of the antipsychotic medicines on thinking and other psychiatric symptoms. It balances the *cholinergic* and *dopamine* systems in the brain.

How Long Does This Medicine Last?

Benztropine is taken two or three times a day.

How Will the Doctor Monitor This Medicine?

The doctor will review your child's medical history and physical examination before starting benztropine. An examination such as the Abnormal Involuntary Movement Scale (AIMS) test may be used to check the child's tongue, legs, and arms for unusual movements that could be helped by the medicine.

After the medicine is started, the doctor will want to have regular appointments with you and your child to see how the medicine is working, to see if a dose change is needed, to watch for side effects, to see if benztropine is still needed, and to see if any other treatment is needed.

What Side Effects Can This Medicine Have?

Any medicine can have side effects, including an allergy to the medicine. Because each patient is different, the doctor will monitor the youth closely, especially when the medicine is started. The doctor will work with you to increase the positive effects and decrease the negative effects of the medicine. Please tell the doctor if any of the listed side effects appear or if you think that the medicine is causing any other problems. Not all of the rare or unusual side effects are listed.

Side effects are most common after starting the medicine or after a dose increase. Many side effects can be avoided or lessened by starting with a very low dose and increasing it slowly—ask the doctor.

Allergic Reaction

Tell the doctor in a day or two (if possible, before the next dose of medicine):

- Hives
- Itching
- Rash

Stop the medicine and get *immediate* medical care:

- Trouble breathing or chest tightness
- Swelling of lips, tongue, or throat

Common Side Effects

Tell the doctor within a week or two:

- Decreased attention or learning in school
- Dry mouth—Have your child try using sugar-free gum or candy.
- Blurred vision
- Constipation—Encourage your child to drink more fluids and eat high-fiber foods; if necessary, the doctor may recommend a fiber medicine such as Benefiber or a stool softener such as Colace or mineral oil.
- Dizziness—When standing up quickly, especially when getting out of bed in the morning; try having the child stand up slowly.
- Loss of appetite, nausea, or upset stomach
- Decreased sweating

Less Common Side Effects

Call the doctor within a day or two:

- Irritability, overactivity
- Rapid heartbeat (pulse) or palpitations
- Difficulty passing urine

Very Rare, but Serious, Side Effects

Call the doctor *immediately*:

- Worsening of asthma or trouble breathing
- Seizure (fit, convulsion)
- Uncontrollable behavior
- Severe confusion, loss of coordination, severe agitation, disorientation

Some Interactions With Other Medicines or Food

Please note that the following are only the most likely interactions with other medicines or food.

Caffeine may increase side effects.

Benztropine may be taken with or without food. Taking it with food may decrease stomach upset.

Tricyclic antidepressants such as imipramine, nortriptyline, or clomipramine also have anticholinergic effects and will increase the side effects of benztropine. Many antipsychotic medications also have anticholinergic effects and increase the side effects of benztropine.

What Could Happen if This Medicine Is Stopped Suddenly?

Stopping benztropine suddenly can cause withdrawal symptoms such as restlessness, anxiety, irritability, nausea, vomiting, diarrhea, headache, and trouble sleeping.

How Long Will This Medicine Be Needed?

Sometimes the benztropine will be needed as long as the person is on the antipsychotic medicine, but sometimes it can be carefully tapered (decreased) and stopped if the person has gotten used to the antipsychotic medicine and there are no longer motor side effects.

What Else Should I Know About This Medicine?

Because benztropine decreases sweating, a person may be more likely to get heatstroke or *hyperthermia* (increase in body temperature). Be sure that your child drinks plenty of fluids in hot weather and does not exercise too much in the sun.

Notes

Use this space to take notes or to write down questions you want to ask the doctor.

_____

_____

_____

_____

_____

_____

_____

_____

_____

_____

_____

_____

_____

_____

From Dulcan MK, Ballard R (editors): *Helping Parents and Teachers Understand Medications for Behavioral and Emotional Problems: A Resource Book of Medication Information Handouts,* Fourth Edition. Washington, DC, American Psychiatric Publishing, 2015

Medication Information for Parents and Teachers

Bupropion—Wellbutrin, Aplenzin, Forfivo

General Information About Medication

Each child and adolescent is different. No one has exactly the same combination of medical and psychological problems. It is a good idea to talk with the doctor or nurse about the reasons a medicine is being used. It is very important to keep all appointments and to be in touch by telephone if you have concerns. It is important to communicate with the doctor, nurse, or therapist. An *advanced practice nurse* (APN) has additional education and training after becoming a registered nurse (RN). Your child's medication may be prescribed by a medical doctor (MD or DO) or an APN. In addition, a *physician assistant* (PA) working with a physician may prescribe certain medications. In this information sheet, "doctor" includes medical doctors as well as APNs and PAs who prescribe medication. Often a nurse (RN) will be part of the team and answer questions and give information.

It is very important that the medicine be taken exactly as the doctor instructs. However, once in a while, everyone forgets to give a medicine on time. It is a good idea to ask the doctor or nurse what to do if this happens. Do not stop or change a medicine without asking the doctor or nurse first.

If the medicine seems to stop working, it may be because it is not being taken regularly. The youth may be "cheeking" or hiding the medicine or forgetting to take it (especially at school). The doses may be too far apart or a different dose or medicine may be needed. Something at school, at home, or in the neighborhood may be upsetting the youth, or he or she may need special help for learning disabilities or tutoring. Please discuss your concerns with the doctor. **Do not just increase the dose.** It is also very important not to decrease the dose or stop the medicine without talking to the doctor first. The problem being treated may come back, or there could be uncomfortable or even dangerous results.

All medicines should be kept in a safe place, out of the reach of children, and should be supervised by an adult. If someone takes too much of a medicine, call the doctor, the poison control center, or a hospital emergency room.

Each medicine has a "generic" or chemical name. Just like laundry detergents or paper towels, some medicines are sold by more than one company under different brand names. The same medicine may be available under a generic name and several brand names. The generic medications are usually less expensive than the brand name ones. The generic medications have the same chemical formula, but they may or may not be exactly the same strength as the brand-name medications. Also, some brands of pills contain dye or other things that can cause allergic reactions. It is a good idea to talk to the doctor and the pharmacist about whether it is important to use a specific brand of medicine.

Any medicine can cause an allergic reaction. Examples are hives, itching, rashes, swelling, and trouble breathing. Even a tiny amount of a medicine can cause a reaction in patients who are allergic to that medicine. Be *sure* to talk to the doctor before restarting a medicine that has caused an allergic reaction and tell the doctor about any reactions to medicine that your child has had before.

Taking more than one medicine at the same time may cause more side effects or cause one of the medicines to not work as well. Always ask the doctor, nurse, or pharmacist before adding another

medicine, either prescription or bought without a prescription in a store or on the Internet. **Be sure that each doctor knows about *all* of the medicines your child is taking. Also tell the doctor about any vitamins, herbal medicines, or supplements your child may be taking.** Some of these may have side effects alone or when taken with this medication. It is a very good idea to keep a list with you of the names and doses of all medicines that your child is taking.

Everyone taking medicine should have a physical examination at least once a year.

If you think that your child may be using drugs or alcohol, please tell the doctor right away.

Pregnancy requires special care in the use of medicine. Some medicines can cause birth defects if taken by a pregnant mother. **Please tell the doctor immediately if you suspect the teenager is at risk of becoming pregnant.** The doctor may wish to discuss sexual behavior and/or birth control with your daughter.

Printed information like this applies to children and adolescents in general. If you have questions about the medicine, or if you notice changes or anything unusual, please ask the doctor or nurse. As scientific research advances, knowledge increases and advice changes. Even experts do not always agree. Many medicines have not been "approved" by the U.S. Food and Drug Administration (FDA) for use in children or use for particular problems. For this reason, use of the medicine for a problem or age group often is not listed in the *Physicians' Desk Reference*. This does not necessarily mean that the medicine is dangerous or does not work, only that the company that makes the medicine has not received permission to advertise the medicine for use in children. Companies often do not apply for this permission because it is expensive to do the tests needed to apply for approval for use in children. Once a medication is approved by the FDA for any purpose, a doctor is allowed to prescribe it according to research and clinical experience.

Note to Teachers

It is a good idea to talk with the parent(s) about the reason(s) that a medication is being used. If the parent(s) sign consent to release information, it is often helpful for you to talk with the doctor. If the parent(s) give permission, the doctor may ask you to fill out rating forms about your experience with the student's behavior, feelings, academic performance, and medication side effects. This information is very useful in selecting and monitoring medication treatment. If you have observations that you think are important, do not hesitate to share these with the student's parent(s) and treating clinicians (with parental consent).

It is very important that the medicine be taken exactly as the doctor instructs. However, everyone forgets to give a medicine on time once in a while. It is a good idea to ask the parent(s) in advance what to do if this happens. Do not stop or change the time you are giving a medicine at school without parental permission. If a medication is to be taken with food, but lunchtime or snack time changes, be sure to notify the parent(s) so appropriate adjustments can be made.

All medicines should be kept in a secure place and should be supervised by an adult. If someone takes too much of a medicine, follow your school procedure for an urgent medical problem.

Taking medicine is a private matter and is best managed discreetly and confidentially. It is important to be sensitive to the student's feelings about taking medicine.

If you suspect that the student is using drugs or alcohol, please tell the parent(s) or a school counselor right away.

Please tell the parent(s) or school nurse if you suspect medication side effects.

Modifications of the classroom environment or assignments may be useful in addition to medication. The student may need to be evaluated for additional help or a 504 plan or an Individualized Education Plan for learning problems or emotional or behavioral issues.

Any expression of suicidal thoughts or feelings or self-harm by a child or adolescent is a signal of distress and should be taken seriously. These behaviors should not be dismissed as "attention seeking." School procedures for safety issues should be followed.

What Is Bupropion (Wellbutrin, Aplenzin, Forfivo)?

Bupropion is called an *antidepressant*, but it is used to treat behavioral problems, including attention-deficit/hyperactivity disorder (ADHD) and conduct problems, as well as depression or seasonal affective disorder (SAD). Bupropion comes in immediate-release tablets (Wellbutrin and generic), sustained-release long-acting tablets (Wellbutrin SR and generic), and very long-acting extended-release tablets (Wellbutrin XL, Aplenzin, Forfivo XL, and generic). Bupropion also comes in brand names Zyban and Buproban, which are used to help people stop smoking.

How Can This Medicine Help?

Bupropion can decrease symptoms of ADHD, impulsive behavior, depression, SAD, and aggression.

How Does This Medicine Work?

Bupropion helps by balancing the levels of certain chemicals that are naturally found in the brain, called *neurotransmitters*. Neurotransmitters are the chemicals that the brain makes for the nerve cells to communicate with each other. Bupropion is sometimes called a *dopamine-norepinephrine reuptake inhibitor*.

How Long Does This Medicine Last?

Immediate-release bupropion must be taken three times a day. The sustained-release form can be taken twice a day, and the extended-release form can be taken only once a day.

How Will the Doctor Monitor This Medicine?

The doctor will review your child's medical history and physical examination before starting bupropion. The doctor may order some tests to be sure your child does not have a hidden medical condition that would make it unsafe to use this medicine. **Bupropion should *not* be used if the child has an eating disorder (anorexia nervosa or bulimia) or a brain problem such as seizures (epilepsy), a head injury, or a brain tumor. Extra caution is needed when using this medicine in children and adolescents with liver or kidney problems.**

The doctor or nurse may measure your child's pulse and blood pressure before starting bupropion.

After the medicine is started, the doctor will want to have regular appointments with you and your child to see how the medicine is working, to see if a dose change is needed, to watch for side effects, to see if bupropion is still needed, and to see if any other treatment is needed. The doctor or nurse may check your child's height, weight, pulse, and blood pressure.

What Side Effects Can This Medicine Have?

Any medicine can have side effects, including an allergy to the medicine. Allergy to bupropion is more common if the patient has had allergic reactions to other medicines. Because each patient is different, the doctor will monitor the youth closely, especially when the medicine is started. The doctor will work with you to increase the positive effects and decrease the negative effects of the medicine. Please tell the doctor if any of the listed side effects appear or if you think that the medicine is causing any other problems. Not all of the rare or unusual side effects are listed.

Side effects are most common after starting the medicine or after a dose increase. Many side effects can be avoided or lessened by starting with a very low dose and increasing it slowly—ask the doctor.

Allergic Reaction

Tell the doctor in a day or two (if possible, before the next dose of medicine):

- Hives (these may appear soon after starting the medicine or up to a month later)
- Itching
- Rash

Stop the medicine and get *immediate* medical care:

- Trouble breathing or chest tightness
- Swelling of lips, tongue, or throat

Common Side Effects

Tell the doctor within a week or two:

- Nervousness or restlessness
- Irritability—Dose may need to be lowered.
- Dry mouth—Have your child try using sugar-free gum or candy.
- Constipation—Encourage your child to drink more fluids and eat high-fiber foods; if necessary, the doctor may recommend a fiber medicine such as Benefiber or a stool softener such as Colace or mineral oil.
- Headache
- Decreased appetite and weight loss
- Nausea—Taking bupropion with food may help.
- Dizziness
- Excessive sweating

Occasional Side Effects

Call the doctor within a day or two if your child experiences any of these side effects:

- Motor tics (fast, repeated movements), muscle twitches (jerking movements), or tremor (shaking)
- Trouble sleeping
- Ringing in the ears

- Yellowing of skin or eyes, dark urine, pale bowel movements, abdominal pain or fullness, unexplained flu-like symptoms, itchy skin—These side effects are extremely rare but could be signs of liver damage.

Less Common, but More Serious, Side Effects

Call the doctor *immediately:*

- Vomiting
- Seizures (fits, convulsions), especially if taking more than 400 mg/day or if drinking alcoholic beverages. This is less common with the longer-acting forms.
- Unusual excitement, decreased need for sleep, rapid speech

Some Interactions With Other Medicines or Food

Please note that the following are only the most likely interactions with other medicines or food.

Bupropion may be taken with or without food.

Carbamazepine (Tegretol) may decrease the positive effect of bupropion.

It can be *very dangerous* to take bupropion at the same time as, or even within several weeks of, taking another type of medicine called a *monoamine oxidase inhibitor* (MAOI), such as selegiline (Eldepryl), phenelzine (Nardil), tranylcypromine (Parnate), or isocarboxazid (Marplan). The combination may cause very high fever, high blood pressure, and extreme excitement and agitation.

Taking bupropion with tramadol can increase the risk of seizures.

The combination of bupropion with atomoxetine (Strattera) may increase levels of atomoxetime and increase side effects.

Caffeine may increase side effects.

What Could Happen if This Medicine Is Stopped Suddenly?

No known medical withdrawal effects occur if bupropion is stopped suddenly. Some people may get a headache as the medicine wears off. If the medicine is stopped, the original problems may come back. Talk to the doctor before stopping the medicine.

How Long Will This Medicine Be Needed?

Bupropion may take up to 4 weeks to reach its full effect. Your child may need to take the medicine for at least several months so that the emotional or behavioral problem does not come back.

What Else Should I Know About This Medicine?

It is *very important* not to chew the sustained-release tablet or to double up doses if one is missed.

Store the medicine away from heat and wetness.

In youth who have bipolar disorder or who are at risk for bipolar disorder, any antidepressant medicine may increase the risk of hypomania or mania (excitement, agitation, increased activity, decreased sleep).

Bupropion is sometimes confused with buspirone. Be sure to check the prescription.

Sometimes the different forms of bupropion are confused. Be sure you know whether the doctor has prescribed the immediate-release, sustained-release, or extended-release form, and check that the pharmacy has dispensed the correct form of medicine. Be sure that the number of "mg" (dose) and the number of times the medicine is taken each day are clear and consistent.

Black Box Antidepressant Warning

In 2004, an advisory committee to the FDA decided that there might be an increased risk of suicidal behavior for some youth taking medicines called *antidepressants*. In the research studies that the committee reviewed, about 3%–4% of youth with depression who took an antidepressant medicine—and 1%–2% of youth with depression who took a placebo (pill without active medicine)—talked about suicidal thoughts (thinking about killing themselves or wishing they were dead) or did something to harm themselves. This means that almost twice as many youth who were taking an antidepressant to treat their depression talked about suicide or had suicidal behavior compared with youth with depression who were taking inactive medicine. There were *no* completed suicides in any of these research studies, which included more than 4,000 children and adolescents. For youth being treated for anxiety, there was no difference in suicidal talking or behavior between those taking antidepressant medication and those taking placebo.

The FDA told drug companies to add a *black box warning* label to all antidepressant medicines. Because of this label, a doctor (or advanced practice nurse) prescribing one of these medicines has to warn youth and their families that there might be more suicidal thoughts and actions in youth taking these medicines.

On the other hand, in places where more youth are taking the newer antidepressant medicines, the number of adolescents who commit suicide has gotten smaller. Also, thinking about or attempting suicide is more common in surveys of teenagers in the community than it is in depressed youth treated in research studies with antidepressant medicine.

If a youth is being treated with this medicine and is doing well, then no changes are needed as a result of this warning. Increased suicidal talk or action is most likely to happen in the first few months of treatment with a medicine. If your child has recently started this medicine, or is about to start, then you and your doctor (or advanced practice nurse) should watch for any changes in behavior. People who are depressed often have suicidal thoughts or actions. It is hard to know whether suicidal thoughts or actions in depressed people are caused by the depression itself or by the medicine. Also, as their depression is getting better, some people talk more about the suicidal thoughts they had before but did not talk about. As young people get better from depression, they might be at higher risk of doing something about suicidal thoughts that they have had for some time, because they have more energy.

What Should a Parent Do?

1. Be honest with your child about possible risks and benefits of medicine.
2. Talk to your child about whether he or she is having any suicidal thoughts, and tell your child to come to you if he or she is having such thoughts.
3. You, your child, and your child's doctor or nurse should develop a safety plan. Pick adults whom your child can tell if he or she is thinking about suicide.
4. Be sure to tell your child's doctor, nurse, or therapist if you suspect that your child is using alcohol or drugs or if something has happened that might make your child feel worse, such as a family separation, breaking up with a boyfriend or girlfriend, someone close dying or attempting suicide, physical or sexual abuse, or failure in school.
5. Be sure that there are no guns in the home and that all medicines (including over-the-counter medicines like Tylenol) are closely supervised by an adult and kept in a safe place.

6. Watch for new or worse thoughts of suicide, self-harm, depression, anxiety (nerves), feeling very agitated or restless, being angry or aggressive, having more trouble sleeping, or anything else that you see for the first time, seems worse, or worries your child or you. If these appear, contact a mental health professional **right away.** Do not just stop or change the dose of the medicine on your own. If the problems are serious, and you cannot reach one of your clinicians, call a 24-hour psychiatry emergency telephone number or take your child to an emergency room.

Youth taking antidepressant medicine should be watched carefully by their parent(s), clinician(s) (doctor, advanced practice nurse, nurse, therapist), and other concerned adults for the first weeks of treatment. It is a good idea to have regular contact with the doctor, APN, nurse, or therapist for the first months to check for feelings of depression or sadness, thoughts of killing or harming himself or herself, and any problems with the medication. If you have questions, be sure to ask the doctor, APN, nurse, or therapist.

For more information, see http://www.parentsmedguide.org.

Notes

Use this space to take notes or to write down questions you want to ask the doctor.

_____

_____

_____

_____

_____

_____

_____

_____

_____

_____

_____

_____

_____

From Dulcan MK, Ballard R (editors): *Helping Parents and Teachers Understand Medications for Behavioral and Emotional Problems: A Resource Book of Medication Information Handouts*, Fourth Edition. Washington, DC, American Psychiatric Publishing, 2015

Medication Information for Parents and Teachers

Buspirone

General Information About Medication

Each child and adolescent is different. No one has exactly the same combination of medical and psychological problems. It is a good idea to talk with the doctor or nurse about the reasons a medicine is being used. It is very important to keep all appointments and to be in touch by telephone if you have concerns. It is important to communicate with the doctor, nurse, or therapist. An *advanced practice nurse* (APN) has additional education and training after becoming a registered nurse (RN). Your child's medication may be prescribed by a medical doctor (MD or DO) or an APN. In addition, a *physician assistant* (PA) working with a physician may prescribe certain medications. In this information sheet, "doctor" includes medical doctors as well as APNs and PAs who prescribe medication. Often a nurse (RN) will be part of the team and answer questions and give information.

It is very important that the medicine be taken exactly as the doctor instructs. However, once in a while, everyone forgets to give a medicine on time. It is a good idea to ask the doctor or nurse what to do if this happens. Do not stop or change a medicine without asking the doctor or nurse first.

If the medicine seems to stop working, it may be because it is not being taken regularly. The youth may be "cheeking" or hiding the medicine or forgetting to take it (especially at school). The doses may be too far apart or a different dose or medicine may be needed. Something at school, at home, or in the neighborhood may be upsetting the youth, or he or she may need special help for learning disabilities or tutoring. Please discuss your concerns with the doctor. **Do not just increase the dose.** It is also very important not to decrease the dose or stop the medicine without talking to the doctor first. The problem being treated may come back, or there could be uncomfortable or even dangerous results.

All medicines should be kept in a safe place, out of the reach of children, and should be supervised by an adult. If someone takes too much of a medicine, call the doctor, the poison control center, or a hospital emergency room.

Each medicine has a "generic" or chemical name. Just like laundry detergents or paper towels, some medicines are sold by more than one company under different brand names. The same medicine may be available under a generic name and several brand names. The generic medications are usually less expensive than the brand name ones. The generic medications have the same chemical formula, but they may or may not be exactly the same strength as the brand-name medications. Also, some brands of pills contain dye or other things that can cause allergic reactions. It is a good idea to talk to the doctor and the pharmacist about whether it is important to use a specific brand of medicine.

Any medicine can cause an allergic reaction. Examples are hives, itching, rashes, swelling, and trouble breathing. Even a tiny amount of a medicine can cause a reaction in patients who are allergic to that medicine. Be *sure* to talk to the doctor before restarting a medicine that has caused an allergic reaction and tell the doctor about any reactions to medicine that your child has had before.

Taking more than one medicine at the same time may cause more side effects or cause one of the medicines to not work as well. Always ask the doctor, nurse, or pharmacist before adding another

77

medicine, either prescription or bought without a prescription in a store or on the Internet. **Be sure that each doctor knows about *all* of the medicines your child is taking. Also tell the doctor about any vitamins, herbal medicines, or supplements your child may be taking.** Some of these may have side effects alone or when taken with this medication. It is a very good idea to keep a list with you of the names and doses of all medicines that your child is taking.

Everyone taking medicine should have a physical examination at least once a year.

If you think that your child may be using drugs or alcohol, please tell the doctor right away.

Pregnancy requires special care in the use of medicine. Some medicines can cause birth defects if taken by a pregnant mother. **Please tell the doctor immediately if you suspect the teenager is at risk of becoming pregnant.** The doctor may wish to discuss sexual behavior and/or birth control with your daughter.

Printed information like this applies to children and adolescents in general. If you have questions about the medicine, or if you notice changes or anything unusual, please ask the doctor or nurse. As scientific research advances, knowledge increases and advice changes. Even experts do not always agree. Many medicines have not been "approved" by the U.S. Food and Drug Administration (FDA) for use in children or use for particular problems. For this reason, use of the medicine for a problem or age group often is not listed in the *Physicians' Desk Reference*. This does not necessarily mean that the medicine is dangerous or does not work, only that the company that makes the medicine has not received permission to advertise the medicine for use in children. Companies often do not apply for this permission because it is expensive to do the tests needed to apply for approval for use in children. Once a medication is approved by the FDA for any purpose, a doctor is allowed to prescribe it according to research and clinical experience.

Note to Teachers

It is a good idea to talk with the parent(s) about the reason(s) that a medication is being used. If the parent(s) sign consent to release information, it is often helpful for you to talk with the doctor. If the parent(s) give permission, the doctor may ask you to fill out rating forms about your experience with the student's behavior, feelings, academic performance, and medication side effects. This information is very useful in selecting and monitoring medication treatment. If you have observations that you think are important, do not hesitate to share these with the student's parent(s) and treating clinicians (with parental consent).

It is very important that the medicine be taken exactly as the doctor instructs. However, everyone forgets to give a medicine on time once in a while. It is a good idea to ask the parent(s) in advance what to do if this happens. Do not stop or change the time you are giving a medicine at school without parental permission. If a medication is to be taken with food, but lunchtime or snack time changes, be sure to notify the parent(s) so appropriate adjustments can be made.

All medicines should be kept in a secure place and should be supervised by an adult. If someone takes too much of a medicine, follow your school procedure for an urgent medical problem.

Taking medicine is a private matter and is best managed discreetly and confidentially. It is important to be sensitive to the student's feelings about taking medicine.

If you suspect that the student is using drugs or alcohol, please tell the parent(s) or a school counselor right away.

Please tell the parent(s) or school nurse if you suspect medication side effects.

Modifications of the classroom environment or assignments may be useful in addition to medication. The student may need to be evaluated for additional help or a 504 plan or an Individualized Education Plan for learning problems or emotional or behavioral issues.

Any expression of suicidal thoughts or feelings or self-harm by a child or adolescent is a signal of distress and should be taken seriously. These behaviors should not be dismissed as "attention seeking." School procedures for safety issues should be followed.

What Is Buspirone?

Buspirone is called an *antianxiety* medicine. It comes in generic tablets. It is not chemically related to the *benzodiazepines*, which are medicines used to decrease anxiety or improve sleep. Buspirone used to come in brand name Buspar, and it is sometimes still called that.

How Can This Medicine Help?

Buspirone can decrease anxiety, nervousness, fears, and excessive worrying. It can help anxious people to be calm enough to learn—with therapy and practice—to understand and tolerate their worries or fears and even to overcome them. Most often, it is used for a short time when symptoms are very uncomfortable or frightening or when they make it hard to do important things such as going to school. Occasionally antianxiety medicines are used for longer periods to treat anxiety that remains after therapy is completed.

How Does This Medicine Work?

Buspirone works by calming the parts of the brain that are too excitable in anxious people. It does this by changing the effects of *neurotransmitters*—the chemicals that the brain makes for brain cells to communicate with each other.

Buspirone does not begin to help immediately. The full effect may not appear for 3–4 weeks.

How Long Does This Medicine Last?

Buspirone usually needs to be taken three times a day.

How Will the Doctor Monitor This Medicine?

The doctor will review your child's medical history and physical examination before starting buspirone. The doctor may order some blood or urine tests to be sure your child does not have a hidden medical condition. The doctor or nurse may measure your child's height, weight, pulse, and blood pressure before starting buspirone.

After the medicine is started, the doctor will want to have regular appointments with you and your child to see how the medicine is working, to see if a dose change is needed, to watch for side effects, to see if buspirone is still needed, and to see if any other treatment is needed. The doctor or nurse may check your child's height, weight, pulse, and blood pressure.

What Side Effects Can This Medicine Have?

Any medicine can have side effects, including an allergy to the medicine. Because each patient is different, the doctor will monitor the youth closely, especially when the medicine is started. The doctor will work with you

to increase the positive effects and decrease the negative effects of the medicine. Please tell the doctor if any of the listed side effects appear or if you think that the medicine is causing any other problems. Not all of the rare or unusual side effects are listed.

Side effects are most common after starting the medicine or after a dose increase. Many side effects can be avoided or lessened by starting with a very low dose and increasing it slowly—ask the doctor.

Allergic Reaction

Tell the doctor in a day or two (if possible, before the next dose of medicine):

- Hives
- Itching
- Rash

Stop the medicine and get *immediate* medical care:

- Trouble breathing or chest tightness
- Swelling of lips, tongue, or throat

Buspirone is usually very safe when used for short periods as the doctor prescribes. Very rarely, buspirone causes excitement, irritability, anger, aggression, nightmares, or uncontrollable behavior. This is called *disinhibition* or a *paradoxical effect.* Stop the medicine and call the doctor if this happens.

Buspirone may cause dizziness, nervousness, nausea, headache, restlessness, or trouble sleeping but does not cause dependence or sleepiness.

There are no known long-term side effects of buspirone.

Some Interactions With Other Medicines or Food

Please note that the following are only the most likely interactions with other medicines or food.

Buspirone may be taken with or without food.

It is important not to drink alcohol or use other sedatives, tranquilizers, or sleeping pills when taking buspirone.

Taking buspirone with certain antibiotics (such as erythromycin) may increase levels of buspirone and increase side effects.

It can be *very dangerous* to take buspirone at the same time as or even within a month of taking another type of medicine called a *monoamine oxidase inhibitor* (MAOI), such as selegiline (Eldepryl), phenelzine (Nardil), tranylcypromine (Parnate), or isocarboxazid (Marplan).

What Could Happen if This Medicine Is Stopped Suddenly?

There are no known problems from stopping buspirone suddenly. There are no withdrawal symptoms, but the anxiety is likely to come back.

How Long Will This Medicine Be Needed?

Buspirone is usually prescribed for only a few weeks to allow the patient to be calm enough to learn new ways to cope with anxiety and to allow the nervous system to become less excitable. Each person is unique, and some people may need these medicines for months or years.

What Else Should I Know About This Medicine?

Buspirone is sometimes confused with bupropion (Wellbutrin, an antidepressant medicine). Be sure that you have the correct medicine from the pharmacy.

Notes

Use this space to take notes or to write down questions you want to ask the doctor.

_____

_____

_____

_____

_____

_____

_____

_____

_____

_____

_____

concerning drug dosages, schedules, routes of administration, and side effects is accurate as of the time of publication and consistent with standards set by the U.S. Food and Drug Administration and the general medical community and accepted child psychiatric practice. The information on this medication sheet does not cover all the possible uses, precautions, side effects, or interactions of this drug. For a complete listing of side effects, see the manufacturer's package insert, which can be obtained from your physician or pharmacist. As medical research and practice advance, therapeutic standards may change. For this reason and because human and mechanical errors sometimes occur, we recommend that readers follow the advice of a physician who is directly involved in their care or the care of a member of their family.

From Dulcan MK, Ballard R (editors): *Helping Parents and Teachers Understand Medications for Behavioral and Emotional Problems: A Resource Book of Medication Information Handouts*, Fourth Edition. Washington, DC, American Psychiatric Publishing, 2015

Medication Information for Parents and Teachers

Carbamazepine—Tegretol, Carbatrol, Epitol, Equetro, Tegretol XR

General Information About Medication

Each child and adolescent is different. No one has exactly the same combination of medical and psychological problems. It is a good idea to talk with the doctor or nurse about the reasons a medicine is being used. It is very important to keep all appointments and to be in touch by telephone if you have concerns. It is important to communicate with the doctor, nurse, or therapist. An *advanced practice nurse* (APN) has additional education and training after becoming a registered nurse (RN). Your child's medication may be prescribed by a medical doctor (MD or DO) or an APN. In addition, a *physician assistant* (PA) working with a physician may prescribe certain medications. In this information sheet, "doctor" includes medical doctors as well as APNs and PAs who prescribe medication. Often a nurse (RN) will be part of the team and answer questions and give information.

It is very important that the medicine be taken exactly as the doctor instructs. However, once in a while, everyone forgets to give a medicine on time. It is a good idea to ask the doctor or nurse what to do if this happens. Do not stop or change a medicine without asking the doctor or nurse first.

If the medicine seems to stop working, it may be because it is not being taken regularly. The youth may be "cheeking" or hiding the medicine or forgetting to take it (especially at school). The doses may be too far apart or a different dose or medicine may be needed. Something at school, at home, or in the neighborhood may be upsetting the youth, or he or she may need special help for learning disabilities or tutoring. Please discuss your concerns with the doctor. **Do not just increase the dose.** It is also very important not to decrease the dose or stop the medicine without talking to the doctor first. The problem being treated may come back, or there could be uncomfortable or even dangerous results.

All medicines should be kept in a safe place, out of the reach of children, and should be supervised by an adult. If someone takes too much of a medicine, call the doctor, the poison control center, or a hospital emergency room.

Each medicine has a "generic" or chemical name. Just like laundry detergents or paper towels, some medicines are sold by more than one company under different brand names. The same medicine may be available under a generic name and several brand names. The generic medications are usually less expensive than the brand name ones. The generic medications have the same chemical formula, but they may or may not be exactly the same strength as the brand-name medications. Also, some brands of pills contain dye or other things that can cause allergic reactions. It is a good idea to talk to the doctor and the pharmacist about whether it is important to use a specific brand of medicine.

Any medicine can cause an allergic reaction. Examples are hives, itching, rashes, swelling, and trouble breathing. Even a tiny amount of a medicine can cause a reaction in patients who are allergic to that medicine. Be *sure* to talk to the doctor before restarting a medicine that has caused an allergic reaction and tell the doctor about any reactions to medicine that your child has had before.

Taking more than one medicine at the same time may cause more side effects or cause one of the medicines to not work as well. Always ask the doctor, nurse, or pharmacist before adding another medicine, either prescription or bought without a prescription in a store or on the Internet. Be sure that each doctor knows about *all* of the medicines your child is taking. Also tell the doctor about any vitamins, herbal medicines, or supplements your child may be taking. Some of these may have side effects alone or when taken with this medication. It is a very good idea to keep a list with you of the names and doses of all medicines that your child is taking.

Everyone taking medicine should have a physical examination at least once a year.

If you think that your child may be using drugs or alcohol, please tell the doctor right away.

Pregnancy requires special care in the use of medicine. Some medicines can cause birth defects if taken by a pregnant mother. **Please tell the doctor immediately if you suspect the teenager is at risk of becoming pregnant.** The doctor may wish to discuss sexual behavior and/or birth control with your daughter.

Printed information like this applies to children and adolescents in general. If you have questions about the medicine, or if you notice changes or anything unusual, please ask the doctor or nurse. As scientific research advances, knowledge increases and advice changes. Even experts do not always agree. Many medicines have not been "approved" by the U.S. Food and Drug Administration (FDA) for use in children or use for particular problems. For this reason, use of the medicine for a problem or age group often is not listed in the *Physicians' Desk Reference*. This does not necessarily mean that the medicine is dangerous or does not work, only that the company that makes the medicine has not received permission to advertise the medicine for use in children. Companies often do not apply for this permission because it is expensive to do the tests needed to apply for approval for use in children. Once a medication is approved by the FDA for any purpose, a doctor is allowed to prescribe it according to research and clinical experience.

Note to Teachers

It is a good idea to talk with the parent(s) about the reason(s) that a medication is being used. If the parent(s) sign consent to release information, it is often helpful for you to talk with the doctor. If the parent(s) give permission, the doctor may ask you to fill out rating forms about your experience with the student's behavior, feelings, academic performance, and medication side effects. This information is very useful in selecting and monitoring medication treatment. If you have observations that you think are important, do not hesitate to share these with the student's parent(s) and treating clinicians (with parental consent).

It is very important that the medicine be taken exactly as the doctor instructs. However, everyone forgets to give a medicine on time once in a while. It is a good idea to ask the parent(s) in advance what to do if this happens. Do not stop or change the time you are giving a medicine at school without parental permission. If a medication is to be taken with food, but lunchtime or snack time changes, be sure to notify the parent(s) so appropriate adjustments can be made.

All medicines should be kept in a secure place and should be supervised by an adult. If someone takes too much of a medicine, follow your school procedure for an urgent medical problem.

Taking medicine is a private matter and is best managed discreetly and confidentially. It is important to be sensitive to the student's feelings about taking medicine.

If you suspect that the student is using drugs or alcohol, please tell the parent(s) or a school counselor right away.

Please tell the parent(s) or school nurse if you suspect medication side effects.

Modifications of the classroom environment or assignments may be useful in addition to medication. The student may need to be evaluated for additional help or a 504 plan or an Individualized Education Plan for learning problems or emotional or behavioral issues.

Any expression of suicidal thoughts or feelings or self-harm by a child or adolescent is a signal of distress and should be taken seriously. These behaviors should not be dismissed as "attention seeking." School procedures for safety issues should be followed.

What Is Carbamazepine (Tegretol, Carbatrol, Epitol, Equetro, Tegretol XR)?

Carbamazepine was first used to treat seizures (fits, convulsions), so it is sometimes called an *anticonvulsant* or *anticonvulsant drug* (AED). Now it is also used for behavioral problems or bipolar disorder whether or not the patient has seizures. It also may be used when the patient has a history of severe mood changes, sometimes called *mood swings*. When used in psychiatry, this medicine is more commonly called a *mood stabilizer*. It is also sometimes used to reduce severe facial nerve pain or nerve pain in people with diabetes.

Carbamazepine comes in brand name Epitol and Tegretol and generic tablets, generic chewable tablets, and Tegretol and generic liquid. Carbamazepine also comes in Tegretol XR and generic extended-release tablets and Carbatrol and Equetro and generic extended-release capsules.

How Can This Medicine Help?

Carbamazepine can reduce aggression, anger, and severe mood swings. It can treat mania or prevent relapse (mania coming back).

How Does This Medicine Work?

Carbamazepine is thought to work by stabilizing a part of the brain cell (the cell membrane or envelope) and by changing the concentrations of certain *neurotransmitters* (chemicals in the brain) such as *GABA* and *glutamate*.

How Long Does This Medicine Last?

Carbamazepine needs to be taken two to four times a day. Tegretol XR and Carbatrol may be taken two times a day.

How Will the Doctor Monitor This Medicine?

The doctor will review your child's medical history and physical examination before starting carbamazepine. The doctor may order some blood or urine tests to be sure your child does not have a hidden medical condition that would make it unsafe to use this medicine. The doctor or nurse may measure your child's pulse and blood pressure before starting carbamazepine. The doctor may order a baseline test counting the blood cells.

After the medicine is started, the doctor will want to have regular appointments with you and your child to see how the medicine is working, to see if a dose change is needed, to watch for side effects, to see if carbamazepine is still needed, and to see if any other treatment is needed. The doctor or nurse may check your child's height, weight, pulse, and blood pressure. The doctor may order blood tests every month or so to make sure that the medicine is at the right dose and to find any side effects on the blood, such as a decrease in the number of white blood cells (the cells that fight infection) or even in all kinds of blood cells. To see if the medicine is at the right dose, blood should be drawn first thing in the morning, 10–12 hours after the last dose and before the morning dose. Many things can change the levels of carbamazepine, so tests may be needed every week when the dose of this or other medicines are being changed.

What Side Effects Can This Medicine Have?

Any medicine can have side effects, including an allergy to the medicine. Because each patient is different, the doctor will monitor the youth closely, especially when the medicine is started. The doctor will work with you to increase the positive effects and decrease the negative effects of the medicine. Please tell the doctor if any of the listed side effects appear or if you think that the medicine is causing any other problems. Not all of the rare or unusual side effects are listed.

Side effects are most common after starting the medicine or after a dose increase. Many side effects can be avoided or lessened by starting with a very low dose and increasing it slowly—ask the doctor.

Allergic Reaction

Tell the doctor in a day or two (if possible, before the next dose of medicine):

- Hives
- Itching
- Rash

Stop the medicine and get *immediate* medical care:

- Trouble breathing or chest tightness
- Swelling of lips, tongue, or throat

General Side Effects

Tell the doctor within a week or two:

The following side effects are more common when first starting the medicine:

- Daytime sleepiness—Do not allow your child to drive, ride a bicycle or motorcycle, or operate machinery if this happens.
- Dizziness
- Clumsiness or decreased coordination
- Nausea or upset stomach—Have your child take medicine with food.

The following side effects are more common at higher doses:

- Double or blurred vision
- Jerky, side-to-side eye movements (*nystagmus*)

Serious Side Effects

Call the doctor within a day or two:

- Anxiety or nervousness
- Agitation or mania
- Impulsive behavior
- Irritability
- Increased aggression
- Hallucinations (hearing voices or seeing things that are not there)
- Motor or vocal tics (fast, repeated movements or sounds)

Very Rare, but Possibly Serious, Side Effects

Call the doctor *immediately*:

- Feeling sick or unusually tired for no reason
- Loss of appetite
- Yellowing of the skin or eyes
- Dark urine or pale bowel movements
- Swelling of the legs or feet
- Greatly increased or decreased frequency of urination
- Unusual bruising or bleeding
- Sore throat or fever
- Mouth ulcers
- Vomiting
- Skin rash, especially with fever
- Severe behavioral problems, including suicidal thinking or behaviors
- Unsteady gait (wobbling or falling when walking)
- New or worse seizures (convulsions)

Some Interactions With Other Medicines or Food

Please note that the following are only the most likely interactions with other medicines or food.

Caffeine may increase side effects.

A large glass of grapefruit juice may increase levels of carbamazepine and increase side effects.

Carbamazepine interacts with many other medicines. Taking it with another medicine may make one or both not work as well or may cause more side effects. Be sure that each doctor knows about *all* of the medicines your child is taking.

The following medicines (and many others) increase the levels of carbamazepine and increase the risk of serious side effects:

- Cimetidine (Tagamet)
- Divalproex (Depakote)

- Erythromycin and similar antibiotics
- Fluoxetine (Prozac)
- Fluvoxamine (Luvox)
- Medicines used to treat fungus infections or tuberculosis (TB)

Carbamazepine may decrease the blood levels of the following medicines (and many others) so that they do not work as well:

- Birth control pills (oral contraceptives)—This combination may lead to accidental pregnancy. An alternative form of birth control may be needed.
- Theophylline

Carbamazepine should not be taken together with clozapine (Clozaril) because of increased risk of severe decrease in blood cells.

Use of carbamazepine with other antiepileptic drugs may increase risk of severe skin rash.

What Could Happen if This Medicine Is Stopped Suddenly?

Stopping carbamazepine suddenly may cause uncomfortable withdrawal symptoms. If the person is taking carbamazepine for epilepsy (seizures), stopping the medicine suddenly could lead to an increase in very dangerous seizures or convulsions.

How Long Will This Medicine Be Needed?

The length of time a person needs to take carbamazepine depends on what problem is being treated. For example, someone with an impulse control disorder usually takes the medicine only until behavioral therapy begins to work. Someone with bipolar disorder may need to take the medicine for many years. Please ask the doctor about the length of treatment needed.

What Else Should I Know About This Medicine?

Carbamazepine increases the risk of sunburn. Be sure that your child wears sunscreen or protective clothing or stays out of the sun.

Taking carbamazepine with food may decrease stomach upset.

Carbamazepine may cause hair loss. The hair usually grows back when the carbamazepine is stopped.

If you are giving the liquid form of carbamazepine, shake it well first and do not give the medicine at the same time as other liquid medicines.

People of Asian descent have a higher risk of developing severe skin rash. Extra blood tests before starting therapy may be needed.

Substitution of brand name form of Tegretol with generic carbamazepine can change (either increase or decrease) carbamazepine levels. Your doctor will monitor carbamazepine levels when switching from one formulation to another.

When taken during pregnancy, carbamazepine may cause birth defects in the baby. Your doctor may consider doing a pregnancy test before your daughter starts this medication. If your daughter is sexually active, or decides to start sexual activity while taking this medication, she should talk with her doctor about birth control and other health issues related to sex. Call the doctor immediately if your daughter becomes pregnant while taking carbamazapine.

Keep the medicine in a safe place under close supervision. **Carbamazepine is very dangerous in overdose.** Keep the pill container tightly closed and in a dry place, away from bathrooms, showers, and humidifiers. If your home is humid in the summer, do not keep large amounts of carbamazepine and do not use carbamazepine past the expiration date.

Notes

Use this space to take notes or to write down questions you want to ask the doctor.

_____

_____

_____

_____

_____

_____

_____

_____

_____

_____

_____

_____

lication and consistent with standards set by the U.S. Food and Drug Administration and the general medical community and accepted child psychiatric practice. The information on this medication sheet does not cover all the possible uses, precautions, side effects, or interactions of this drug. For a complete listing of side effects, see the manufacturer's package insert, which can be obtained from your physician or pharmacist. As medical research and practice advance, therapeutic standards may change. For this reason and because human and mechanical errors sometimes occur, we recommend that readers follow the advice of a physician who is directly involved in their care or the care of a member of their family.

From Dulcan MK, Ballard R (editors): *Helping Parents and Teachers Understand Medications for Behavioral and Emotional Problems: A Resource Book of Medication Information Handouts*, Fourth Edition. Washington, DC, American Psychiatric Publishing, 2015

Medication Information for Parents and Teachers

Chlorpromazine

General Information About Medication

Each child and adolescent is different. No one has exactly the same combination of medical and psychological problems. It is a good idea to talk with the doctor or nurse about the reasons a medicine is being used. It is very important to keep all appointments and to be in touch by telephone if you have concerns. It is important to communicate with the doctor, nurse, or therapist. An *advanced practice nurse* (APN) has additional education and training after becoming a registered nurse (RN). Your child's medication may be prescribed by a medical doctor (MD or DO) or an APN. In addition, a *physician assistant* (PA) working with a physician may prescribe certain medications. In this information sheet, "doctor" includes medical doctors as well as APNs and PAs who prescribe medication. Often a nurse (RN) will be part of the team and answer questions and give information.

It is very important that the medicine be taken exactly as the doctor instructs. However, once in a while, everyone forgets to give a medicine on time. It is a good idea to ask the doctor or nurse what to do if this happens. Do not stop or change a medicine without asking the doctor or nurse first.

If the medicine seems to stop working, it may be because it is not being taken regularly. The youth may be "cheeking" or hiding the medicine or forgetting to take it (especially at school). The doses may be too far apart or a different dose or medicine may be needed. Something at school, at home, or in the neighborhood may be upsetting the youth, or he or she may need special help for learning disabilities or tutoring. Please discuss your concerns with the doctor. **Do not just increase the dose.** It is also very important not to decrease the dose or stop the medicine without talking to the doctor first. The problem being treated may come back, or there could be uncomfortable or even dangerous results.

All medicines should be kept in a safe place, out of the reach of children, and should be supervised by an adult. If someone takes too much of a medicine, call the doctor, the poison control center, or a hospital emergency room.

Each medicine has a "generic" or chemical name. Just like laundry detergents or paper towels, some medicines are sold by more than one company under different brand names. The same medicine may be available under a generic name and several brand names. The generic medications are usually less expensive than the brand name ones. The generic medications have the same chemical formula, but they may or may not be exactly the same strength as the brand-name medications. Also, some brands of pills contain dye or other things that can cause allergic reactions. It is a good idea to talk to the doctor and the pharmacist about whether it is important to use a specific brand of medicine.

Any medicine can cause an allergic reaction. Examples are hives, itching, rashes, swelling, and trouble breathing. Even a tiny amount of a medicine can cause a reaction in patients who are allergic to that medicine. Be *sure* to talk to the doctor before restarting a medicine that has caused an allergic reaction and tell the doctor about any reactions to medicine that your child has had before.

Taking more than one medicine at the same time may cause more side effects or cause one of the medicines to not work as well. Always ask the doctor, nurse, or pharmacist before adding another

91

medicine, either prescription or bought without a prescription in a store or on the Internet. **Be sure that each doctor knows about *all* of the medicines your child is taking. Also tell the doctor about any vitamins, herbal medicines, or supplements your child may be taking.** Some of these may have side effects alone or when taken with this medication. It is a very good idea to keep a list with you of the names and doses of all medicines that your child is taking.

Everyone taking medicine should have a physical examination at least once a year.

If you think that your child may be using drugs or alcohol, please tell the doctor right away.

Pregnancy requires special care in the use of medicine. Some medicines can cause birth defects if taken by a pregnant mother. **Please tell the doctor immediately if you suspect the teenager is at risk of becoming pregnant.** The doctor may wish to discuss sexual behavior and/or birth control with your daughter.

Printed information like this applies to children and adolescents in general. If you have questions about the medicine, or if you notice changes or anything unusual, please ask the doctor or nurse. As scientific research advances, knowledge increases and advice changes. Even experts do not always agree. Many medicines have not been "approved" by the U.S. Food and Drug Administration (FDA) for use in children or use for particular problems. For this reason, use of the medicine for a problem or age group often is not listed in the *Physicians' Desk Reference*. This does not necessarily mean that the medicine is dangerous or does not work, only that the company that makes the medicine has not received permission to advertise the medicine for use in children. Companies often do not apply for this permission because it is expensive to do the tests needed to apply for approval for use in children. Once a medication is approved by the FDA for any purpose, a doctor is allowed to prescribe it according to research and clinical experience.

Note to Teachers

It is a good idea to talk with the parent(s) about the reason(s) that a medication is being used. If the parent(s) sign consent to release information, it is often helpful for you to talk with the doctor. If the parent(s) give permission, the doctor may ask you to fill out rating forms about your experience with the student's behavior, feelings, academic performance, and medication side effects. This information is very useful in selecting and monitoring medication treatment. If you have observations that you think are important, do not hesitate to share these with the student's parent(s) and treating clinicians (with parental consent).

It is very important that the medicine be taken exactly as the doctor instructs. However, everyone forgets to give a medicine on time once in a while. It is a good idea to ask the parent(s) in advance what to do if this happens. Do not stop or change the time you are giving a medicine at school without parental permission. If a medication is to be taken with food, but lunchtime or snack time changes, be sure to notify the parent(s) so appropriate adjustments can be made.

All medicines should be kept in a secure place and should be supervised by an adult. If someone takes too much of a medicine, follow your school procedure for an urgent medical problem.

Taking medicine is a private matter and is best managed discreetly and confidentially. It is important to be sensitive to the student's feelings about taking medicine.

If you suspect that the student is using drugs or alcohol, please tell the parent(s) or a school counselor right away.

Please tell the parent(s) or school nurse if you suspect medication side effects.

Modifications of the classroom environment or assignments may be useful in addition to medication. The student may need to be evaluated for additional help or a 504 plan or an Individualized Education Plan for learning problems or emotional or behavioral issues.

Any expression of suicidal thoughts or feelings or self-harm by a child or adolescent is a signal of distress and should be taken seriously. These behaviors should not be dismissed as "attention seeking." School procedures for safety issues should be followed.

What Is Chlorpromazine?

Chlorpromazine is sometimes called a *typical, conventional,* or *first-generation antipsychotic* medicine. It is also called a *neuroleptic* or *phenothiazine.* It used to be called a *major tranquilizer.* It comes in generic tablets and shots (injections). It used to come in brand name Thorazine, and sometimes it is still called that.

How Can This Medicine Help?

Chlorpromazine is used to treat psychosis, such as in schizophrenia, mania, or very severe depression. It can reduce hallucinations (hearing voices or seeing things that are not there) and delusions (troubling beliefs that other people do not share). It can help the patient be less upset and agitated. It can improve the patient's ability to think clearly.

Sometimes chlorpromazine is used for a short time to decrease severe aggression or very serious behavioral problems in young people with intellectual disability or autism spectrum disorder.

It is sometimes used together with other medicines to help with sleep in people with psychosis.

This medicine is very powerful and should be used to treat very serious problems or symptoms that other medicines do not help.

In medical settings, chlorpromazine is also used to treat severe nausea and vomiting or severe, long-lasting attacks of hiccups.

How Does This Medicine Work?

Cells in the brain (neurons) communicate using chemicals called *neurotransmitters.* Too much or too little of these substances in certain parts of the brain can cause problems. Chlorpromazine reduces the activity of one of these neurotransmitters, *dopamine.* Blocking the effect of dopamine in certain parts of the brain reduces what have been called *positive symptoms* of psychosis: delusions; hallucinations; disorganized and unusual thinking, speaking, and behavior; excessive activity (agitation); and lack of activity (catatonia). Reducing dopamine action in other parts of the brain may lead to the side effects of this medicine.

How Long Does This Medicine Last?

Chlorpromazine may be taken only once a day, but divided doses are often used to lessen side effects. Sometimes it is used at bedtime only. Sometimes it is used as needed *(prn)* for immediate help with agitation or aggression.

How Will the Doctor Monitor This Medicine?

The doctor will review your child's medical history and physical examination before starting chlorpromazine. The doctor may order some blood or urine tests to be sure your child does not have a hidden medical condition. The doctor or nurse may measure your child's pulse and blood pressure before starting chlorpromazine.

Be sure to tell the doctor if anyone in the family is hearing impaired or has had heart problems or died suddenly.

Before starting chlorpromazine and every so often afterward, a test such as the Abnormal Involuntary Movement Scale (AIMS) may be used to check your child's tongue, legs, and arms for unusual movements that could be caused by the medicine.

After the medicine is started, the doctor will want to have regular appointments with you and your child to see how the medicine is working, to see if a dose change is needed, to watch for side effects, to see if chlorpromazine is still needed, and to see if any other treatment is needed. The doctor or nurse may check your child's height, weight, pulse, and blood pressure and watch for abnormal movements.

What Side Effects Can This Medicine Have?

Any medicine can have side effects, including an allergy to the medicine. Because each patient is different, the doctor will monitor the youth closely, especially when the medicine is started. The doctor will work with you to increase the positive effects and decrease the negative effects of the medicine. Please tell the doctor if any of the listed side effects appear or if you think that the medicine is causing any other problems. Not all of the rare or unusual side effects are listed.

Side effects are most common after starting the medicine or after a dose increase. Many side effects can be avoided or lessened by starting with a very low dose and increasing it slowly—ask the doctor.

Allergic Reaction

Tell the doctor in a day or two (if possible, before the next dose of medicine):

- Hives
- Itching
- Rash

Stop the medicine and get *immediate* medical care:

- Trouble breathing or chest tightness
- Swelling of lips, tongue, or throat

Common, but Not Usually Serious, Side Effects

Discuss the following side effects with your child's doctor within a week or two. They often can be helped if the doctor lowers the dose of medicine or changes the times medicine is taken.

- Dry mouth—Have your child try using sugar-free gum or candy.
- Daytime sleepiness or tiredness—Do not allow your child to drive, ride a bicycle or motorcycle, or operate machinery if this happens. This problem may be lessened by taking the medicine at bedtime.
- Constipation—Encourage your child to drink more fluids and eat high-fiber foods; if necessary, the doctor may recommend a fiber medicine such as Benefiber or a stool softener such as Colace or mineral oil.
- Increased risk of sunburn—Have your child wear sunscreen or protective clothing or stay out of the sun.
- Mild trouble urinating
- Blurred vision

- Dizziness—This side effect is worse when the child stands up quickly, especially when getting out of bed in the morning; try having the child stand up slowly.
- Weight gain—Seek nutritional counseling; provide your child with low-calorie snacks and encourage regular exercise.
- Decreased sexual interest or ability
- Changes in menstrual cycle
- Increase in breast size or discharge from the breasts (in both boys and girls)—This may go away with time.

Less Common, but Not Usually Serious, Side Effects

Discuss the following side effects with your child's doctor within a week or two. They often can be helped if the doctor lowers the dose of medicine or changes the times medicine is taken.

- Restlessness or inability to sit still
- Shaking of hands and fingers
- Drooling
- Decreased movement and decreased facial expressions
- Decreased coordination

Less Common, but Potentially Serious, Side Effects

Call the doctor or go to an emergency room *right away:*

- Overheating or heatstroke—Prevent by decreasing activity in hot weather, staying out of the sun, and drinking water.
- Seizure (fit, convulsion)—This is more likely in people with a history of seizures or head injury.
- Severe confusion
- Stiffness of the tongue, jaw, neck, back, or legs

Very Rare, but Serious, Side Effects

- Extreme stiffness or lack of movement, very high fever, mental confusion, irregular pulse rate, or eye pain—**This is a medical emergency. Go to an emergency room** *right away.*
- Sudden stiffness and inability to breathe or swallow—**Go to an emergency room or call 911.** Tell the paramedics, nurses, and doctors that the patient is taking chlorpromazine. Other medicines can be used to treat this problem fast.
- Increased thirst, frequent urination, lethargy, tiredness, dizziness—These could be signs of diabetes (especially if your child is overweight or there is a family history of diabetes). **Talk to a doctor within a day.**
- Yellowing of skin or eyes, dark urine, pale bowel movements, abdominal pain or fullness, unexplained flu-like symptoms, itchy skin (this could be a sign of liver damage—extremely rare). **Talk to a doctor within a day.**

What Else Should I Know About Side Effects?

Most side effects lessen over time. If they are troublesome, talk with your child's doctor. Some side effects can be decreased by taking a smaller dose of medicine, by stopping the medicine, by changing to another medicine, or by adding another medicine.

One side effect that may not go away is *tardive dyskinesia* (or TD). Patients with tardive dyskinesia have involuntary movements of the body, especially the mouth and tongue. The patient may look as though he or she is making faces over and over again. Jerky movements of the arms, legs, or body may occur. There may be fine, wormlike, or sudden repeated movements of the tongue, or the person may appear to be chewing something or smacking or puckering his or her lips. The fingers may look as though they are rolling something. If you notice any unusual movements, be sure to tell the doctor. The doctor may use the AIMS test to look for these movements.

Heart problems are more common if other medicines are also being taken. Be sure to tell all your child's doctors and your pharmacist about all medications your child is taking.

Neuroleptic malignant syndrome is a very rare side effect that can lead to death. The symptoms are severe muscle stiffness, high fever, increased heart rate and blood pressure, irregular heartbeat (pulse), and sweating. It may lead to unconsciousness. If you suspect this, **call 911 or go to an emergency room right away.**

Some Interactions With Other Medicines or Food

Please note that the following are only the most likely interactions with other medicines or food.

Chlorpromazine may be taken with or without food.

Combining chlorpromazine with medicines such as benztropin (Cogentin), trihexyphenidyl, or diphenhydramine (Benadryl) may increase the side effects of both medicines. Chlorpromazine should not be taken with some antibiotics or antifungal medications because together they can increase the risk for abnormal heart rhythms. Be sure to talk with your child's doctor about any new medication prescribed while taking chlorpromazine.

It is better to limit drinks with caffeine (coffee, tea, soft drinks) because caffeine works in the opposite way from this medicine, and the positive effects might be decreased.

What Could Happen if This Medicine Is Stopped Suddenly?

Involuntary movements, or *withdrawal dyskinesias*, may appear within 1–4 weeks of lowering the dose or stopping the medicine. Usually these go away, but they can last for days to months. If chlorpromazine is stopped suddenly, emotional problems, such as irritability, nervousness, or moodiness; behavior problems; or physical problems such as stomachache, loss of appetite, nausea, vomiting, diarrhea, sweating, indigestion, trouble sleeping, trembling, or shaking may appear. These problems usually last only a few days to a few weeks. If they happen, tell your child's doctor. The medicine dose may need to be lowered more slowly (tapered). Always check with the doctor before stopping a medicine.

How Long Will This Medicine Be Needed?

How long your child will need to be on chlorpromazine depends partly on the reason that it was prescribed. Some problems last for only a few months, whereas others last much longer. It is especially important with medicines as powerful as this one to ask the doctor whether it is still needed. Every few months, you should discuss with your child's doctor the reasons for using chlorpromazine and whether it is time to try lowering the dose.

What Else Should I Know About This Medicine?

There are many newer medicines that are used for the same kinds of problems. If your child is having bad side effects or the medicine does not seem to be working, ask the doctor if another medicine might work as well or better and have fewer side effects for your child.

Notes

Use this space to take notes or to write down questions you want to ask the doctor.

_____

_____

_____

_____

_____

_____

_____

_____

_____

_____

_____

_____

_____

see the manufacturer's package insert, which can be obtained from your physician or pharmacist. As medical research and practice advance, therapeutic standards may change. For this reason and because human and mechanical errors sometimes occur, we recommend that readers follow the advice of a physician who is directly involved in their care or the care of a member of their family.

From Dulcan MK, Ballard R (editors): *Helping Parents and Teachers Understand Medications for Behavioral and Emotional Problems: A Resource Book of Medication Information Handouts*, Fourth Edition. Washington, DC, American Psychiatric Publishing, 2015

Medication Information for Parents and Teachers

Citalopram—Celexa

General Information About Medication

Each child and adolescent is different. No one has exactly the same combination of medical and psychological problems. It is a good idea to talk with the doctor or nurse about the reasons a medicine is being used. It is very important to keep all appointments and to be in touch by telephone if you have concerns. It is important to communicate with the doctor, nurse, or therapist. An *advanced practice nurse* (APN) has additional education and training after becoming a registered nurse (RN). Your child's medication may be prescribed by a medical doctor (MD or DO) or an APN. In addition, a *physician assistant* (PA) working with a physician may prescribe certain medications. In this information sheet, "doctor" includes medical doctors as well as APNs and PAs who prescribe medication. Often a nurse (RN) will be part of the team and answer questions and give information.

It is very important that the medicine be taken exactly as the doctor instructs. However, once in a while, everyone forgets to give a medicine on time. It is a good idea to ask the doctor or nurse what to do if this happens. Do not stop or change a medicine without asking the doctor or nurse first.

If the medicine seems to stop working, it may be because it is not being taken regularly. The youth may be "cheeking" or hiding the medicine or forgetting to take it (especially at school). The doses may be too far apart or a different dose or medicine may be needed. Something at school, at home, or in the neighborhood may be upsetting the youth, or he or she may need special help for learning disabilities or tutoring. Please discuss your concerns with the doctor. **Do not just increase the dose.** It is also very important not to decrease the dose or stop the medicine without talking to the doctor first. The problem being treated may come back, or there could be uncomfortable or even dangerous results.

All medicines should be kept in a safe place, out of the reach of children, and should be supervised by an adult. If someone takes too much of a medicine, call the doctor, the poison control center, or a hospital emergency room.

Each medicine has a "generic" or chemical name. Just like laundry detergents or paper towels, some medicines are sold by more than one company under different brand names. The same medicine may be available under a generic name and several brand names. The generic medications are usually less expensive than the brand name ones. The generic medications have the same chemical formula, but they may or may not be exactly the same strength as the brand-name medications. Also, some brands of pills contain dye or other things that can cause allergic reactions. It is a good idea to talk to the doctor and the pharmacist about whether it is important to use a specific brand of medicine.

Any medicine can cause an allergic reaction. Examples are hives, itching, rashes, swelling, and trouble breathing. Even a tiny amount of a medicine can cause a reaction in patients who are allergic to that medicine. Be *sure* to talk to the doctor before restarting a medicine that has caused an allergic reaction and tell the doctor about any reactions to medicine that your child has had before.

Taking more than one medicine at the same time may cause more side effects or cause one of the medicines to not work as well. Always ask the doctor, nurse, or pharmacist before adding another

medicine, either prescription or bought without a prescription in a store or on the Internet. **Be sure that each doctor knows about *all* of the medicines your child is taking. Also tell the doctor about any vitamins, herbal medicines, or supplements your child may be taking.** Some of these may have side effects alone or when taken with this medication. It is a very good idea to keep a list with you of the names and doses of all medicines that your child is taking.

Everyone taking medicine should have a physical examination at least once a year.

If you think that your child may be using drugs or alcohol, please tell the doctor right away.

Pregnancy requires special care in the use of medicine. Some medicines can cause birth defects if taken by a pregnant mother. **Please tell the doctor immediately if you suspect the teenager is at risk of becoming pregnant.** The doctor may wish to discuss sexual behavior and/or birth control with your daughter.

Printed information like this applies to children and adolescents in general. If you have questions about the medicine, or if you notice changes or anything unusual, please ask the doctor or nurse. As scientific research advances, knowledge increases and advice changes. Even experts do not always agree. Many medicines have not been "approved" by the U.S. Food and Drug Administration (FDA) for use in children or use for particular problems. For this reason, use of the medicine for a problem or age group often is not listed in the *Physicians' Desk Reference*. This does not necessarily mean that the medicine is dangerous or does not work, only that the company that makes the medicine has not received permission to advertise the medicine for use in children. Companies often do not apply for this permission because it is expensive to do the tests needed to apply for approval for use in children. Once a medication is approved by the FDA for any purpose, a doctor is allowed to prescribe it according to research and clinical experience.

Note to Teachers

It is a good idea to talk with the parent(s) about the reason(s) that a medication is being used. If the parent(s) sign consent to release information, it is often helpful for you to talk with the doctor. If the parent(s) give permission, the doctor may ask you to fill out rating forms about your experience with the student's behavior, feelings, academic performance, and medication side effects. This information is very useful in selecting and monitoring medication treatment. If you have observations that you think are important, do not hesitate to share these with the student's parent(s) and treating clinicians (with parental consent).

It is very important that the medicine be taken exactly as the doctor instructs. However, everyone forgets to give a medicine on time once in a while. It is a good idea to ask the parent(s) in advance what to do if this happens. Do not stop or change the time you are giving a medicine at school without parental permission. If a medication is to be taken with food, but lunchtime or snack time changes, be sure to notify the parent(s) so appropriate adjustments can be made.

All medicines should be kept in a secure place and should be supervised by an adult. If someone takes too much of a medicine, follow your school procedure for an urgent medical problem.

Taking medicine is a private matter and is best managed discreetly and confidentially. It is important to be sensitive to the student's feelings about taking medicine.

If you suspect that the student is using drugs or alcohol, please tell the parent(s) or a school counselor right away.

Please tell the parent(s) or school nurse if you suspect medication side effects.

Modifications of the classroom environment or assignments may be useful in addition to medication. The student may need to be evaluated for additional help or a 504 plan or an Individualized Education Plan for learning problems or emotional or behavioral issues.

Any expression of suicidal thoughts or feelings or self-harm by a child or adolescent is a signal of distress and should be taken seriously. These behaviors should not be dismissed as "attention seeking." School procedures for safety issues should be followed.

What Is Citalopram (Celexa)?

Citalopram (brand name Celexa) is an antidepressant known as a *selective serotonin reuptake inhibitor* (SSRI). It comes in generic and brand name tablets and generic liquid form.

How Can This Medicine Help?

Citalopram is used to treat depression and anxiety disorders such as obsessive-compulsive disorder (OCD), posttraumatic stress disorder (PTSD), panic disorder, separation anxiety disorder, selective mutism, social anxiety disorder, and generalized anxiety disorder.

How Does This Medicine Work?

Citalopram increases the amount of a *neurotransmitter* called *serotonin* in certain parts of the brain. People with emotional and behavioral problems, such as depression and anxiety, may have low levels of serotonin in certain parts of the brain. SSRIs such as citalopram help by increasing the action of brain serotonin to more normal levels.

How Long Does This Medicine Last?

Citalopram can be taken only once a day for most people.

How Will the Doctor Monitor This Medicine?

The doctor will review your child's medical history and physical examination before starting citalopram. The doctor may order some blood or urine tests to be sure your child does not have a hidden medical condition that would make it unsafe to use this medicine. Extra care is needed when using SSRIs in youth with seizures (epilepsy); heart, liver, or kidney problems; or diabetes. The doctor or nurse may measure your child's pulse, blood pressure, and weight before starting the medicine.

Be sure to tell the doctor if your child or anyone in the family has bipolar disorder or has tried to kill himself or herself.

After the medicine is started, the doctor will want to have regular appointments with you and your child to see how the medicine is working, to see if a dose change is needed, to watch for side effects, to see if citalopram is still needed, and to see if any other treatment is needed. The doctor or nurse may check your child's height, weight, pulse, and blood pressure.

Before using medicine and at times afterward, the doctor may ask your child to fill out a rating scale about depression or anxiety to help see how your child is doing.

What Side Effects Can This Medicine Have?

Any medicine can have side effects, including an allergy to the medicine. Because each patient is different, the doctor will monitor the youth closely, especially when the medicine is started. The doctor will work with you to increase the positive effects and decrease the negative effects of the medicine. Please tell the doctor if any of the listed side effects appear or if you think that the medicine is causing any other problems. Not all of the rare or unusual side effects are listed.

Side effects are most common after starting the medicine or after a dose increase. Many side effects can be avoided or lessened by starting with a very low dose and increasing it slowly—ask the doctor.

Allergic Reaction

Tell the doctor in a day or two (if possible, before the next dose of medicine):

- Hives
- Itching
- Rash

Stop the medicine and get *immediate* medical care:

- Trouble breathing or chest tightness
- Swelling of lips, tongue, or throat

Common Side Effects

Tell the doctor within a week or two, or sooner if the problems are getting worse:

- Nausea, upset stomach, vomiting
- Diarrhea or excessive gas
- Dry mouth—Have your child try using sugar-free gum or candy.
- Constipation—Encourage your child to drink more fluids and eat high-fiber foods; if necessary, the doctor may recommend a fiber medicine such as Benefiber or a stool softener such as Colace or mineral oil.
- Headache
- Anxiety or nervousness
- Insomnia (trouble sleeping)
- Restlessness, increased activity level
- Daytime sleepiness or tiredness—Do not allow your child to drive, ride a bicycle or motorcycle, or operate machinery if this side effect is present.
- Dizziness—This side effect is worse when the child stands up quickly, especially when getting out of bed in the morning; try having the child stand up slowly.
- Tremor (shakiness)
- Excessive sweating
- Apathy, lack of interest in school or friends—This may happen after an initial good response to treatment.
- Decreased sexual interest, trouble with sexual functioning
- Weight gain
- Weight loss

Less Common, but More Serious, Side Effects

Call the doctor within a day or two:

- Significant suicidal thoughts or self-injurious behavior
- Increased activity, rapid speech, feeling "speeded up," decreased need for sleep, being very excited or irritable (cranky), agitation, acting out of character
- Bleeding, such as bruising or nosebleeds, or bleeding with surgery

Serious Side Effects

Call the doctor *immediately* or go to the nearest emergency room:

- Seizure (fit, convulsion)
- Stiffness, high fever, confusion, tremors (shaking)
- Overheating or heatstroke—Prevent by decreasing activity in hot weather, staying out of the sun, and drinking water.

Serotonin Syndrome

A very serious side effect called *serotonin syndrome* can happen when certain kinds of medicines (including SSRI antidepressants and other medicines, such as triptans [which are given for migraines] or linezolid) are taken by the same person. *Very* rarely, it can happen at high doses of just one medicine. The early signs are restlessness, confusion, shaking, skin turning red, muscle stiffness, sweating, and jerking of muscles. If you see these symptoms, stop the medicine and send or take the youth to an emergency room right away.

Some Interactions With Other Medicines or Food

Please note that the following are only the most likely interactions with other medicines or food.

Citalopram interacts with many other prescription and over-the-counter medicines, including some antibiotics and other psychiatric medicines. It is especially important to tell the doctor and pharmacist about all of the medicines your child is taking or has taken in the past few months, including over-the-counter and herbal medicines. Sometimes one medicine can increase or decrease the blood level of another medicine, so that different doses are needed. Erythromycin and similar antibiotics, as well as antifungal agents such as ketoconazole, may increase levels of citalopram and increase side effects. Citalopram may increase the heart side effects of pimozide (Orap), so those two medicines should not be taken by the same person. Tryptophan or the herbal medicine St. John's Wort also increases serotonin and can cause serious side effects if taken with citalopram. Taking citalopram with aspirin, nonsteroidal anti-inflammatory drugs (NSAIDs) (medications including ibuprofen or naproxen), or anticoagulant medications (including warfarin) increases risk of abnormal bleeding.

It can be *very dangerous* to take an SSRI at the same time as or even within a month of taking another type of medicine called a *monoamine oxidase inhibitor* (MAOI), such as selegiline (Eldepryl), phenelzine (Nardil), tranylcypromine (Parnate), or isocarboxazid (Marplan).

Citalopram can be taken with or without food.

Caffeine may increase side effects of citalopram.

What Could Happen if This Medicine Is Stopped Suddenly?

No known serious medical effects occur if citalopram is stopped suddenly, but there may be uncomfortable feelings, which should be avoided if possible. Your child might have trouble sleeping, nervousness, irritability, dizziness, and flu-like symptoms. Ask the doctor before stopping citalopram or if these symptoms happen while the dose is being decreased.

How Long Will This Medicine Be Needed?

Citalopram may take up to 1–2 months to reach its full effect. If your child has a good response to citalopram, it is a good idea to continue the medicine for at least 6–12 months. It is important to review this with your doctor.

What Else Should I Know About This Medicine?

In youth who have bipolar disorder or who may be at risk for bipolar disorder, any antidepressant medicine may increase the risk of hypomania or mania (excitement, agitation, increased activity, decreased sleep).

In hot weather, make sure your child drinks enough water or other liquids and does not get overheated.

Sometimes, after a person has improved while taking citalopram, he or she loses interest in school or friends or just stops trying. Please tell your child's doctor if this happens—it may be a side effect of the medicine. A lower dose or a different medicine may be needed.

Store the medicine away from sunlight, heat, moisture, and humidity.

In 2011, the Food and Drug Administration issued a warning that citalopram should not be used at doses greater than 40 mg per day because it might cause dangerous heart rhythms. There is no evidence that this has happened in children. Talk with your doctor if your child needs doses of citalopram higher than 40 mg.

Black Box Antidepressant Warning

In 2004, an advisory committee to the FDA decided that there might be an increased risk of suicidal behavior for some youth taking medicines called *antidepressants*. In the research studies that the committee reviewed, about 3%–4% of youth with depression who took an antidepressant medicine—and 1%–2% of youth with depression who took a placebo (pill without active medicine)—talked about suicidal thoughts (thinking about killing themselves or wishing they were dead) or did something to harm themselves. This means that almost twice as many youth who were taking an antidepressant to treat their depression talked about suicide or had suicidal behavior compared with youth with depression who were taking inactive medicine. There were *no* completed suicides in any of these research studies, which included more than 4,000 children and adolescents. For youth being treated for anxiety, there was no difference in suicidal talking or behavior between those taking antidepressant medication and those taking placebo.

The FDA told drug companies to add a *black box warning* label to all antidepressant medicines. Because of this label, a doctor (or advanced practice nurse) prescribing one of these medicines has to warn youth and their families that there might be more suicidal thoughts and actions in youth taking these medicines.

On the other hand, in places where more youth are taking the newer antidepressant medicines, the number of adolescents who commit suicide has gotten smaller. Also, thinking about or attempting suicide is more common in surveys of teenagers in the community than it is in depressed youth treated in research studies with antidepressant medicine.

If a youth is being treated with this medicine and is doing well, then no changes are needed as a result of this warning. Increased suicidal talk or action is most likely to happen in the first few months of treatment with a medicine. If your child has recently started this medicine or is about to start, then you and your doctor (or advanced practice nurse) should watch for any changes in behavior. People who are depressed often have suicidal thoughts or actions. It is hard to know whether suicidal thoughts or actions in depressed people are caused by the depression itself or by the medicine. Also, as their depression is getting better, some people talk more about the suicidal thoughts that they had before but did not talk about. As young people get better from depression, they might be at higher risk of doing something about suicidal thoughts that they have had for some time, because they have more energy.

What Should a Parent Do?

1. Be honest with your child about possible risks and benefits of medicine.
2. Talk to your child about whether he or she is having any suicidal thoughts, and tell your child to come to you if he or she is having such thoughts.
3. You, your child, and your child's doctor or nurse should develop a safety plan. Pick adults whom your child can tell if he or she is thinking about suicide.
4. Be sure to tell your child's doctor, nurse, or therapist if you suspect that your child is using alcohol or drugs or if something has happened that might make your child feel worse, such as a family separation, breaking up with a boyfriend or girlfriend, someone close dying or attempting suicide, physical or sexual abuse, or failure in school.
5. Be sure that there are no guns in the home and that all medicines (including over-the-counter medicines like Tylenol) are closely supervised by an adult and kept in a safe place.
6. Watch for new or worse thoughts of suicide, self-harm, depression, anxiety (nerves), feeling very agitated or restless, being angry or aggressive, having more trouble sleeping, or anything else that you see for the first time, seems worse, or worries your child or you. If these appear, contact a mental health professional **right away.** Do not just stop or change the dose of the medicine on your own. If the problems are serious, and you cannot reach one of your clinicians, call a 24-hour psychiatry emergency telephone number or take your child to an emergency room.

Youth taking antidepressant medicine should be watched carefully by their parent(s), clinician(s) (doctor, advanced practice nurse, nurse, therapist), and other concerned adults for the first weeks of treatment. It is a good idea to have regular contact with the doctor, APN, nurse, or therapist for the first months to check for feelings of depression or sadness, thoughts of killing or harming himself or herself, and any problems with the medication. If you have questions, be sure to ask the doctor, APN, nurse, or therapist.

For more information, see http://www.parentsmedguide.org/.

Notes

Use this space to take notes or to write down questions you want to ask the doctor.

_____

_____

_____

_____

_____

_____

_____

_____

_____

_____

_____

_____

_____

From Dulcan MK, Ballard R (editors): _Helping Parents and Teachers Understand Medications for Behavioral and Emotional Problems: A Resource Book of Medication Information Handouts_, Fourth Edition. Washington, DC, American Psychiatric Publishing, 2015

Medication Information for Parents and Teachers

Clomipramine—Anafranil

General Information About Medication

Each child and adolescent is different. No one has exactly the same combination of medical and psychological problems. It is a good idea to talk with the doctor or nurse about the reasons a medicine is being used. It is very important to keep all appointments and to be in touch by telephone if you have concerns. It is important to communicate with the doctor, nurse, or therapist. An *advanced practice nurse* (APN) has additional education and training after becoming a registered nurse (RN). Your child's medication may be prescribed by a medical doctor (MD or DO) or an APN. In addition, a *physician assistant* (PA) working with a physician may prescribe certain medications. In this information sheet, "doctor" includes medical doctors as well as APNs and PAs who prescribe medication. Often a nurse (RN) will be part of the team and answer questions and give information.

It is very important that the medicine be taken exactly as the doctor instructs. However, once in a while, everyone forgets to give a medicine on time. It is a good idea to ask the doctor or nurse what to do if this happens. Do not stop or change a medicine without asking the doctor or nurse first.

If the medicine seems to stop working, it may be because it is not being taken regularly. The youth may be "cheeking" or hiding the medicine or forgetting to take it (especially at school). The doses may be too far apart or a different dose or medicine may be needed. Something at school, at home, or in the neighborhood may be upsetting the youth, or he or she may need special help for learning disabilities or tutoring. Please discuss your concerns with the doctor. **Do not just increase the dose.** It is also very important not to decrease the dose or stop the medicine without talking to the doctor first. The problem being treated may come back, or there could be uncomfortable or even dangerous results.

All medicines should be kept in a safe place, out of the reach of children, and should be supervised by an adult. If someone takes too much of a medicine, call the doctor, the poison control center, or a hospital emergency room.

Each medicine has a "generic" or chemical name. Just like laundry detergents or paper towels, some medicines are sold by more than one company under different brand names. The same medicine may be available under a generic name and several brand names. The generic medications are usually less expensive than the brand name ones. The generic medications have the same chemical formula, but they may or may not be exactly the same strength as the brand-name medications. Also, some brands of pills contain dye or other things that can cause allergic reactions. It is a good idea to talk to the doctor and the pharmacist about whether it is important to use a specific brand of medicine.

Any medicine can cause an allergic reaction. Examples are hives, itching, rashes, swelling, and trouble breathing. Even a tiny amount of a medicine can cause a reaction in patients who are allergic to that medicine. Be *sure* to talk to the doctor before restarting a medicine that has caused an allergic reaction and tell the doctor about any reactions to medicine that your child has had before.

Taking more than one medicine at the same time may cause more side effects or cause one of the medicines to not work as well. Always ask the doctor, nurse, or pharmacist before adding another medicine, either prescription or bought without a prescription in a store or on the Internet. Be sure

107

that each doctor knows about *all* of the medicines your child is taking. **Also tell the doctor about any vitamins, herbal medicines, or supplements your child may be taking.** Some of these may have side effects alone or when taken with this medication. It is a very good idea to keep a list with you of the names and doses of all medicines that your child is taking.

Everyone taking medicine should have a physical examination at least once a year.

If you think that your child may be using drugs or alcohol, please tell the doctor right away.

Pregnancy requires special care in the use of medicine. Some medicines can cause birth defects if taken by a pregnant mother. **Please tell the doctor immediately if you suspect the teenager is at risk of becoming pregnant.** The doctor may wish to discuss sexual behavior and/or birth control with your daughter.

Printed information like this applies to children and adolescents in general. If you have questions about the medicine, or if you notice changes or anything unusual, please ask the doctor or nurse. As scientific research advances, knowledge increases and advice changes. Even experts do not always agree. Many medicines have not been "approved" by the U.S. Food and Drug Administration (FDA) for use in children or use for particular problems. For this reason, use of the medicine for a problem or age group often is not listed in the *Physicians' Desk Reference*. This does not necessarily mean that the medicine is dangerous or does not work, only that the company that makes the medicine has not received permission to advertise the medicine for use in children. Companies often do not apply for this permission because it is expensive to do the tests needed to apply for approval for use in children. Once a medication is approved by the FDA for any purpose, a doctor is allowed to prescribe it according to research and clinical experience.

Note to Teachers

It is a good idea to talk with the parent(s) about the reason(s) that a medication is being used. If the parent(s) sign consent to release information, it is often helpful for you to talk with the doctor. If the parent(s) give permission, the doctor may ask you to fill out rating forms about your experience with the student's behavior, feelings, academic performance, and medication side effects. This information is very useful in selecting and monitoring medication treatment. If you have observations that you think are important, do not hesitate to share these with the student's parent(s) and treating clinicians (with parental consent).

It is very important that the medicine be taken exactly as the doctor instructs. However, everyone forgets to give a medicine on time once in a while. It is a good idea to ask the parent(s) in advance what to do if this happens. Do not stop or change the time you are giving a medicine at school without parental permission. If a medication is to be taken with food, but lunchtime or snack time changes, be sure to notify the parent(s) so appropriate adjustments can be made.

All medicines should be kept in a secure place and should be supervised by an adult. If someone takes too much of a medicine, follow your school procedure for an urgent medical problem.

Taking medicine is a private matter and is best managed discreetly and confidentially. It is important to be sensitive to the student's feelings about taking medicine.

If you suspect that the student is using drugs or alcohol, please tell the parent(s) or a school counselor right away.

Please tell the parent(s) or school nurse if you suspect medication side effects.

Modifications of the classroom environment or assignments may be useful in addition to medication. The student may need to be evaluated for additional help or a 504 plan or an Individualized Education Plan for learning problems or emotional or behavioral issues.

Any expression of suicidal thoughts or feelings or self-harm by a child or adolescent is a signal of distress and should be taken seriously. These behaviors should not be dismissed as "attention seeking." School procedures for safety issues should be followed.

You may notice the following side effects at school:

Common Side Effects

- Dry mouth—Allow the student to chew sugar-free gum, carry a water bottle, or make extra trips to the water fountain.
- Constipation—Allow the student to drink more fluids or to use the bathroom more often.
- Daytime sleepiness—The student should not drive, ride a bicycle or motorcycle, or operate machinery.
- Dizziness (especially when standing up quickly)—This may happen in the classroom or during physical education. Suggest that the student stand up more slowly.
- Irritability

Occasional Side Effects

- Stuttering
- Increased risk of sunburn (this may be a problem if recess or physical education is outdoors in warm weather)—The student should wear sunscreen or protective clothing or stay out of the sun.

Less Common Side Effects

- Nausea—The student may need to take the medicine after a meal or snack.
- Trouble urinating—The student may need more time in the bathroom.
- Blurred vision—The student may have trouble seeing the blackboard.
- Motor tics (fast, repeated movements) or muscle twitches (jerking movements) of parts of the body
- Increased activity, rapid speech, feeling "speeded up," decreased need for sleep, being very excited or irritable (cranky)
- Skin rash

Rare, but Potentially Serious, Side Effects

Call the parent(s) or follow your school's emergency procedures *immediately* **if the student experiences any of the following side effects:**

- Seizure (fit, convulsion) (**This is a medical emergency.**)
- Very fast or irregular heartbeat (**This is a medical emergency.**)
- Fainting
- Hallucinations (hearing voices or seeing things that are not there)
- Inability to urinate
- Confusion
- Severe change in behavior

What Is Clomipramine (Anafranil)?

Clomipramine is called a *tricyclic antidepressant*. It is used to treat obsessive-compulsive disorder (OCD) and trichotillomania (compulsive hair pulling). It comes in brand name Anafranil and generic capsules.

How Can This Medicine Help?

Clomipramine can decrease anxiety (nervousness), obsessions and compulsions, or severe habits such as hair pulling (trichotillomania). The medicine may take several weeks to work.

How Does This Medicine Work?

Tricyclic antidepressants affect the natural substances called *neurotransmitters* that are needed for certain parts of the brain to work more normally. Clomipramine primarily increases the activity of the neurotransmitter called *serotonin*.

How Long Does This Medicine Last?

Although a dose lasts for a whole day in adults and older teenagers, in younger children several doses a day may be needed.

How Will the Doctor Monitor This Medicine?

The doctor will review your child's medical history and physical examination, paying special attention to pulse rate, blood pressure, weight, and height, before starting clomipramine. These measurements will be taken when the dose is increased and occasionally as long as the medicine is continued. The doctor may order some blood or urine tests to be sure your child does not have a hidden medical condition that would make it unsafe to use this medicine.

Tricyclic antidepressants can slow the speed at which signals move through the heart. This effect is not dangerous if the heart is normal, which is why an ECG (electrocardiogram or heart rhythm test) is done before starting the medicine. The ECG may be repeated as the dose is increased and occasionally while the medicine is being taken. Changes in the heart from the medicine usually can be seen on the ECG before they become a problem, so your child's doctor will order an ECG every so often. To find possible hidden heart risks, it is especially important to tell the doctor if your child or anyone in the family has a history of fainting, palpitations, or irregular heartbeat or if anyone in the family died suddenly.

Be sure to tell the doctor if your child or anyone in the family has bipolar disorder or has tried to kill himself or herself.

Because clomipramine may increase the risk of seizures (fits, convulsions), the doctor will want to know whether your child has ever had a seizure or a head injury and\ if there is any family history of epilepsy. Your child's doctor may want to order an EEG (electroencephalogram or brain wave test) before starting the medicine.

Experts do not agree on whether blood tests are needed to measure the level of this medicine. Blood levels seem to be most useful when your doctor suspects that the dose of medicine is too high or too low. The most accurate level is obtained by drawing blood first thing in the morning, after at least 5 days on the same dose, approximately 12 hours after the evening dose of medicine and before the morning dose.

After the medicine is started, the doctor will want to have regular appointments with you and your child to see how the medicine is working, to see if a dose change is needed, to watch for side effects, to see if clomipramine is still needed, and to see if any other treatment is needed. The doctor or nurse may check your child's height, weight, pulse, and blood pressure or order tests, such as an ECG or blood level.

Before using medicine and at times afterward, the doctor may ask your child to fill out a rating scale about anxiety or symptoms of OCD, to help see how your child is doing.

What Side Effects Can This Medicine Have?

Any medicine can have side effects, including an allergy to the medicine. Because each patient is different, the doctor will monitor the youth closely, especially when the medicine is started. The doctor will work with you to increase the positive effects and decrease the negative effects of the medicine. Please tell the doctor if any of the listed side effects appear or if you think that the medicine is causing any other problems. Not all of the rare or unusual side effects are listed.

Side effects are most common after starting the medicine or after a dose increase. Many side effects can be avoided or lessened by starting with a very low dose and increasing it slowly—ask the doctor.

Allergic Reaction

Tell the doctor in a day or two (if possible, before the next dose of medicine):

- Hives
- Itching
- Rash—This may be caused by an allergy to the medicine or to a dye in the specific brand of pill.

Stop the medicine and get *immediate* medical care:

- Trouble breathing or chest tightness
- Swelling of lips, tongue, or throat

Common Side Effects

Tell the doctor within a week or two:

- Dry mouth—Have your child try using sugar-free gum or candy.
- Constipation—Encourage your child to drink more fluids and eat high-fiber foods; if necessary, the doctor may recommend a fiber medicine such as Benefiber or a stool softener such as Colace or mineral oil.
- Daytime sleepiness—Do not allow your child to drive, ride a bicycle or motorcycle, or operate machinery if this happens.
- Dizziness—This side effect is worse when the child stands up quickly, especially when getting out of bed in the morning; try having the child stand up slowly.
- Weight gain
- Loss of appetite and weight loss
- Irritability
- Acne

Occasional Side Effects

Tell the doctor within a week or two:

- Nightmares
- Stuttering
- Blurred vision
- Increase in breast size, nipple discharge, or both (in girls)
- Increase in breast size (in boys)

Less Common, but More Serious, Side Effects

Call the doctor within a day or two:

- High or low blood pressure
- Nausea
- Trouble urinating
- Motor tics (fast, repeated movements) or muscle twitches (jerking movements)
- Increased activity, rapid speech, feeling "speeded up," decreased need for sleep, being very excited or irritable (cranky)

Rare, but Potentially Serious, Side Effects

Call the doctor *immediately*:

- Seizure (fit, convulsion)—**Go to an emergency room.**
- Very fast or irregular heartbeat—**Go to an emergency room.**
- Fainting
- Hallucinations (hearing voices or seeing things that are not there)
- Inability to pass urine
- Confusion
- Severe change in behavior

Serotonin Syndrome

A very serious side effect called *serotonin syndrome* can happen when certain kinds of medicines (including SSRI antidepressants, clomipramine, and other medicines, such as triptans for migraine headaches, buspirone, linezolid, tramadol, or St. John's wort) are taken by the same person. Very rarely, serotonin syndrome can happen at high doses of just one medicine. The early signs are restlessness, confusion, shaking, skin turning red, sweating, muscle stiffness, sweating, and jerking of muscles. If you see these symptoms, stop the medicine and send or take the youth to an emergency room right away.

Some Interactions With Other Medicines or Food

Please note that the following are only the most likely interactions with other medicines or food.

Check with your child's doctor before giving your child decongestants or over-the-counter cold medicine.

Another antidepressant may increase the level of clomipramine and increase side effects.

It can be *very dangerous* to take clomipramine at the same time as or even within a month of taking another type of medicine called a *monoamine oxidase inhibitor* (MAOI), such as selegiline (Eldepryl), phenelzine (Nardil), tranylcypromine (Parnate), or isocarboxazid (Marplan).

Caffeine may worsen side effects on the heart or symptoms of anxiety. It is best not to drink coffee, tea, or soft drinks with caffeine while taking this medicine. A large glass of grapefruit juice may increase the levels and side effects of clomipramine.

What Could Happen if This Medicine Is Stopped Suddenly?

Stopping the medicine suddenly or skipping a dose is not dangerous but can be very uncomfortable. Your child may feel like he or she has the flu—with a headache, muscle aches, stomachache, and upset stomach. Behavioral problems, sadness, nervousness, or trouble sleeping also may occur. If these feelings appear every day, the medicine may need to be given more often during each day.

How Long Will This Medicine Be Needed?

There is no way to know how long a person will need to take this medicine. Parents work together with the doctor to determine what is right for each child. When used to treat obsessive-compulsive disorder, the medicine may be needed for a long time. Some people may need to take the medicine even as adults.

What Else Should I Know About This Medicine?

In youth who have bipolar disorder or who are at risk for bipolar disorder, any antidepressant medicine may increase the risk of hypomania or mania (excitement, agitation, increased activity, decreased sleep).

An overdose by accident or on purpose with this medicine is very dangerous! You must closely supervise the medicine. You may have to lock up the medicine if your child or teenager is suicidal or if young children live in or visit your home.

Tricyclic antidepressants may cause dry mouth, which could increase the chance of tooth decay. Regular brushing of teeth and checkups with the dentist are especially important.

This medicine causes increased risk of sunburn. Be sure that your child wears sunscreen or protective clothing or stays out of the sun.

People who take tricyclic antidepressants must not drink alcohol or use tranquilizers. Severe sleepiness, loss of consciousness, or even death may result.

Black Box Antidepressant Warning

In 2004, an advisory committee to the FDA decided that there might be an increased risk of suicidal behavior for some youth taking medicines called *antidepressants*. In the research studies that the committee reviewed, about 3%–4% of youth with depression who took an antidepressant medicine—and 1%–2% of youth with depression who took a placebo (pill without active medicine)—talked about suicidal thoughts (thinking about killing themselves or wishing they were dead) or did something to harm themselves. This means that almost twice as many youth who were taking an antidepressant to treat their depression talked about suicide or had suicidal behavior compared with youth with depression who were taking inactive medicine. There were *no* completed suicides in any of these research studies, which included more than 4,000 children and adolescents. For youth being treated for anxiety, there was no difference in suicidal talking or behavior between those taking antidepressant medication and those taking placebo.

The FDA told drug companies to add a *black box warning* label to all antidepressant medicines. Because of this label, a doctor (or advanced practice nurse) prescribing one of these medicines has to warn youth and their families that there might be more suicidal thoughts and actions in youth taking these medicines.

On the other hand, in places where more youth are taking the newer antidepressant medicines, the number of adolescents who commit suicide has gotten smaller. Also, thinking about or attempting suicide is more common in surveys of teenagers in the community than it is in depressed youth treated in research studies with antidepressant medicine.

If a youth is being treated with this medicine and is doing well, then no changes are needed as a result of this warning. Increased suicidal talk or action is most likely to happen in the first few months of treatment with a medicine. If your child has recently started this medicine or is about to start, then you and your doctor (or advanced practice nurse) should watch for any changes in behavior. People who are depressed often have suicidal thoughts or actions. It is hard to know whether suicidal thoughts or actions in depressed people are caused by the depression itself or by the medicine. Also, as their depression is getting better, some people talk more about the suicidal thoughts that they had before but did not talk about. As young people get better from depression, they might be at higher risk of doing something about suicidal thoughts that they have had for some time, because they have more energy.

What Should a Parent Do?

1. Be honest with your child about possible risks and benefits of medicine.

2. Talk to your child about whether he or she is having any suicidal thoughts, and tell your child to come to you if he or she is having such thoughts.

3. You, your child, and your child's doctor or nurse should develop a safety plan. Pick adults whom your child can tell if he or she is thinking about suicide.

4. Be sure to tell your child's doctor, nurse, or therapist if you suspect that your child is using alcohol or drugs or if something has happened that might make your child feel worse, such as a family separation, breaking up with a boyfriend or girlfriend, someone close dying or attempting suicide, physical or sexual abuse, or failure in school.

5. Be sure that there are no guns in the home and that all medicines (including over-the-counter medicines like Tylenol) are closely supervised by an adult and kept in a safe place.

6. Watch for new or worse thoughts of suicide, self-harm, depression, anxiety (nerves), feeling very agitated or restless, being angry or aggressive, having more trouble sleeping, or anything else that you see for the first time, seems worse, or worries your child or you. If these appear, contact a mental health professional **right away.** Do not just stop or change the dose of the medicine on your own. If the problems are serious, and you cannot reach one of your clinicians, call a 24-hour psychiatry emergency telephone number or take your child to an emergency room.

Youth taking antidepressant medicine should be watched carefully by their parent(s), clinician(s) (doctor, advanced practice nurse, nurse, therapist), and other concerned adults for the first weeks of treatment. It is a good idea to have regular contact with the doctor, APN, nurse, or therapist for the first months to check for feelings of depression or sadness, thoughts of killing or harming himself or herself, and any problems with the medication. If you have questions, be sure to ask the doctor, APN, nurse, or therapist.

For more information, see http://www.parentsmedguide.org/.

Notes

Use this space to take notes or to write down questions you want to ask the doctor.

_____

_____

_____

_____

_____

_____

_____

_____

_____

_____

_____

_____

_____

_____

From Dulcan MK, Ballard R (editors): _Helping Parents and Teachers Understand Medications for Behavioral and Emotional Problems: A Resource Book of Medication Information Handouts_, Fourth Edition. Washington, DC, American Psychiatric Publishing, 2015

Medication Information for Parents and Teachers

Clonazepam—Klonopin

General Information About Medication

Each child and adolescent is different. No one has exactly the same combination of medical and psychological problems. It is a good idea to talk with the doctor or nurse about the reasons a medicine is being used. It is very important to keep all appointments and to be in touch by telephone if you have concerns. It is important to communicate with the doctor, nurse, or therapist. An *advanced practice nurse* (APN) has additional education and training after becoming a registered nurse (RN). Your child's medication may be prescribed by a medical doctor (MD or DO) or an APN. In addition, a *physician assistant* (PA) working with a physician may prescribe certain medications. In this information sheet, "doctor" includes medical doctors as well as APNs and PAs who prescribe medication. Often a nurse (RN) will be part of the team and answer questions and give information.

It is very important that the medicine be taken exactly as the doctor instructs. However, once in a while, everyone forgets to give a medicine on time. It is a good idea to ask the doctor or nurse what to do if this happens. Do not stop or change a medicine without asking the doctor or nurse first.

If the medicine seems to stop working, it may be because it is not being taken regularly. The youth may be "cheeking" or hiding the medicine or forgetting to take it (especially at school). The doses may be too far apart or a different dose or medicine may be needed. Something at school, at home, or in the neighborhood may be upsetting the youth, or he or she may need special help for learning disabilities or tutoring. Please discuss your concerns with the doctor. **Do not just increase the dose.** It is also very important not to decrease the dose or stop the medicine without talking to the doctor first. The problem being treated may come back, or there could be uncomfortable or even dangerous results.

All medicines should be kept in a safe place, out of the reach of children, and should be supervised by an adult. If someone takes too much of a medicine, call the doctor, the poison control center, or a hospital emergency room.

Each medicine has a "generic" or chemical name. Just like laundry detergents or paper towels, some medicines are sold by more than one company under different brand names. The same medicine may be available under a generic name and several brand names. The generic medications are usually less expensive than the brand name ones. The generic medications have the same chemical formula, but they may or may not be exactly the same strength as the brand-name medications. Also, some brands of pills contain dye or other things that can cause allergic reactions. It is a good idea to talk to the doctor and the pharmacist about whether it is important to use a specific brand of medicine.

Any medicine can cause an allergic reaction. Examples are hives, itching, rashes, swelling, and trouble breathing. Even a tiny amount of a medicine can cause a reaction in patients who are allergic to that medicine. Be *sure* to talk to the doctor before restarting a medicine that has caused an allergic reaction and tell the doctor about any reactions to medicine that your child has had before.

Taking more than one medicine at the same time may cause more side effects or cause one of the medicines to not work as well. Always ask the doctor, nurse, or pharmacist before adding another

117

medicine, either prescription or bought without a prescription in a store or on the Internet. Be sure that each doctor knows about *all* of the medicines your child is taking. Also tell the doctor about any vitamins, herbal medicines, or supplements your child may be taking. Some of these may have side effects alone or when taken with this medication. It is a very good idea to keep a list with you of the names and doses of all medicines that your child is taking.

Everyone taking medicine should have a physical examination at least once a year.

If you think that your child may be using drugs or alcohol, please tell the doctor right away.

Pregnancy requires special care in the use of medicine. Some medicines can cause birth defects if taken by a pregnant mother. **Please tell the doctor immediately if you suspect the teenager is at risk of becoming pregnant.** The doctor may wish to discuss sexual behavior and/or birth control with your daughter.

Printed information like this applies to children and adolescents in general. If you have questions about the medicine, or if you notice changes or anything unusual, please ask the doctor or nurse. As scientific research advances, knowledge increases and advice changes. Even experts do not always agree. Many medicines have not been "approved" by the U.S. Food and Drug Administration (FDA) for use in children or use for particular problems. For this reason, use of the medicine for a problem or age group often is not listed in the *Physicians' Desk Reference.* This does not necessarily mean that the medicine is dangerous or does not work, only that the company that makes the medicine has not received permission to advertise the medicine for use in children. Companies often do not apply for this permission because it is expensive to do the tests needed to apply for approval for use in children. Once a medication is approved by the FDA for any purpose, a doctor is allowed to prescribe it according to research and clinical experience.

Note to Teachers

It is a good idea to talk with the parent(s) about the reason(s) that a medication is being used. If the parent(s) sign consent to release information, it is often helpful for you to talk with the doctor. If the parent(s) give permission, the doctor may ask you to fill out rating forms about your experience with the student's behavior, feelings, academic performance, and medication side effects. This information is very useful in selecting and monitoring medication treatment. If you have observations that you think are important, do not hesitate to share these with the student's parent(s) and treating clinicians (with parental consent).

It is very important that the medicine be taken exactly as the doctor instructs. However, everyone forgets to give a medicine on time once in a while. It is a good idea to ask the parent(s) in advance what to do if this happens. Do not stop or change the time you are giving a medicine at school without parental permission. If a medication is to be taken with food, but lunchtime or snack time changes, be sure to notify the parent(s) so appropriate adjustments can be made.

All medicines should be kept in a secure place and should be supervised by an adult. If someone takes too much of a medicine, follow your school procedure for an urgent medical problem.

Taking medicine is a private matter and is best managed discreetly and confidentially. It is important to be sensitive to the student's feelings about taking medicine.

If you suspect that the student is using drugs or alcohol, please tell the parent(s) or a school counselor right away.

Please tell the parent(s) or school nurse if you suspect medication side effects.

Modifications of the classroom environment or assignments may be useful in addition to medication. The student may need to be evaluated for additional help or a 504 plan or an Individualized Education Plan for learning problems or emotional or behavioral issues.

Any expression of suicidal thoughts or feelings or self-harm by a child or adolescent is a signal of distress and should be taken seriously. These behaviors should not be dismissed as "attention seeking." School procedures for safety issues should be followed.

What Is Clonazepam (Klonopin)?

Clonazepam is a *benzodiazepine*. It comes in brand name Klonopin and generic tablets and Klonopin Wafers (rapid-dissolving tablets).

How Can This Medicine Help?

Clonazepam is used to treat epilepsy (seizures, convulsions), tremors (shaking), and panic disorder. It can also help decrease anxiety in social anxiety disorder or posttraumatic stress disorder (PTSD). It can help calm people who have mania or acute psychosis. The rapid-dissolving tablets can be held in the mouth and work very fast.

Clonazepam also can be used for sleep problems, such as night terrors (sudden waking up from sleep with great fear) or sleepwalking, when these problems put the youth at risk of an accident or make it impossible for other family members to get enough sleep.

How Does This Medicine Work?

Clonazepam works on special places *(receptors)* in brain cells to increase the action of the brain chemical *GABA* (a *neurotransmitter*) in parts of the brain.

How Long Does This Medicine Last?

Clonazepam needs to be taken two or three times a day if taken regularly. The rapid-dissolving tablet may be taken as needed to prevent or stop a panic attack.

How Will the Doctor Monitor This Medicine?

The doctor will review your child's medical history and physical examination before starting clonazepam. The doctor may order some blood or urine tests to be sure your child does not have a hidden medical condition. The doctor or nurse may measure your child's pulse and blood pressure before starting clonazepam. Blood tests are not usually needed before starting clonazepam.

After the medicine is started, the doctor will want to have regular appointments with you and your child to see how the medicine is working, to see if a dose change is needed, to watch for side effects, to see if clonazepam is still needed, and to see if any other treatment is needed. The doctor or nurse may check your child's height, weight, pulse, and blood pressure.

What Side Effects Can This Medicine Have?

Any medicine can have side effects, including an allergy to the medicine. Because each patient is different, the doctor will monitor the youth closely, especially when the medicine is started. The doctor will work with you

to increase the positive effects and decrease the negative effects of the medicine. Please tell the doctor if any of the listed side effects appear or if you think that the medicine is causing any other problems. Not all of the rare or unusual side effects are listed.

Side effects are most common after starting the medicine or after a dose increase. Many side effects can be avoided or lessened by starting with a very low dose and increasing it slowly—ask the doctor.

Allergic Reaction

Tell the doctor in a day or two (if possible, before the next dose of medicine):

- Hives
- Itching
- Rash

Stop the medicine and get *immediate* medical care:

- Trouble breathing or chest tightness
- Swelling of lips, tongue, or throat

Common Side Effects

The following side effects are more common when first starting the medicine:

Tell the doctor within a week or two:

- Difficulty with balance
- Daytime drowsiness or sleepiness—Do not allow your child to drive, ride a bicycle or motorcycle, or operate machinery if this happens.

Behavioral and Emotional Side Effects

Call the doctor within a day or two:

- Irritability
- Excitement
- Increased anger or aggression
- Severe change in behavior
- Trouble sleeping or nightmares
- Decreased concentration
- Memory loss
- Feeling "spacey"

Serious Side Effects

- **Call the doctor or go to an emergency room immediately if your child exhibits uncontrollable behavior.**
- **People who take clonazepam must not drink alcohol. Severe sleepiness, loss of consciousness, or even death may result.**

Some Interactions With Other Medicines or Food

Please note that the following are only the most likely interactions with other medicines or food.

Clonazepam may be taken with or without food.

Taking clonazepam with alcohol and/or other sedative medicines or antihistamines (such as Benadryl) increases sleepiness, decreases muscle coordination, and may even decrease breathing.

It is better to limit drinks with caffeine (coffee, tea, soft drinks) because caffeine works in the opposite way from this medicine, and the positive effects might be decreased.

What Could Happen if This Medicine Is Stopped Suddenly?

Stopping clonazepam suddenly could cause seizures (fits, convulsions), especially if your child is being treated for seizures. Other symptoms caused by stopping suddenly could be headache, vomiting, decreased concentration, confusion, tremor (shaking), and muscle cramps.

How Long Will This Medicine Be Needed?

When being used for anxiety, agitation, or mania, clonazepam is usually used for a relatively short time, until other medications and/or behavioral treatments can start to work.

What Else Should I Know About This Medicine?

Because benzodiazepines can be abused (especially by people who abuse alcohol or drugs) and can cause psychological dependence or physical dependence (addiction), they are regulated by special state and federal laws as *controlled substances*. These laws place limitations on telephone prescriptions and refills.

Use of clonazepam for a long time may lead to dependence on the medicine.

People with sleep apnea (breathing stops while they are asleep) should not take clonazepam. Tell the doctor if your child snores very loudly.

Clonazepam should be avoided during pregnancy, especially in the first 3 months, because it may cause birth defects in the baby.

Klonopin may be confused with clonidine. Be sure to check the prescription when you get it from the pharmacy.

Notes

Use this space to take notes or to write down questions you want to ask the doctor.

_____

_____

_____

_____

_____

_____

_____

_____

_____

_____

_____

From Dulcan MK, Ballard R (editors): *Helping Parents and Teachers Understand Medications for Behavioral and Emotional Problems: A Resource Book of Medication Information Handouts,* Fourth Edition. Washington, DC, American Psychiatric Publishing, 2015

Medication Information for Parents and Teachers

Clonidine—Catapres, Catapres-TTS, Kapvay

General Information About Medication

Each child and adolescent is different. No one has exactly the same combination of medical and psychological problems. It is a good idea to talk with the doctor or nurse about the reasons a medicine is being used. It is very important to keep all appointments and to be in touch by telephone if you have concerns. It is important to communicate with the doctor, nurse, or therapist. An *advanced practice nurse* (APN) has additional education and training after becoming a registered nurse (RN). Your child's medication may be prescribed by a medical doctor (MD or DO) or an APN. In addition, a *physician assistant* (PA) working with a physician may prescribe certain medications. In this information sheet, "doctor" includes medical doctors as well as APNs and PAs who prescribe medication. Often a nurse (RN) will be part of the team and answer questions and give information.

It is very important that the medicine be taken exactly as the doctor instructs. However, once in a while, everyone forgets to give a medicine on time. It is a good idea to ask the doctor or nurse what to do if this happens. Do not stop or change a medicine without asking the doctor or nurse first.

If the medicine seems to stop working, it may be because it is not being taken regularly. The youth may be "cheeking" or hiding the medicine or forgetting to take it (especially at school). The doses may be too far apart or a different dose or medicine may be needed. Something at school, at home, or in the neighborhood may be upsetting the youth, or he or she may need special help for learning disabilities or tutoring. Please discuss your concerns with the doctor. **Do not just increase the dose.** It is also very important not to decrease the dose or stop the medicine without talking to the doctor first. The problem being treated may come back, or there could be uncomfortable or even dangerous results.

All medicines should be kept in a safe place, out of the reach of children, and should be supervised by an adult. If someone takes too much of a medicine, call the doctor, the poison control center, or a hospital emergency room.

Each medicine has a "generic" or chemical name. Just like laundry detergents or paper towels, some medicines are sold by more than one company under different brand names. The same medicine may be available under a generic name and several brand names. The generic medications are usually less expensive than the brand name ones. The generic medications have the same chemical formula, but they may or may not be exactly the same strength as the brand-name medications. Also, some brands of pills contain dye or other things that can cause allergic reactions. It is a good idea to talk to the doctor and the pharmacist about whether it is important to use a specific brand of medicine.

Any medicine can cause an allergic reaction. Examples are hives, itching, rashes, swelling, and trouble breathing. Even a tiny amount of a medicine can cause a reaction in patients who are allergic to that medicine. Be *sure* to talk to the doctor before restarting a medicine that has caused an allergic reaction and tell the doctor about any reactions to medicine that your child has had before.

Taking more than one medicine at the same time may cause more side effects or cause one of the medicines to not work as well. Always ask the doctor, nurse, or pharmacist before adding another medicine, either prescription or bought without a prescription in a store or on the Internet. Be sure that each doctor knows about *all* of the medicines your child is taking. Also tell the doctor about any vitamins, herbal medicines, or supplements your child may be taking. Some of these may have side effects alone or when taken with this medication. It is a very good idea to keep a list with you of the names and doses of all medicines that your child is taking.

Everyone taking medicine should have a physical examination at least once a year.

If you think that your child may be using drugs or alcohol, please tell the doctor right away.

Pregnancy requires special care in the use of medicine. Some medicines can cause birth defects if taken by a pregnant mother. **Please tell the doctor immediately if you suspect the teenager is at risk of becoming pregnant.** The doctor may wish to discuss sexual behavior and/or birth control with your daughter.

Printed information like this applies to children and adolescents in general. If you have questions about the medicine, or if you notice changes or anything unusual, please ask the doctor or nurse. As scientific research advances, knowledge increases and advice changes. Even experts do not always agree. Many medicines have not been "approved" by the U.S. Food and Drug Administration (FDA) for use in children or use for particular problems. For this reason, use of the medicine for a problem or age group often is not listed in the *Physicians' Desk Reference*. This does not necessarily mean that the medicine is dangerous or does not work, only that the company that makes the medicine has not received permission to advertise the medicine for use in children. Companies often do not apply for this permission because it is expensive to do the tests needed to apply for approval for use in children. Once a medication is approved by the FDA for any purpose, a doctor is allowed to prescribe it according to research and clinical experience.

Note to Teachers

It is a good idea to talk with the parent(s) about the reason(s) that a medication is being used. If the parent(s) sign consent to release information, it is often helpful for you to talk with the doctor. If the parent(s) give permission, the doctor may ask you to fill out rating forms about your experience with the student's behavior, feelings, academic performance, and medication side effects. This information is very useful in selecting and monitoring medication treatment. If you have observations that you think are important, do not hesitate to share these with the student's parent(s) and treating clinicians (with parental consent).

It is very important that the medicine be taken exactly as the doctor instructs. However, everyone forgets to give a medicine on time once in a while. It is a good idea to ask the parent(s) in advance what to do if this happens. Do not stop or change the time you are giving a medicine at school without parental permission. If a medication is to be taken with food, but lunchtime or snack time changes, be sure to notify the parent(s) so appropriate adjustments can be made.

All medicines should be kept in a secure place and should be supervised by an adult. If someone takes too much of a medicine, follow your school procedure for an urgent medical problem.

Taking medicine is a private matter and is best managed discreetly and confidentially. It is important to be sensitive to the student's feelings about taking medicine.

If you suspect that the student is using drugs or alcohol, please tell the parent(s) or a school counselor right away.

Please tell the parent(s) or school nurse if you suspect medication side effects.

Modifications of the classroom environment or assignments may be useful in addition to medication. The student may need to be evaluated for additional help or a 504 plan or an Individualized Education Plan for learning problems or emotional or behavioral issues.

Any expression of suicidal thoughts or feelings or self-harm by a child or adolescent is a signal of distress and should be taken seriously. These behaviors should not be dismissed as "attention seeking." School procedures for safety issues should be followed.

What Is Clonidine (Catapres, Catapres-TTS, Kapvay)?

Clonidine was first used to treat high blood pressure, so it is sometimes called an *antihypertensive*. Now it is being used to treat symptoms of attention-deficit/hyperactivity disorder (ADHD), Tourette's disorder, or chronic tics (fast, repeated movements) and to reduce symptoms of withdrawal from cigarettes or narcotics. It is sometimes used to treat aggression, posttraumatic stress disorder (PTSD), anxiety (nervousness), or panic disorder in children and adolescents. It may be used at bedtime to treat severe sleep problems in youth with ADHD, intellectual disability, or autism spectrum disorder. It comes in brand name Catapres and generic tablets, a skin patch (transdermal form, Catapres-TTS) that releases medicine slowly for 5 days in children (7 days in adults), and a brand name Kapvay or generic extended-release tablet that can be used by itself or in addition to a stimulant medication for the treatment of ADHD.

How Can This Medicine Help?

Clonidine can decrease symptoms of hyperactivity, impulsivity, anxiety, irritability, temper tantrums, explosive anger, and tics. It can increase patience and frustration tolerance as well as improve self-control and cooperation with adults. Clonidine may be used by itself or together with a stimulant medication (methylphenidate or amphetamine) for ADHD or by itself for Tourette's disorder. The positive effects usually do not start for 2 weeks after a stable dose is reached. The full benefit may not be seen for 2–4 months.

How Does This Medicine Work?

Clonidine works by decreasing the level of excitement in parts of the brain. It is sometimes called an *alpha-adrenergic agonist*. It affects the levels of *norepinephrine*, one of the *neurotransmitters* (chemicals that the brain makes for nerve cells to communicate with each other). This effect helps people with tic disorders to stop moving or making noises when they do not want to and helps people with ADHD to slow down and think before doing something. It calms parts of the brain that are too excited in people with severe anxiety. This medicine is chemically different from sedatives or tranquilizers, even though it may make your child sleepy, especially when he or she first starts taking it.

How Long Does This Medicine Last?

When children take clonidine for problems with emotions or behavior, it must be taken three to four times a day. The extended-release version, Kapvay, is taken up to twice a day. When clonidine is taken for high blood pressure, a single dose lasts for 6–10 hours. When taken for sleep, it may be used at bedtime only. Sometimes the sleepiness lasts into the next day. The clonidine effect may not last the whole night, and the youth wakes up in the middle of the night. This problem is less likely with extended-release forms of clonidine.

How Will the Doctor Monitor This Medicine?

The doctor will review your child's medical history and physical examination before starting clonidine. The doctor may order some blood or urine tests to be sure your child does not have a hidden medical condition. Be sure to tell the doctor if your child or anyone in the family has high blood pressure, heart disease, fainting, diabetes, or kidney problems. Tell the doctor if your child cannot swallow whole pills. The doctor also may want to obtain an ECG (electrocardiogram or heart rhythm test) before starting the medicine. The doctor or nurse will measure your child's height, weight, pulse, and blood pressure before starting clonidine.

After the medicine is started, the doctor will want to have regular appointments with you and your child to see how the medicine is working, to see if a dose change is needed, to watch for side effects, to see if clonidine is still needed, and to see if any other treatment is needed. The doctor or nurse will check your child's height, weight, pulse, and blood pressure.

What Side Effects Can This Medicine Have?

Any medicine can have side effects, including an allergy to the medicine. Because each patient is different, the doctor will monitor the youth closely, especially when the medicine is started. The doctor will work with you to increase the positive effects and decrease the negative effects of the medicine. Please tell the doctor if any of the listed side effects appear or if you think that the medicine is causing any other problems. Not all of the rare or unusual side effects are listed.

Side effects are most common after starting the medicine or after a dose increase. Many side effects can be avoided or lessened by starting with a very low dose and increasing it slowly—ask the doctor.

Allergic Reaction

Tell the doctor in a day or two (if possible, before the next dose of medicine):

- Hives
- Itching
- Rash

Stop the medicine and get *immediate* medical care:

- Trouble breathing or chest tightness
- Swelling of lips, tongue, or throat

Common, but Usually Mild, Side Effects

The following side effects are more common when starting clonidine or when the dose is increased. If these effects do not go away after a week or two, ask the doctor about lowering the dose.

- Daytime sleepiness, especially when bored or not doing anything—This is usually worst in the first 2–4 weeks. Do not allow your child to drive, ride a bicycle or motorcycle, or operate machinery if this happens.
- Fatigue or tiredness
- Low blood pressure (rarely a serious problem in children and adolescents)
- Dizziness or light-headedness—This side effect is worse when the child stands up quickly, especially when getting out of bed in the morning; try having the child stand up slowly.

126

- Headache
- Stomachache

If one of the following side effects appears, call the doctor within a day or two:

- Slow pulse rate (heartbeat)
- Insomnia (trouble sleeping)—This may be caused by the medicine wearing off.
- Ringing in the ears
- Redness and itching under the skin patch

Less Common Side Effects

Call the doctor within a day or two:

- Depression or increased irritability
- Confusion
- Bed-wetting
- Muscle cramps
- Itching
- Runny nose

Less Common, but Serious, Side Effects

Call the doctor *immediately*:

- Severe or increased dizziness or light-headedness
- Sleepiness that worsens or returns after the initial sleepiness has stopped from getting used to the current dose of the medicine.

Very Rare, but Serious, Side Effects

Call the doctor *immediately*:

- Fainting
- Irregular heartbeat
- Trouble breathing
- Decreased frequency of urination; rapid, puffy swelling of the body (especially the legs and feet); sudden headaches with nausea and vomiting—These could be signs of kidney failure.

Side Effects Reported in Adults but Rare in Children

Tell the doctor within a week:

- Dry mouth—Have your child try using sugar-free gum or candy.
- Constipation—Encourage your child to drink more fluids and eat high-fiber foods; if necessary, the doctor may recommend a fiber medicine such as Benefiber or a stool softener such as Colace or mineral oil.
- Low blood pressure

- Weakness
- Nightmares
- Increased blood sugar (mainly in persons with diabetes)
- Sensation of cold or pain in fingers or toes
- Weight gain

Some Interactions With Other Medicines or Food

Please note that the following are only the most likely interactions with other medicines or food.

Clonidine may be taken with or without food.

Increased sleepiness will occur in combination with medications for anxiety (sedatives or tranquilizers), sleep (hypnotics), allergy or colds (antihistamines), psychosis, or seizures (anticonvulsants).

An increased risk for a slow heart rate or a serious change in the heart's rhythm can occur if taking clonidine with other medications known to affect heart rhythm (such as digitalis, calcium-channel blockers, or beta-blockers).

What Could Happen if This Medicine Is Stopped Suddenly?

It is important not to stop clonidine suddenly but to decrease it slowly (taper) as directed by the doctor. Stopping clonidine suddenly may result in

- Very high blood pressure, even if blood pressure was normal before starting the medicine (rebound hypertension)
- Temporary worsening of behavioral problems or tics
- Nervousness or anxiety
- Rapid or irregular heartbeat
- Chest pain
- Headache
- Stomach cramps, nausea, vomiting
- Trouble sleeping

It is also very important not to miss a dose of clonidine, because withdrawal symptoms such as heart or blood pressure problems may occur. **Be sure not to let the prescription run out!** It is especially important not to miss any clonidine doses if methylphenidate is also being taken.

How Long Will This Medicine Be Needed?

There is no way to know how long a person will need to take clonidine. The parent(s), the doctor, and the school will work together to determine what is right for each patient. Some people need the medicine for a few years; some people may need it longer.

What Else Should I Know About This Medicine?

If a child is sleepy from the clonidine, something active or interesting to do will help the child to stay awake. Sleeping extra hours will not help. Sleepiness usually decreases as the child gets used to the medicine. If the youth is still sleepy in the daytime after 4 weeks at the same dose, a lower dose or a different medicine may be needed.

If the skin patch is being used, it should be applied on an area of the body without hair that is difficult for the child to reach. First, wash the skin with soap and water, then dry. The patch is applied like an adhesive bandage. The child can take a shower or bath with the patch on, but the patch may need to be replaced after swimming or heavy sweating. A protective cover may be placed on top of the patch, but the cover may worsen skin irritation. Do not cut the patch, because that may change the speed at which the medicine is absorbed through the skin. The patch may contain conducting metal (such as aluminum), so remove the patch before getting an MRI (magnetic resonance imaging) test.

Kapvay must be taken whole and swallowed. It should not be chewed, crushed, or broken.

If you miss a dose of Kapvay, give the next dose at the regular time. Do not try to make up for the missed dose.

It is very important not to drink alcohol or take drugs while on clonidine.

Clonidine may be confused with clonazepam, clozapine, Klonopin, or quinidine. Be sure to check the prescription when you get it from the pharmacy.

If your child is taking the extended-release form of clonidine, Kapvay, your doctor will tell you how to gradually increase the number of pills per day to the right dose. If your child stops taking the medication for several days, you should not restart right away at the same dose. Talk with your doctor about the best way to restart the medication.

It is very important that all forms of clonidine are kept locked away from small children and from anyone who might take an overdose. Taking more clonidine than prescribed can cause severe side effects or even death.

Notes

Use this space to take notes or to write down questions you want to ask the doctor.

_____

_____

_____

_____

_____

_____

_____

_____

_____

_____

_____

_____

_____

From Dulcan MK, Ballard R (editors): *Helping Parents and Teachers Understand Medications for Behavioral and Emotional Problems: A Resource Book of Medication Information Handouts*, Fourth Edition. Washington, DC, American Psychiatric Publishing, 2015

Medication Information for Parents and Teachers

Clozapine—Clozaril, FazaClo, Versacloz

General Information About Medication

Each child and adolescent is different. No one has exactly the same combination of medical and psychological problems. It is a good idea to talk with the doctor or nurse about the reasons a medicine is being used. It is very important to keep all appointments and to be in touch by telephone if you have concerns. It is important to communicate with the doctor, nurse, or therapist. An *advanced practice nurse* (APN) has additional education and training after becoming a registered nurse (RN). Your child's medication may be prescribed by a medical doctor (MD or DO) or an APN. In addition, a *physician assistant* (PA) working with a physician may prescribe certain medications. In this information sheet, "doctor" includes medical doctors as well as APNs and PAs who prescribe medication. Often a nurse (RN) will be part of the team and answer questions and give information.

It is very important that the medicine be taken exactly as the doctor instructs. However, once in a while, everyone forgets to give a medicine on time. It is a good idea to ask the doctor or nurse what to do if this happens. Do not stop or change a medicine without asking the doctor or nurse first.

If the medicine seems to stop working, it may be because it is not being taken regularly. The youth may be "cheeking" or hiding the medicine or forgetting to take it (especially at school). The doses may be too far apart or a different dose or medicine may be needed. Something at school, at home, or in the neighborhood may be upsetting the youth, or he or she may need special help for learning disabilities or tutoring. Please discuss your concerns with the doctor. **Do not just increase the dose.** It is also very important not to decrease the dose or stop the medicine without talking to the doctor first. The problem being treated may come back, or there could be uncomfortable or even dangerous results.

All medicines should be kept in a safe place, out of the reach of children, and should be supervised by an adult. If someone takes too much of a medicine, call the doctor, the poison control center, or a hospital emergency room.

Each medicine has a "generic" or chemical name. Just like laundry detergents or paper towels, some medicines are sold by more than one company under different brand names. The same medicine may be available under a generic name and several brand names. The generic medications are usually less expensive than the brand name ones. The generic medications have the same chemical formula, but they may or may not be exactly the same strength as the brand-name medications. Also, some brands of pills contain dye or other things that can cause allergic reactions. It is a good idea to talk to the doctor and the pharmacist about whether it is important to use a specific brand of medicine.

Any medicine can cause an allergic reaction. Examples are hives, itching, rashes, swelling, and trouble breathing. Even a tiny amount of a medicine can cause a reaction in patients who are allergic to that medicine. Be *sure* to talk to the doctor before restarting a medicine that has caused an allergic reaction and tell the doctor about any reactions to medicine that your child has had before.

Taking more than one medicine at the same time may cause more side effects or cause one of the medicines to not work as well. Always ask the doctor, nurse, or pharmacist before adding another

medicine, either prescription or bought without a prescription in a store or on the Internet. **Be sure that each doctor knows about *all* of the medicines your child is taking. Also tell the doctor about any vitamins, herbal medicines, or supplements your child may be taking.** Some of these may have side effects alone or when taken with this medication. It is a very good idea to keep a list with you of the names and doses of all medicines that your child is taking.

Everyone taking medicine should have a physical examination at least once a year.

If you think that your child may be using drugs or alcohol, please tell the doctor right away.

Pregnancy requires special care in the use of medicine. Some medicines can cause birth defects if taken by a pregnant mother. **Please tell the doctor immediately if you suspect the teenager is at risk of becoming pregnant.** The doctor may wish to discuss sexual behavior and/or birth control with your daughter.

Printed information like this applies to children and adolescents in general. If you have questions about the medicine, or if you notice changes or anything unusual, please ask the doctor or nurse. As scientific research advances, knowledge increases and advice changes. Even experts do not always agree. Many medicines have not been "approved" by the U.S. Food and Drug Administration (FDA) for use in children or use for particular problems. For this reason, use of the medicine for a problem or age group often is not listed in the *Physicians' Desk Reference.* This does not necessarily mean that the medicine is dangerous or does not work, only that the company that makes the medicine has not received permission to advertise the medicine for use in children. Companies often do not apply for this permission because it is expensive to do the tests needed to apply for approval for use in children. Once a medication is approved by the FDA for any purpose, a doctor is allowed to prescribe it according to research and clinical experience.

Note to Teachers

It is a good idea to talk with the parent(s) about the reason(s) that a medication is being used. If the parent(s) sign consent to release information, it is often helpful for you to talk with the doctor. If the parent(s) give permission, the doctor may ask you to fill out rating forms about your experience with the student's behavior, feelings, academic performance, and medication side effects. This information is very useful in selecting and monitoring medication treatment. If you have observations that you think are important, do not hesitate to share these with the student's parent(s) and treating clinicians (with parental consent).

It is very important that the medicine be taken exactly as the doctor instructs. However, everyone forgets to give a medicine on time once in a while. It is a good idea to ask the parent(s) in advance what to do if this happens. Do not stop or change the time you are giving a medicine at school without parental permission. If a medication is to be taken with food, but lunchtime or snack time changes, be sure to notify the parent(s) so appropriate adjustments can be made.

All medicines should be kept in a secure place and should be supervised by an adult. If someone takes too much of a medicine, follow your school procedure for an urgent medical problem.

Taking medicine is a private matter and is best managed discreetly and confidentially. It is important to be sensitive to the student's feelings about taking medicine.

If you suspect that the student is using drugs or alcohol, please tell the parent(s) or a school counselor right away.

Please tell the parent(s) or school nurse if you suspect medication side effects.

Modifications of the classroom environment or assignments may be useful in addition to medication. The student may need to be evaluated for additional help or a 504 plan or an Individualized Education Plan for learning problems or emotional or behavioral issues.

Any expression of suicidal thoughts or feelings or self-harm by a child or adolescent is a signal of distress and should be taken seriously. These behaviors should not be dismissed as "attention seeking." School procedures for safety issues should be followed.

What Is Clozapine (Clozaril, FazaClo, Versacloz)?

Clozapine is called an *atypical* or *second-generation antipsychotic*. It is sometimes called an *atypical psychotropic agent*, or simply an *atypical*. It comes in brand name Clozaril and generic tablets and FazaClo and generic orally disintegrating (dissolves in the mouth) tablets as well as a liquid form (Versacloz).

How Can This Medicine Help?

Clozapine is used to treat psychosis, such as in schizophrenia, mania, or very severe depression, if other antipsychotic medicines have not helped enough. It can reduce *positive symptoms* such as hallucinations (hearing voices or seeing things that are not there); delusions (troubling beliefs that other people do not share); agitation; and very unusual thinking, speech, and behavior. It is also used to lessen the *negative symptoms* of schizophrenia, such as lack of interest in doing things (apathy), lack of motivation, social withdrawal, and lack of energy.

This medicine is very powerful and is used to treat very serious problems or symptoms that other medicines do not help. Be patient; the positive effects of this medicine may not appear for 4–6 weeks, and the full positive effect may not be seen for 6–12 months.

How Does This Medicine Work?

Cells in the brain communicate using chemicals called *neurotransmitters*. Too much or too little of these substances in parts of the brain can cause problems. Clozapine works by blocking the action of two of these neurotransmitters—*dopamine* and *serotonin*—in certain areas of the brain.

How Long Does This Medicine Last?

Clozapine can usually be taken only once a day, although at higher doses, dividing into two doses may be needed to decrease side effects.

How Will the Doctor Monitor This Medicine?

The doctor will review your child's medical history and physical examination before starting clozapine. The doctor may order some blood or urine tests to be sure your child does not have a hidden medical condition that would make it unsafe to use this medicine. The doctor or nurse may measure your child's pulse and blood pressure before starting clozapine. The doctor may order other tests, such as baseline tests for blood sugar and cholesterol. A blood test to count the different kinds of blood cells must be done before starting clozapine. An EEG (electroencephalogram or brain wave test) may be done before starting clozapine to see if there is an increased risk of seizures (convulsions).

Be sure to tell the doctor if anyone in the family has diabetes, high blood pressure, high cholesterol, or heart disease.

After the medicine is started, the doctor will want to have regular appointments with you and your child to see how the medicine is working, to see if a dose change is needed, to watch for side effects, to see if clozapine is still needed, and to see if any other treatment is needed. The doctor or nurse will check your child's height, weight, pulse, and blood pressure, and watch for abnormal movements. The FDA has a required schedule of blood tests to watch for a decrease in the number of white blood cells (see "What Else Should I Know About Side Effects?"). Sometimes blood tests are needed to watch for diabetes or increased cholesterol.

What Side Effects Can This Medicine Have?

Any medicine can have side effects, including an allergy to the medicine. Because each patient is different, the doctor will monitor the youth closely, especially when the medicine is started. The doctor will work with you to increase the positive effects and decrease the negative effects of the medicine. Please tell the doctor if any of the listed side effects appear or if you think that the medicine is causing any other problems. Not all of the rare or unusual side effects are listed.

Side effects are most common after starting the medicine or after a dose increase. Many side effects can be avoided or lessened by starting with a very low dose and increasing it slowly—ask the doctor.

Allergic Reaction

Tell the doctor in a day or two (if possible, before the next dose of medicine):

- Hives
- Itching
- Rash

Stop the medicine and get *immediate* medical care:

- Trouble breathing or chest tightness
- Swelling of lips, tongue, or throat

Common, but Not Usually Serious, Side Effects

Discuss the following side effects with your child's doctor when convenient. These side effects often can be helped by lowering the dose of medicine, changing the times medicine is taken, or adding another medicine.

- Daytime sleepiness or tiredness—Do not allow your child to drive, ride a bicycle or motorcycle, or operate machinery if this happens. This problem may be lessened by taking the medicine at bedtime.
- Dry mouth—Have your child try using sugar-free gum or candy.
- Trouble urinating
- Constipation—Encourage your child to drink more fluids and eat high-fiber foods; if necessary, the doctor may recommend a fiber medicine such as Benefiber or a stool softener such as Colace or mineral oil.
- Blurred vision
- Dizziness—This side effect is worse when the child stands up quickly, especially when getting out of bed in the morning; try having the child stand up slowly.
- Increased appetite
- Weight gain—Seek nutritional counseling; provide your child with low-calorie snacks and encourage regular exercise.
- Nausea

- Vomiting
- Stomach pain
- Headache
- Bed-wetting

Very Rare, but Not Usually Serious, Side Effects

Discuss the following side effects with your child's doctor when convenient. These side effects often can be helped by lowering the dose of medicine, changing the times medicine is taken, or adding another medicine.

- Drooling
- Increased restlessness or inability to sit still
- Shaking of hands and fingers
- Decreased or slowed movement and decreased facial expressions

Less Common, but Potentially Serious, Side Effects

Call the doctor *immediately*:

- Stiffness of the tongue, jaw, neck, back, or legs
- Seizure (fit, convulsion)—This is more common in people with a history of seizures or head injury and at higher doses of clozapine.

Talk to a doctor within a day:

- Increased thirst, frequent urination (having to go to the bathroom often), lethargy, tiredness, dizziness, and blurred vision—These could be signs of diabetes (especially if your child is overweight or there is a family history of diabetes).
- Fast or irregular heartbeat (pulse)

Very Rare, but Serious, Side Effects

- Fever, chills, sore throat, or skin bruising or small spots—This may mean a decrease in the number of blood cells. **Call the doctor within a day or two.**
- Extreme stiffness or lack of movement, very high fever, mental confusion, irregular pulse rate, or eye pain—**This is a medical emergency. Go to an emergency room *right away*.**
- Sudden stiffness and inability to breathe or swallow—**Go to an emergency room or call 911.** Tell the paramedics, nurses, and doctors that the patient is taking clozapine. Other medicines can be used to treat this problem fast.
- Heart problems have been reported in adults and young people taking clozapine. If your child is extremely tired all of the time, has changes in breathing, a rapid heartbeat, or chest pain, **call the doctor right away.**

What Else Should I Know About Side Effects?

Most side effects lessen over time. If they are troublesome, talk with your child's doctor. Some side effects can be decreased by taking a smaller dose of medicine, by stopping the medicine, by changing to another medicine, or by adding another medicine. Clozapine is often increased very slowly to reduce the risk of side effects.

Most people who take clozapine gain weight. Children seem to have more problems with this than adults. The weight gain may be from increased appetite and from ways that the medicine changes how the body processes food. Clozapine may also change the way that the body handles glucose (sugar) and may cause high levels of blood sugar (*hyperglycemia*). People who take clozapine, especially those who gain a lot of weight, are at increased risk of developing *diabetes* and of having increased fats (*lipids—cholesterol* and *triglycerides*) in their blood. Over time, both diabetes and increased fats in the blood may lead to heart disease, stroke, and other complications. The FDA has put warnings on all atypical agents about the increased risks of hyperglycemia, diabetes, and increased blood cholesterol and triglycerides when taking one of these medicines. It is much easier to prevent weight gain than to lose weight later. When your child first starts taking clozapine, it is a good idea to be sure that he or she eats a well-balanced diet without "junk food" and with healthy snacks like fruits and vegetables, not sweets or fried foods. He or she should drink water or skim milk, not pop, sodas, soft drinks, or sugary juices. Regular exercise is important for maintaining a healthy weight (and may also help with sleep).

Because clozapine may cause a rare but very dangerous decrease in the white blood cells (*agranulocytosis*), people taking this medicine must be registered by the pharmacy to be sure that the white cells in the blood are measured as required. The pharmacy is allowed to dispense the medicine only after being sure that the white blood cell count (WBC) is normal. This must be done every week for the first 6 months, then every 2 weeks for 6 months, and then once a month for as long as clozapine is taken.

One very rare side effect that may not go away is *tardive dyskinesia* (or TD). Patients with tardive dyskinesia have involuntary movements (movements that they cannot help making) of the body, especially the mouth and tongue. The patient may look as though he or she is making faces over and over again. Jerky movements of the arms, legs, or body may occur. There may be fine, wormlike, or sudden repeated movements of the tongue, or the person may appear to be chewing something or smacking or puckering his or her lips. The fingers may look as though they are rolling something. If you notice any unusual movements, be sure to tell the doctor. The doctor may use the AIMS test to look for these movements. Clozapine is less likely than other antipsychotic medicines to cause tardive dyskinesia and may even decrease the symptoms of tardive dyskinesia that are caused by other antipsychotic medicines.

Sometimes this medicine can cause a *dystonic reaction*. This is a sudden stiffening of the muscles, most often in the jaw, neck, tongue, face, or shoulders. If this happens, and your child is not having trouble breathing, you may give a dose of diphenhydramine (Benadryl). Follow the dose instructions on the package for your child's age. This should relax the muscles in a few minutes. Then call your doctor to tell him or her what happened. If the muscles do not relax, take your child to the emergency department.

Neuroleptic malignant syndrome is a very rare side effect that can lead to death. The symptoms are severe muscle stiffness, high fever, increased heart rate and blood pressure, irregular heartbeat (pulse), and sweating. It may lead to unconsciousness. If you suspect this, **call 911 or go to an emergency room right away.**

Some Interactions With Other Medicines or Food

Please note that the following are only the most likely interactions with other medicines or food.

Clozapine may be taken with or without food.

It is better to limit drinks with caffeine (coffee, tea, soft drinks) because caffeine works in the opposite way from clozapine, may increase the side effects of the medicine, and might decrease the positive effects.

Carbamazepine (Tegretol) should not be taken with clozapine because of increased risk of decreased white blood cells.

Antidepressants (selective serotonin reuptake inhibitors or SSRIs) such as fluoxetine (Prozac), citalopram (Celexa), fluvoxamine (Luvox CR), sertraline (Zoloft), and paroxetine (Paxil); antibiotics such as erythromycin; and antifungal agents such as ketoconazole may increase blood levels of clozapine and cause increased side effects, especially sedation or seizures.

What Could Happen if This Medicine Is Stopped Suddenly?

Involuntary movements, or *withdrawal dyskinesias*, may appear within 1–4 weeks of lowering the dose or stopping the medicine. Usually these go away, but they can last for days to months. If this medicine is stopped suddenly, emotional disturbance (such as irritability, nervousness, moodiness, or oppositional behavior) or physical problems (such as stomachache, loss of appetite, nausea, vomiting, diarrhea, sweating, indigestion, trouble sleeping, trembling, or shaking) may appear. These problems usually last only a few days to a few weeks. If they happen, you should tell your child's doctor. The medicine dose may need to be lowered more slowly (tapered). Always check with the doctor before stopping a medicine.

How Long Will This Medicine Be Needed?

How long your child will need to take this medicine depends partly on the reason that it was prescribed. Some problems last for only a few months, whereas others last much longer. It is important to ask the doctor whether medicine is still needed, especially with medicines as powerful as this one. Every few months, you should discuss with your child's doctor the reasons for using the medicine and whether the medicine may be stopped or the dose lowered.

What Else Should I Know About This Medicine?

There are other medicines that are used for the same kinds of problems. If your child is having bad side effects or the medicine does not seem to be working, ask the doctor if another medicine might work as well or better and have fewer side effects for your child. Each person reacts differently to medicines.

The orally disintegrating tablet should be removed from the package by peeling apart, just before use. The tablet should be melted in the mouth and swallowed with saliva. If the tablet needs to be split, throw away the part not taken.

Notes

Use this space to take notes or to write down questions you want to ask the doctor.

_____

_____

_____

_____

_____

_____

_____

_____

_____

_____

_____

_____

_____

_____

Cyproheptadine

General Information About Medication

Each child and adolescent is different. No one has exactly the same combination of medical and psychological problems. It is a good idea to talk with the doctor or nurse about the reasons a medicine is being used. It is very important to keep all appointments and to be in touch by telephone if you have concerns. It is important to communicate with the doctor, nurse, or therapist. An *advanced practice nurse* (APN) has additional education and training after becoming a registered nurse (RN). Your child's medication may be prescribed by a medical doctor (MD or DO) or an APN. In addition, a *physician assistant* (PA) working with a physician may prescribe certain medications. In this information sheet, "doctor" includes medical doctors as well as APNs and PAs who prescribe medication. Often a nurse (RN) will be part of the team and answer questions and give information.

It is very important that the medicine be taken exactly as the doctor instructs. However, once in a while, everyone forgets to give a medicine on time. It is a good idea to ask the doctor or nurse what to do if this happens. Do not stop or change a medicine without asking the doctor or nurse first.

If the medicine seems to stop working, it may be because it is not being taken regularly. The youth may be "cheeking" or hiding the medicine or forgetting to take it (especially at school). The doses may be too far apart or a different dose or medicine may be needed. Something at school, at home, or in the neighborhood may be upsetting the youth, or he or she may need special help for learning disabilities or tutoring. Please discuss your concerns with the doctor. **Do not just increase the dose.** It is also very important not to decrease the dose or stop the medicine without talking to the doctor first. The problem being treated may come back, or there could be uncomfortable or even dangerous results.

All medicines should be kept in a safe place, out of the reach of children, and should be supervised by an adult. If someone takes too much of a medicine, call the doctor, the poison control center, or a hospital emergency room.

Each medicine has a "generic" or chemical name. Just like laundry detergents or paper towels, some medicines are sold by more than one company under different brand names. The same medicine may be available under a generic name and several brand names. The generic medications are usually less expensive than the brand name ones. The generic medications have the same chemical formula, but they may or may not be exactly the same strength as the brand-name medications. Also, some brands of pills contain dye or other things that can cause allergic reactions. It is a good idea to talk to the doctor and the pharmacist about whether it is important to use a specific brand of medicine.

Any medicine can cause an allergic reaction. Examples are hives, itching, rashes, swelling, and trouble breathing. Even a tiny amount of a medicine can cause a reaction in patients who are allergic to that medicine. Be *sure* to talk to the doctor before restarting a medicine that has caused an allergic reaction and tell the doctor about any reactions to medicine that your child has had before.

Taking more than one medicine at the same time may cause more side effects or cause one of the medicines to not work as well. Always ask the doctor, nurse, or pharmacist before adding another

medicine, either prescription or bought without a prescription in a store or on the Internet. **Be sure that each doctor knows about** *all* **of the medicines your child is taking. Also tell the doctor about any vitamins, herbal medicines, or supplements your child may be taking.** Some of these may have side effects alone or when taken with this medication. It is a very good idea to keep a list with you of the names and doses of all medicines that your child is taking.

Everyone taking medicine should have a physical examination at least once a year.

If you think that your child may be using drugs or alcohol, please tell the doctor right away.

Pregnancy requires special care in the use of medicine. Some medicines can cause birth defects if taken by a pregnant mother. **Please tell the doctor immediately if you suspect the teenager is at risk of becoming pregnant.** The doctor may wish to discuss sexual behavior and/or birth control with your daughter.

Printed information like this applies to children and adolescents in general. If you have questions about the medicine, or if you notice changes or anything unusual, please ask the doctor or nurse. As scientific research advances, knowledge increases and advice changes. Even experts do not always agree. Many medicines have not been "approved" by the U.S. Food and Drug Administration (FDA) for use in children or use for particular problems. For this reason, use of the medicine for a problem or age group often is not listed in the *Physicians' Desk Reference*. This does not necessarily mean that the medicine is dangerous or does not work, only that the company that makes the medicine has not received permission to advertise the medicine for use in children. Companies often do not apply for this permission because it is expensive to do the tests needed to apply for approval for use in children. Once a medication is approved by the FDA for any purpose, a doctor is allowed to prescribe it according to research and clinical experience.

Note to Teachers

It is a good idea to talk with the parent(s) about the reason(s) that a medication is being used. If the parent(s) sign consent to release information, it is often helpful for you to talk with the doctor. If the parent(s) give permission, the doctor may ask you to fill out rating forms about your experience with the student's behavior, feelings, academic performance, and medication side effects. This information is very useful in selecting and monitoring medication treatment. If you have observations that you think are important, do not hesitate to share these with the student's parent(s) and treating clinicians (with parental consent).

It is very important that the medicine be taken exactly as the doctor instructs. However, everyone forgets to give a medicine on time once in a while. It is a good idea to ask the parent(s) in advance what to do if this happens. Do not stop or change the time you are giving a medicine at school without parental permission. If a medication is to be taken with food, but lunchtime or snack time changes, be sure to notify the parent(s) so appropriate adjustments can be made.

All medicines should be kept in a secure place and should be supervised by an adult. If someone takes too much of a medicine, follow your school procedure for an urgent medical problem.

Taking medicine is a private matter and is best managed discreetly and confidentially. It is important to be sensitive to the student's feelings about taking medicine.

If you suspect that the student is using drugs or alcohol, please tell the parent(s) or a school counselor right away.

Please tell the parent(s) or school nurse if you suspect medication side effects.

Modifications of the classroom environment or assignments may be useful in addition to medication. The student may need to be evaluated for additional help or a 504 plan or an Individualized Education Plan for learning problems or emotional or behavioral issues.

Any expression of suicidal thoughts or feelings or self-harm by a child or adolescent is a signal of distress and should be taken seriously. These behaviors should not be dismissed as "attention seeking." School procedures for safety issues should be followed.

What Is Cyproheptadine?

Cyproheptadine is called an *antihistamine*. Antihistamines were developed to treat allergies. Cyproheptadine is sometimes used to treat anxiety (nervousness) or insomnia (difficulty falling asleep). It may be used to increase appetite in people who do not eat enough food and to prevent cluster and migraine headaches. Cyproheptadine comes in generic tablets and syrup.

How Can This Medicine Help?

Cyproheptadine may decrease nervousness. When used for anxiety, it works best when used for a short time along with psychotherapy. Cyproheptadine can help with insomnia when used for a short time along with a behavioral program, such as regular soothing routines at bedtime and increased exercise in the daytime. In people who are not eating enough and are too thin, it can increase appetite and help to gain weight.

How Does This Medicine Work?

Cyproheptadine can help decrease anxiety and help falling asleep because of its sedative effect—that is, it makes people a little sleepy so that they feel less nervous and fall asleep more easily. It works on the *serotonin* system as well as the *cholinergic* and *histamine* systems.

How Long Does This Medicine Last?

Cyproheptadine lasts for 4–7 hours.

How Will the Doctor Monitor This Medicine?

The doctor will review your child's medical history and physical examination before starting cyproheptadine. Be sure to tell the doctor if your child or anyone in the family has a history of asthma or of heart rhythm problems, palpitations, or fainting. The doctor or nurse may measure your child's height, weight, pulse, and blood pressure before starting the medicine.

After the medicine is started, the doctor will want to have regular appointments with you and your child to see how the medicine is working, to see if a dose change is needed, to watch for side effects, to see if cyproheptadine is still needed, and to see if any other treatment is needed. The doctor or nurse may check your child's height, weight, pulse, and blood pressure.

What Side Effects Can This Medicine Have?

Any medicine can have side effects, including an allergy to the medicine. Because each patient is different, the doctor will monitor the youth closely, especially when the medicine is started. The doctor will work with you

to increase the positive effects and decrease the negative effects of the medicine. Please tell the doctor if any of the listed side effects appear or if you think that the medicine is causing any other problems. Not all of the rare or unusual side effects are listed.

Side effects are most common after starting the medicine or after a dose increase. Many side effects can be avoided or lessened by starting with a very low dose and increasing it slowly—ask the doctor.

Allergic Reaction

Tell the doctor in a day or two (if possible, before the next dose of medicine):

- Hives
- Itching
- Rash

Stop the medicine and get *immediate* medical care:

- Trouble breathing or chest tightness
- Swelling of lips, tongue, or throat

Common Side Effects

Tell the doctor within a week or two:

- Daytime sleepiness—Do not allow your child to drive, ride a bicycle or motorcycle, or operate machinery if this happens.
- Decreased attention, memory, or learning in school
- Increased appetite and weight gain
- Dry mouth—Have your child try using sugar-free gum or candy.
- Headache
- Blurred vision
- Constipation—Encourage your child to drink more fluids and eat high-fiber foods; if necessary, the doctor may recommend a fiber medicine such as Benefiber or a stool softener such as Colace or mineral oil.
- Trouble passing urine
- Dizziness or light-headedness—This side effect is worse when the child stands up quickly, especially when getting out of bed in the morning; try having the child stand up slowly.
- Nausea or upset stomach

Less Common Side Effects

Call the doctor within a day or two:

- Poor coordination
- Motor tics (fast, repeated movements)
- Unusual muscle movements
- Irritability, increased overactivity
- Waking up after sleeping for a short time and being unable to get back to sleep

- Exposure to sunlight may cause severe sunburn, skin rash, redness, or itching; have the child stay out of the sun or use sunscreen or protective clothing.

Very Rare, but Serious, Side Effects

Call the doctor *immediately*:

- Worsening of asthma or trouble breathing
- Seizure (fit, convulsion)
- Uncontrollable behavior
- Hallucinations (seeing things that are not really there)
- Severe muscle stiffness
- Irregular heartbeat (pulse), fainting, palpitations

Some Interactions With Other Medicines or Food

Please note that the following are only the most likely interactions with other medicines or food.

If other medicines that can cause sleepiness are taken with cyproheptadine, severe sleepiness can result.

It can be *very dangerous* to take cyproheptadine at the same time as or even within a month of taking another type of medicine called a *monoamine oxidase inhibitor* (MAOI), such as selegiline (Eldepryl), phenelzine (Nardil), tranylcypromine (Parnate), or isocarboxazid (Marplan).

What Could Happen if This Medicine Is Stopped Suddenly?

Stopping this medicine suddenly does not usually cause problems, but diarrhea or feeling sick may result if it has been taken for a long time. The problem being treated may come back. Always ask the doctor whether a medicine can be stopped suddenly or must be decreased slowly (tapered).

How Long Will This Medicine Be Needed?

When used for nervousness or sleep, cyproheptadine is usually prescribed for a very short time to allow the patient to be calm enough to learn new ways to cope. If the person needs treatment for a longer time, another medicine is usually prescribed.

What Else Should I Know About This Medicine?

The medicine should be given with milk or food.

People who take cyproheptadine must not drink alcohol. Severe sleepiness or even loss of consciousness may result.

Notes

Use this space to take notes or to write down questions you want to ask the doctor.

_____

_____

_____

_____

_____

_____

_____

_____

_____

_____

_____

_____

From Dulcan MK, Ballard R (editors): *Helping Parents and Teachers Understand Medications for Behavioral and Emotional Problems: A Resource Book of Medication Information Handouts*, Fourth Edition. Washington, DC, American Psychiatric Publishing, 2015

Medication Information for Parents and Teachers

Desipramine—Norpramin

General Information About Medication

Each child and adolescent is different. No one has exactly the same combination of medical and psychological problems. It is a good idea to talk with the doctor or nurse about the reasons a medicine is being used. It is very important to keep all appointments and to be in touch by telephone if you have concerns. It is important to communicate with the doctor, nurse, or therapist. An *advanced practice nurse* (APN) has additional education and training after becoming a registered nurse (RN). Your child's medication may be prescribed by a medical doctor (MD or DO) or an APN. In addition, a *physician assistant* (PA) working with a physician may prescribe certain medications. In this information sheet, "doctor" includes medical doctors as well as APNs and PAs who prescribe medication. Often a nurse (RN) will be part of the team and answer questions and give information.

It is very important that the medicine be taken exactly as the doctor instructs. However, once in a while, everyone forgets to give a medicine on time. It is a good idea to ask the doctor or nurse what to do if this happens. Do not stop or change a medicine without asking the doctor or nurse first.

If the medicine seems to stop working, it may be because it is not being taken regularly. The youth may be "cheeking" or hiding the medicine or forgetting to take it (especially at school). The doses may be too far apart or a different dose or medicine may be needed. Something at school, at home, or in the neighborhood may be upsetting the youth, or he or she may need special help for learning disabilities or tutoring. Please discuss your concerns with the doctor. **Do not just increase the dose.** It is also very important not to decrease the dose or stop the medicine without talking to the doctor first. The problem being treated may come back, or there could be uncomfortable or even dangerous results.

All medicines should be kept in a safe place, out of the reach of children, and should be supervised by an adult. If someone takes too much of a medicine, call the doctor, the poison control center, or a hospital emergency room.

Each medicine has a "generic" or chemical name. Just like laundry detergents or paper towels, some medicines are sold by more than one company under different brand names. The same medicine may be available under a generic name and several brand names. The generic medications are usually less expensive than the brand name ones. The generic medications have the same chemical formula, but they may or may not be exactly the same strength as the brand-name medications. Also, some brands of pills contain dye or other things that can cause allergic reactions. It is a good idea to talk to the doctor and the pharmacist about whether it is important to use a specific brand of medicine.

Any medicine can cause an allergic reaction. Examples are hives, itching, rashes, swelling, and trouble breathing. Even a tiny amount of a medicine can cause a reaction in patients who are allergic to that medicine. Be *sure* to talk to the doctor before restarting a medicine that has caused an allergic reaction and tell the doctor about any reactions to medicine that your child has had before.

Taking more than one medicine at the same time may cause more side effects or cause one of the medicines to not work as well. Always ask the doctor, nurse, or pharmacist before adding another medicine, either prescription or bought without a prescription in a store or on the Internet. Be sure

145

that each doctor knows about *all* of the medicines your child is taking. Also tell the doctor about any vitamins, herbal medicines, or supplements your child may be taking. Some of these may have side effects alone or when taken with this medication. It is a very good idea to keep a list with you of the names and doses of all medicines that your child is taking.

Everyone taking medicine should have a physical examination at least once a year.

If you think that your child may be using drugs or alcohol, please tell the doctor right away.

Pregnancy requires special care in the use of medicine. Some medicines can cause birth defects if taken by a pregnant mother. **Please tell the doctor immediately if you suspect the teenager is at risk of becoming pregnant.** The doctor may wish to discuss sexual behavior and/or birth control with your daughter.

Printed information like this applies to children and adolescents in general. If you have questions about the medicine, or if you notice changes or anything unusual, please ask the doctor or nurse. As scientific research advances, knowledge increases and advice changes. Even experts do not always agree. Many medicines have not been "approved" by the U.S. Food and Drug Administration (FDA) for use in children or use for particular problems. For this reason, use of the medicine for a problem or age group often is not listed in the *Physicians' Desk Reference*. This does not necessarily mean that the medicine is dangerous or does not work, only that the company that makes the medicine has not received permission to advertise the medicine for use in children. Companies often do not apply for this permission because it is expensive to do the tests needed to apply for approval for use in children. Once a medication is approved by the FDA for any purpose, a doctor is allowed to prescribe it according to research and clinical experience.

Note to Teachers

It is a good idea to talk with the parent(s) about the reason(s) that a medication is being used. If the parent(s) sign consent to release information, it is often helpful for you to talk with the doctor. If the parent(s) give permission, the doctor may ask you to fill out rating forms about your experience with the student's behavior, feelings, academic performance, and medication side effects. This information is very useful in selecting and monitoring medication treatment. If you have observations that you think are important, do not hesitate to share these with the student's parent(s) and treating clinicians (with parental consent).

It is very important that the medicine be taken exactly as the doctor instructs. However, everyone forgets to give a medicine on time once in a while. It is a good idea to ask the parent(s) in advance what to do if this happens. Do not stop or change the time you are giving a medicine at school without parental permission. If a medication is to be taken with food, but lunchtime or snack time changes, be sure to notify the parent(s) so appropriate adjustments can be made.

All medicines should be kept in a secure place and should be supervised by an adult. If someone takes too much of a medicine, follow your school procedure for an urgent medical problem.

Taking medicine is a private matter and is best managed discreetly and confidentially. It is important to be sensitive to the student's feelings about taking medicine.

If you suspect that the student is using drugs or alcohol, please tell the parent(s) or a school counselor right away.

Please tell the parent(s) or school nurse if you suspect medication side effects.

Modifications of the classroom environment or assignments may be useful in addition to medication. The student may need to be evaluated for additional help or a 504 plan or an Individualized Education Plan for learning problems or emotional or behavioral issues.

Any expression of suicidal thoughts or feelings or self-harm by a child or adolescent is a signal of distress and should be taken seriously. These behaviors should not be dismissed as "attention seeking." School procedures for safety issues should be followed.

You may notice the following side effects at school:

Common Side Effects

- Dry mouth—Allow the student to chew sugar-free gum, carry a water bottle, or make extra trips to the water fountain.
- Constipation—Allow the student to drink more fluids or to use the bathroom more often.
- Daytime sleepiness—The student should not drive, ride a bicycle or motorcycle, or operate machinery.
- Dizziness (especially when standing up quickly)—This may happen in the classroom or during physical education. Suggest that the student stand up more slowly.
- Irritability

Occasional Side Effects

- Stuttering
- Increased risk of sunburn (this may be a problem if recess or physical education is outdoors in warm weather)—The student should wear sunscreen or protective clothing or stay out of the sun.

Less Common Side Effects

- Nausea—The student may need to take the medicine after a meal or snack.
- Trouble urinating—The student may need more time in the bathroom.
- Motor tics (fast, repeated movements) or muscle twitches (jerking movements) of parts of the body.
- Increased activity, rapid speech, feeling "speeded up," being very excited or irritable (cranky)
- Skin rash

Rare, but Potentially Serious, Side Effects

Call the parent(s) or follow your school's emergency procedures *immediately* **if the student experiences any of the following side effects:**

- Seizure (fit, convulsion)—**(This is a medical emergency.)**
- Very fast or irregular heartbeat—**(This is a medical emergency.)**
- Fainting
- Hallucinations (hearing voices or seeing things that are not there)
- Inability to urinate
- Confusion
- Severe change in behavior

What Is Desipramine (Norpramin)?

Desipramine is called a *tricyclic antidepressant*. It was first used to treat depression but is now used to treat attention-deficit/hyperactivity disorder (ADHD), school phobia, separation anxiety, panic disorder, and some sleep disorders (such as night terrors or sleepwalking). It comes in brand name Norpramin and generic tablets.

How Can This Medicine Help?

Desipramine can decrease symptoms of ADHD, anxiety (nervousness), panic, bed-wetting, and night terrors or sleepwalking. The medicine may take several weeks to work.

How Does This Medicine Work?

Tricyclic antidepressants affect the natural substances (*neurotransmitters*) that are needed for certain parts of the brain to work more normally. They increase the activity of *serotonin* and *norepinephrine*.

How Long Does This Medicine Last?

Although in adults and older teenagers a dose lasts for a whole day, in younger children several doses a day may be needed.

How Will the Doctor Monitor This Medicine?

The doctor will review your child's medical history and physical examination, paying special attention to pulse rate, blood pressure, weight, and height, before starting desipramine. These measurements will be taken when the dose is increased and occasionally as long as the medicine is continued. The doctor may order some blood or urine tests to be sure your child does not have a hidden medical condition.

Tricyclic antidepressants can slow the speed at which signals move through the heart. This effect is not dangerous if the heart is normal, which is why an ECG (electrocardiogram or heart rhythm test) is done before starting the medicine. The ECG may be repeated as the dose is increased and occasionally while the medicine is being taken. Changes in the heart from the medicine usually can be seen on the ECG before they become a problem, so your child's doctor will order an ECG every so often. To find possible hidden heart risks, it is especially important to tell the doctor if your child or anyone in the family has a history of fainting, palpitations, or irregular heartbeat or if anyone in the family died suddenly.

Be sure to tell the doctor if your child or anyone in the family has bipolar disorder or has tried to kill himself or herself.

Because desipramine may increase the risk of seizures (fits, convulsions), the doctor will want to know whether your child has ever had a seizure or a head injury and if there is any family history of epilepsy. Your child's doctor may want to order an EEG (electroencephalogram or brain wave test) before starting the medicine.

Experts do not agree on whether blood tests are needed to measure the level of this medicine. Blood levels seem to be most useful when your doctor suspects that the dose of medicine is too high or too low. The most accurate level is obtained by drawing blood first thing in the morning, after at least 5 days on the same dose, approximately 12 hours after the evening dose of medicine and before the morning dose.

After the medicine is started, the doctor will want to have regular appointments with you and your child to see how the medicine is working, to see if a dose change is needed, to watch for side effects, to see if desipramine is still needed, and to see if any other treatment is needed. The doctor or nurse may check your child's height, weight, pulse, and blood pressure or order tests, such as an ECG or blood level.

If desipramine is being used for ADHD, the doctor may ask for your child's teacher to fill out reports on your child's learning and behavior at school. Before using medicine and at times afterward, the doctor may ask your child to fill out a rating scale about anxiety and depression, to help see how your child is doing.

What Side Effects Can This Medicine Have?

Any medicine can have side effects, including an allergy to the medicine. Because each patient is different, the doctor will monitor the youth closely, especially when the medicine is started. The doctor will work with you to increase the positive effects and decrease the negative effects of the medicine. Please tell the doctor if any of the listed side effects appear or if you think that the medicine is causing any other problems. Not all of the rare or unusual side effects are listed.

Side effects are most common after starting the medicine or after a dose increase. Many side effects can be avoided or lessened by starting with a very low dose and increasing it slowly—ask the doctor.

Allergic Reaction

Tell the doctor in a day or two (if possible, before the next dose of medicine):

- Hives
- Itching
- Rash

Stop the medicine and get *immediate* medical care:

- Trouble breathing or chest tightness
- Swelling of lips, tongue, or throat

Common Side Effects

Tell the doctor within a week or two:

- Dry mouth—Have your child try using sugar-free gum or candy.
- Constipation—Encourage your child to drink more fluids and eat high-fiber foods; if necessary, the doctor may recommend a fiber medicine such as Benefiber or a stool softener such as Colace or mineral oil.
- Daytime sleepiness—Do not allow your child to drive, ride a bicycle or motorcycle, or operate machinery if this happens.
- Dizziness—This side effect is worse when the child stands up quickly, especially when getting out of bed in the morning; try having the child stand up slowly.
- Weight gain
- Loss of appetite and weight loss
- Irritability

Occasional Side Effects

Tell the doctor within a week or two:

- Nightmares
- Stuttering

- Blurred vision
- Increase in breast size, nipple discharge, or both (in girls)
- Increase in breast size (in boys)

Less Common, but More Serious, Side Effects

Call the doctor within a day or two:

- High or low blood pressure
- Nausea
- Trouble urinating
- Motor tics (fast, repeated movements) or muscle twitches (jerking movements)
- Increased activity, rapid speech, feeling "speeded up," decreased need for sleep, being very excited or irritable (cranky)

Rare, but Potentially Serious, Side Effects

Call the doctor *immediately*:

- Seizure (fit, convulsion)—**Go to an emergency room.**
- Very fast or irregular heartbeat—**Go to an emergency room.**
- Fainting
- Hallucinations (hearing voices or seeing things that are not there)
- Inability to pass urine
- Confusion
- Severe change in behavior

Some Interactions With Other Medicines or Food

Please note that the following are only the most likely interactions with other medicines or food.

Check with your child's doctor before giving your child decongestants or over-the-counter cold medicine.

Taking another antidepressant or valproate with desipramine may increase the level of desipramine and increase side effects.

Taking carbamazepine (Tegretol) with desipramine may decrease the positive effects of desipramine and increase the side effects of carbamazepine.

It can be *very dangerous* to take desipramine at the same time as or even within a month of taking another type of medicine called a *monoamine oxidase inhibitor* (MAOI), such as selegiline (Eldepryl), phenelzine (Nardil), tranylcypromine (Parnate), or isocarboxazid (Marplan).

Caffeine may worsen side effects on the heart or symptoms of anxiety. It is best not to drink coffee, tea, or soft drinks with caffeine while taking this medicine.

What Could Happen if This Medicine Is Stopped Suddenly?

Stopping the medicine suddenly or skipping a dose is not dangerous but can be very uncomfortable. Your child may feel like he or she has the flu—with a headache, muscle aches, stomachache, and upset stomach. Behavioral problems, sadness, nervousness, or trouble sleeping also may occur. If these feelings appear every day, the medicine may need to be given more often during each day.

How Long Will This Medicine Be Needed?

There is no way to know how long a person will need to take this medicine. Parents work together with the doctor to determine what is right for each child. The medicine may be needed for a long time. Some people may need to take the medicine even as adults.

What Else Should I Know About This Medicine?

In youth who have bipolar disorder or who are at risk for bipolar disorder, any antidepressant medicine may increase the risk of hypomania or mania (excitement, agitation, increased activity, decreased sleep).

An overdose by accident or on purpose with this medicine is very dangerous! You must closely supervise the medicine. You may have to lock up the medicine if your child or teenager is suicidal or if young children live in or visit your home.

Tricyclic antidepressants may cause dry mouth, which could increase the chance of tooth decay. Regular brushing of teeth and checkups with the dentist are especially important.

This medicine causes increased risk of sunburn. Be sure that your child wears sunscreen or protective clothing or stays out of the sun.

People who take tricyclic antidepressants must not drink alcohol or use tranquilizers. Severe sleepiness, loss of consciousness, or even death may result.

Black Box Antidepressant Warning

In 2004, an advisory committee to the FDA decided that there might be an increased risk of suicidal behavior for some youth taking medicines called *antidepressants*. In the research studies that the committee reviewed, about 3%–4% of youth with depression who took an antidepressant medicine—and 1%–2% of youth with depression who took a placebo (pill without active medicine)—talked about suicidal thoughts (thinking about killing themselves or wishing they were dead) or did something to harm themselves. This means that almost twice as many youth who were taking an antidepressant to treat their depression talked about suicide or had suicidal behavior compared with youth with depression who were taking inactive medicine. There were *no* completed suicides in any of these research studies, which included more than 4,000 children and adolescents. For youth being treated for anxiety, there was no difference in suicidal talking or behavior between those taking antidepressant medication and those taking placebo.

The FDA told drug companies to add a *black box warning* label to all antidepressant medicines. Because of this label, a doctor (or advanced practice nurse) prescribing one of these medicines has to warn youth and their families that there might be more suicidal thoughts and actions in youth taking these medicines.

On the other hand, in places where more youth are taking the newer antidepressant medicines, the number of adolescents who commit suicide has gotten smaller. Also, thinking about or attempting suicide is more common in surveys of teenagers in the community than it is in depressed youth treated in research studies with antidepressant medicine.

If a youth is being treated with this medicine and is doing well, then no changes are needed as a result of this warning. Increased suicidal talk or action is most likely to happen in the first few months of treatment with a medicine. If your child has recently started this medicine or is about to start, then you and your doctor (or advanced practice nurse) should watch for any changes in behavior. People who are depressed often have suicidal thoughts or actions. It is hard to know whether suicidal thoughts or actions in depressed people are caused by the depression itself or by the medicine. Also, as their depression is getting better, some people talk more about the suicidal thoughts that they had before but did not talk about. As young people get better from depression, they might be at higher risk of doing something about suicidal thoughts that they have had for some time, because they have more energy.

What Should a Parent Do?

1. Be honest with your child about possible risks and benefits of medicine.

2. Talk to your child about whether he or she is having any suicidal thoughts, and tell your child to come to you if he or she is having such thoughts.

3. You, your child, and your child's doctor or nurse should develop a safety plan. Pick adults whom your child can tell if he or she is thinking about suicide.

4. Be sure to tell your child's doctor, nurse, or therapist if you suspect that your child is using alcohol or drugs or if something has happened that might make your child feel worse, such as a family separation, breaking up with a boyfriend or girlfriend, someone close dying or attempting suicide, physical or sexual abuse, or failure in school.

5. Be sure that there are no guns in the home and that all medicines (including over-the-counter medicines like Tylenol) are closely supervised by an adult and kept in a safe place.

6. Watch for new or worse thoughts of suicide, self-harm, depression, anxiety (nerves), feeling very agitated or restless, being angry or aggressive, having more trouble sleeping, or anything else that you see for the first time, seems worse, or worries your child or you. If these appear, contact a mental health professional **right away.** Do not just stop or change the dose of the medicine on your own. If the problems are serious, and you cannot reach one of your clinicians, call a 24-hour psychiatry emergency telephone number or take your child to an emergency room.

Youth taking antidepressant medicine should be watched carefully by their parent(s), clinician(s) (doctor, advanced practice nurse, nurse, therapist), and other concerned adults for the first weeks of treatment. It is a good idea to have regular contact with the doctor, APN, nurse, or therapist for the first months to check for feelings of depression or sadness, thoughts of killing or harming himself or herself, and any problems with the medication. If you have questions, be sure to ask the doctor, APN, nurse, or therapist.

For more information, see http://www.parentsmedguide.org/.

Notes

Use this space to take notes or to write down questions you want to ask the doctor.

_____

_____

———————————————————————————————

———————————————————————————————

———————————————————————————————

———————————————————————————————

———————————————————————————————

———————————————————————————————

———————————————————————————————

———————————————————————————————

———————————————————————————————

———————————————————————————————

———————————————————————————————

———————————————————————————————

Medication Information for Parents and Teachers

Desmopressin Acetate—DDAVP, Stimate

General Information About Medication

Each child and adolescent is different. No one has exactly the same combination of medical and psychological problems. It is a good idea to talk with the doctor or nurse about the reasons a medicine is being used. It is very important to keep all appointments and to be in touch by telephone if you have concerns. It is important to communicate with the doctor, nurse, or therapist. An *advanced practice nurse* (APN) has additional education and training after becoming a registered nurse (RN). Your child's medication may be prescribed by a medical doctor (MD or DO) or an APN. In addition, a *physician assistant* (PA) working with a physician may prescribe certain medications. In this information sheet, "doctor" includes medical doctors as well as APNs and PAs who prescribe medication. Often a nurse (RN) will be part of the team and answer questions and give information.

It is very important that the medicine be taken exactly as the doctor instructs. However, once in a while, everyone forgets to give a medicine on time. It is a good idea to ask the doctor or nurse what to do if this happens. Do not stop or change a medicine without asking the doctor or nurse first.

If the medicine seems to stop working, it may be because it is not being taken regularly. The youth may be "cheeking" or hiding the medicine or forgetting to take it (especially at school). The doses may be too far apart or a different dose or medicine may be needed. Something at school, at home, or in the neighborhood may be upsetting the youth, or he or she may need special help for learning disabilities or tutoring. Please discuss your concerns with the doctor. **Do not just increase the dose.** It is also very important not to decrease the dose or stop the medicine without talking to the doctor first. The problem being treated may come back, or there could be uncomfortable or even dangerous results.

All medicines should be kept in a safe place, out of the reach of children, and should be supervised by an adult. If someone takes too much of a medicine, call the doctor, the poison control center, or a hospital emergency room.

Each medicine has a "generic" or chemical name. Just like laundry detergents or paper towels, some medicines are sold by more than one company under different brand names. The same medicine may be available under a generic name and several brand names. The generic medications are usually less expensive than the brand name ones. The generic medications have the same chemical formula, but they may or may not be exactly the same strength as the brand-name medications. Also, some brands of pills contain dye or other things that can cause allergic reactions. It is a good idea to talk to the doctor and the pharmacist about whether it is important to use a specific brand of medicine.

Any medicine can cause an allergic reaction. Examples are hives, itching, rashes, swelling, and trouble breathing. Even a tiny amount of a medicine can cause a reaction in patients who are allergic to that medicine. Be *sure* to talk to the doctor before restarting a medicine that has caused an allergic reaction and tell the doctor about any reactions to medicine that your child has had before.

155

Taking more than one medicine at the same time may cause more side effects or cause one of the medicines to not work as well. **Always ask the doctor, nurse, or pharmacist before adding another medicine, either prescription or bought without a prescription in a store or on the Internet. Be sure that each doctor knows about *all* of the medicines your child is taking. Also tell the doctor about any vitamins, herbal medicines, or supplements your child may be taking.** Some of these may have side effects alone or when taken with this medication. It is a very good idea to keep a list with you of the names and doses of all medicines that your child is taking.

Everyone taking medicine should have a physical examination at least once a year.

If you think that your child may be using drugs or alcohol, please tell the doctor right away.

Pregnancy requires special care in the use of medicine. Some medicines can cause birth defects if taken by a pregnant mother. **Please tell the doctor immediately if you suspect the teenager is at risk of becoming pregnant.** The doctor may wish to discuss sexual behavior and/or birth control with your daughter.

Printed information like this applies to children and adolescents in general. If you have questions about the medicine, or if you notice changes or anything unusual, please ask the doctor or nurse. As scientific research advances, knowledge increases and advice changes. Even experts do not always agree. Many medicines have not been "approved" by the U.S. Food and Drug Administration (FDA) for use in children or use for particular problems. For this reason, use of the medicine for a problem or age group often is not listed in the *Physicians' Desk Reference.* This does not necessarily mean that the medicine is dangerous or does not work, only that the company that makes the medicine has not received permission to advertise the medicine for use in children. Companies often do not apply for this permission because it is expensive to do the tests needed to apply for approval for use in children. Once a medication is approved by the FDA for any purpose, a doctor is allowed to prescribe it according to research and clinical experience.

Note to Teachers

It is a good idea to talk with the parent(s) about the reason(s) that a medication is being used. If the parent(s) sign consent to release information, it is often helpful for you to talk with the doctor. If the parent(s) give permission, the doctor may ask you to fill out rating forms about your experience with the student's behavior, feelings, academic performance, and medication side effects. This information is very useful in selecting and monitoring medication treatment. If you have observations that you think are important, do not hesitate to share these with the student's parent(s) and treating clinicians (with parental consent).

It is very important that the medicine be taken exactly as the doctor instructs. However, everyone forgets to give a medicine on time once in a while. It is a good idea to ask the parent(s) in advance what to do if this happens. Do not stop or change the time you are giving a medicine at school without parental permission. If a medication is to be taken with food, but lunchtime or snack time changes, be sure to notify the parent(s) so appropriate adjustments can be made.

All medicines should be kept in a secure place and should be supervised by an adult. If someone takes too much of a medicine, follow your school procedure for an urgent medical problem.

Taking medicine is a private matter and is best managed discreetly and confidentially. It is important to be sensitive to the student's feelings about taking medicine.

If you suspect that the student is using drugs or alcohol, please tell the parent(s) or a school counselor right away.

Desmopressin (DDAVP, Stimate) may cause increased urination in the daytime. The student may need extra trips to the bathroom.

Please tell the parent(s) or school nurse if you suspect medication side effects.

Modifications of the classroom environment or assignments may be useful in addition to medication. The student may need to be evaluated for additional help or a 504 plan or an Individualized Education Plan for learning problems or emotional or behavioral issues.

Any expression of suicidal thoughts or feelings or self-harm by a child or adolescent is a signal of distress and should be taken seriously. These behaviors should not be dismissed as "attention seeking." School procedures for safety issues should be followed.

What Is Desmopressin (DDAVP, Stimate)?

Desmopressin is a man-made version of a naturally occurring hormone—the antidiuretic hormone *vasopressin*, which is made by the *pituitary gland*. Desmopressin comes in two forms: a nasal (nose) spray (DDAVP, Stimate, and generic) and DDAVP and generic tablets. Only the tablets are used now to treat bed-wetting.

How Can This Medicine Help?

When given at bedtime, desmopressin can prevent bed-wetting (also called nocturnal enuresis). It may be used every night or only for nights when the youth is sleeping away from home (camp, sleepovers) and would be embarrassed by wetting the bed.

How Does This Medicine Work?

Desmopressin temporarily stops or slows the kidney from making urine. After the medicine wears off, there is an increase in urine the next day.

How Long Does This Medicine Last?

Desmopressin lasts for about 10 hours, only for nights on which it is given (at bedtime). When the medicine is stopped, bed-wetting usually returns. If desmopressin is being used regularly, several times a year it may be stopped to see if the youth has grown out of bed-wetting.

How Will the Doctor Monitor This Medicine?

The doctor will review your child's medical history and physical examination before starting desmopressin. The doctor may order blood or urine tests to be sure your child does not have a hidden medical condition that would make it unsafe to use this medicine. The doctor or nurse may measure your child's pulse and blood pressure before starting desmopressin.

After the medicine is started, the doctor will want to have regular appointments with you and your child to see how the medicine is working, to see if a dose change is needed, to watch for side effects, to see if desmopressin is still needed, and to see if any other treatment is needed. The doctor or nurse may check your child's height, weight, pulse, and blood pressure, or order a blood or urine test to see how much water and salt is in your child's body.

157

What Side Effects Can This Medicine Have?

Any medicine can have side effects, including an allergy to the medicine. Because each patient is different, the doctor will monitor the youth closely, especially when the medicine is started. The doctor will work with you to increase the positive effects and decrease the negative effects of the medicine. Please tell the doctor if any of the listed side effects appear or if you think that the medicine is causing any other problems. Not all of the rare or unusual side effects are listed.

Side effects are most common after starting the medicine or after a dose increase. Many side effects can be avoided or lessened by starting with a very low dose and increasing it slowly—ask the doctor.

Allergic Reaction

Tell the doctor in a day or two (if possible, before the next dose of medicine):

- Hives
- Itching
- Rash

Stop the medicine and get *immediate* medical care:

- Trouble breathing or chest tightness
- Swelling of lips, tongue, or throat

Common Side Effects

Tell the doctor within a week or two:

- Headaches
- Nausea (upset stomach)
- Dizziness

Very Rare, but Serious, Side Effect

If the youth drinks too much water or takes medicines that increase the action of desmopressin, "water poisoning" (hyponatremia) and a seizure (convulsion) may result. This can also occur if the child has been sick in a way that upsets his or her salt and water balance in the body. If your child is sick with vomiting, diarrhea, the flu, or high fever, desmopressin should not be given until the illness is over. Your child should not take desmopressin on days when he or she does very heavy exercise, especially in the heat. Symptoms of hyponatremia include nausea, vomiting, fatigue, muscle cramps, or weakness. If these occur, **seek medical attention** *immediately.*

Some Interactions With Other Medicines or Food

Please note that the following are only the most likely interactions with other medicines or food.

Taking carbamazepine (Tegretol) with desmopressin may dangerously increase the action of desmopressin.

Medications that can cause increased thirst and increased water consumption such as antidepressants can increase the risk of hyponatremia.

What Could Happen if This Medicine Is Stopped Suddenly?

There are no known medical withdrawal effects, but the bed-wetting could return.

How Long Will This Medicine Be Needed?

Most young people who wet the bed grow out of it sooner or later. That is why it is a good idea to try stopping the desmopressin every so often to see if the bed-wetting has gone away on its own.

What Else Should I Know About This Medicine?

Because desmopressin blocks the usual way the body corrects for amounts of water, drinking of fluids (especially water) should be limited in the evening and night.

This medicine is very expensive. Many families prefer to try using behavior therapy or the "bell and pad" system to stop bed-wetting. If these methods work, the positive effects last longer than when medicine is used.

Notes

Use this space to take notes or to write down questions you want to ask the doctor.

_____

_____

_____

_____

_____

_____

_____

_____

_____

_____

_____

_____

_____

_____

Medication Information for Parents and Teachers

Diazepam—Valium

General Information About Medication

Each child and adolescent is different. No one has exactly the same combination of medical and psychological problems. It is a good idea to talk with the doctor or nurse about the reasons a medicine is being used. It is very important to keep all appointments and to be in touch by telephone if you have concerns. It is important to communicate with the doctor, nurse, or therapist. An *advanced practice nurse* (APN) has additional education and training after becoming a registered nurse (RN). Your child's medication may be prescribed by a medical doctor (MD or DO) or an APN. In addition, a *physician assistant* (PA) working with a physician may prescribe certain medications. In this information sheet, "doctor" includes medical doctors as well as APNs and PAs who prescribe medication. Often a nurse (RN) will be part of the team and answer questions and give information.

It is very important that the medicine be taken exactly as the doctor instructs. However, once in a while, everyone forgets to give a medicine on time. It is a good idea to ask the doctor or nurse what to do if this happens. Do not stop or change a medicine without asking the doctor or nurse first.

If the medicine seems to stop working, it may be because it is not being taken regularly. The youth may be "cheeking" or hiding the medicine or forgetting to take it (especially at school). The doses may be too far apart or a different dose or medicine may be needed. Something at school, at home, or in the neighborhood may be upsetting the youth, or he or she may need special help for learning disabilities or tutoring. Please discuss your concerns with the doctor. **Do not just increase the dose.** It is also very important not to decrease the dose or stop the medicine without talking to the doctor first. The problem being treated may come back, or there could be uncomfortable or even dangerous results.

All medicines should be kept in a safe place, out of the reach of children, and should be supervised by an adult. If someone takes too much of a medicine, call the doctor, the poison control center, or a hospital emergency room.

Each medicine has a "generic" or chemical name. Just like laundry detergents or paper towels, some medicines are sold by more than one company under different brand names. The same medicine may be available under a generic name and several brand names. The generic medications are usually less expensive than the brand name ones. The generic medications have the same chemical formula, but they may or may not be exactly the same strength as the brand-name medications. Also, some brands of pills contain dye or other things that can cause allergic reactions. It is a good idea to talk to the doctor and the pharmacist about whether it is important to use a specific brand of medicine.

Any medicine can cause an allergic reaction. Examples are hives, itching, rashes, swelling, and trouble breathing. Even a tiny amount of a medicine can cause a reaction in patients who are allergic to that medicine. Be *sure* to talk to the doctor before restarting a medicine that has caused an allergic reaction and tell the doctor about any reactions to medicine that your child has had before.

Taking more than one medicine at the same time may cause more side effects or cause one of the medicines to not work as well. Always ask the doctor, nurse, or pharmacist before adding another

medicine, either prescription or bought without a prescription in a store or on the Internet. **Be sure that each doctor knows about *all* of the medicines your child is taking. Also tell the doctor about any vitamins, herbal medicines, or supplements your child may be taking.** Some of these may have side effects alone or when taken with this medication. It is a very good idea to keep a list with you of the names and doses of all medicines that your child is taking.

Everyone taking medicine should have a physical examination at least once a year.

If you think that your child may be using drugs or alcohol, please tell the doctor right away.

Pregnancy requires special care in the use of medicine. Some medicines can cause birth defects if taken by a pregnant mother. **Please tell the doctor immediately if you suspect the teenager is at risk of becoming pregnant.** The doctor may wish to discuss sexual behavior and/or birth control with your daughter.

Printed information like this applies to children and adolescents in general. If you have questions about the medicine, or if you notice changes or anything unusual, please ask the doctor or nurse. As scientific research advances, knowledge increases and advice changes. Even experts do not always agree. Many medicines have not been "approved" by the U.S. Food and Drug Administration (FDA) for use in children or use for particular problems. For this reason, use of the medicine for a problem or age group often is not listed in the *Physicians' Desk Reference.* This does not necessarily mean that the medicine is dangerous or does not work, only that the company that makes the medicine has not received permission to advertise the medicine for use in children. Companies often do not apply for this permission because it is expensive to do the tests needed to apply for approval for use in children. Once a medication is approved by the FDA for any purpose, a doctor is allowed to prescribe it according to research and clinical experience.

Note to Teachers

It is a good idea to talk with the parent(s) about the reason(s) that a medication is being used. If the parent(s) sign consent to release information, it is often helpful for you to talk with the doctor. If the parent(s) give permission, the doctor may ask you to fill out rating forms about your experience with the student's behavior, feelings, academic performance, and medication side effects. This information is very useful in selecting and monitoring medication treatment. If you have observations that you think are important, do not hesitate to share these with the student's parent(s) and treating clinicians (with parental consent).

It is very important that the medicine be taken exactly as the doctor instructs. However, everyone forgets to give a medicine on time once in a while. It is a good idea to ask the parent(s) in advance what to do if this happens. Do not stop or change the time you are giving a medicine at school without parental permission. If a medication is to be taken with food, but lunchtime or snack time changes, be sure to notify the parent(s) so appropriate adjustments can be made.

All medicines should be kept in a secure place and should be supervised by an adult. If someone takes too much of a medicine, follow your school procedure for an urgent medical problem.

Taking medicine is a private matter and is best managed discreetly and confidentially. It is important to be sensitive to the student's feelings about taking medicine.

If you suspect that the student is using drugs or alcohol, please tell the parent(s) or a school counselor right away.

Please tell the parent(s) or school nurse if you suspect medication side effects.

Modifications of the classroom environment or assignments may be useful in addition to medication. The student may need to be evaluated for additional help or a 504 plan or an Individualized Education Plan for learning problems or emotional or behavioral issues.

Any expression of suicidal thoughts or feelings or self-harm by a child or adolescent is a signal of distress and should be taken seriously. These behaviors should not be dismissed as "attention seeking." School procedures for safety issues should be followed.

What Is Diazepam (Valium)?

Diazepam is a *benzodiazepine*, or *antianxiety* medicine. It used to be called a *minor tranquilizer*. It is sometimes called an *anxiolytic* or *sedative*. It comes in brand name Valium and generic tablets and liquid. There are other forms used for medical problems.

How Can This Medicine Help?

Diazepam can decrease anxiety, nervousness, fears, and excessive worrying. It can help anxious people to be calm enough to learn—with therapy and practice (exposure to feared things or situations)—to understand and tolerate their worries or fears and even to overcome them. People with generalized anxiety disorder, social phobia, posttraumatic stress disorder (PTSD), or panic disorder can be helped by diazepam. Most often, it is used for a short time when symptoms are very uncomfortable or frightening or when they make it hard to do important things such as going to school. Diazepam can decrease the severe physical symptoms (rapid heart-beat, trouble breathing, dizziness, sweating) of panic attacks and phobias.

Diazepam also can be used for sleep problems, such as night terrors (sudden waking up from sleep with great fear) or sleepwalking, when these problems put the youth at risk of an accident or make it impossible for other family members to get enough sleep. Diazepam can help with insomnia (difficulty falling asleep) when used for a short time along with a behavioral program.

Sometimes diazepam is used for a few days to treat agitation in mania or psychosis until other medicines start to work.

Diazepam may also be prescribed for some neurological or muscle conditions.

How Does This Medicine Work?

Diazepam works by calming the parts of the brain that are too excitable in anxious people. The medicine does this by working on *receptors* (special places on brain cells) in certain parts of the brain to change the action of *GABA*, a *neurotransmitter*—a chemical that the brain makes for brain cells to communicate with each other.

How Long Does This Medicine Last?

Diazepam usually needs to be taken twice a day. For acute symptoms of anxiety or agitation, it can be taken occasionally as needed. When used for sleep, it is taken at bedtime. There may still be some effects in the morning, because it lasts a long time.

How Will the Doctor Monitor This Medicine?

The doctor will review your child's medical history and physical examination before starting diazepam. The doctor may order some blood or urine tests or an ECG (electrocardiogram or heart rhythm test) to be sure your child does not have a hidden medical condition. The doctor or nurse may measure your child's height, weight, pulse, and blood pressure before starting diazepam.

After the medicine is started, the doctor will want to have regular appointments with you and your child to see how the medicine is working, to see if a dose change is needed, to watch for side effects, to see if diazepam is still needed, and to see if any other treatment is needed. The doctor or nurse may check your child's height, weight, pulse, and blood pressure.

What Side Effects Can This Medicine Have?

Any medicine can have side effects, including an allergy to the medicine. Because each patient is different, the doctor will monitor the youth closely, especially when the medicine is started. The doctor will work with you to increase the positive effects and decrease the negative effects of the medicine. Please tell the doctor if any of the listed side effects appear or if you think that the medicine is causing any other problems. Not all of the rare or unusual side effects are listed.

Side effects are most common after starting the medicine or after a dose increase. Many side effects can be avoided or lessened by starting with a very low dose and increasing it slowly—ask the doctor.

Allergic Reaction

Tell the doctor in a day or two (if possible, before the next dose of medicine):

- Hives
- Itching
- Rash

Stop the medicine and get *immediate* medical care:

- Trouble breathing or chest tightness
- Swelling of lips, tongue, or throat

Diazepam is usually very safe when used for short periods as the doctor prescribes. The most common side effect is daytime sleepiness. Diazepam can also cause dizziness, feeling "spacey," or decreased coordination. If the medicine is causing any of these problems it is very important not to drive a car, ride a bicycle or motorcycle, or operate machinery.

Diazepam can cause decreased concentration and memory. These problems, along with daytime sleepiness, may decrease learning and performance in school.

People who take diazepam must not drink alcohol. Severe sleepiness or even loss of consciousness may result.

It is possible to become psychologically and physically dependent on diazepam, but that is not a common problem for patients who see their doctors regularly. Because some people abuse benzodiazepines, it is illegal to give or sell these medicines to someone other than the patient for whom they were prescribed.

Very rarely, diazepam causes excitement, irritability, anger, aggression, trouble sleeping, nightmares, uncontrollable behavior, or memory loss. This is called *disinhibition* or a *paradoxical effect*. Stop the medicine and call the doctor if this happens.

Some Interactions With Other Medicines or Food

Please note that the following are only the most likely interactions with other medicines or food.

Diazepam may be taken with or without food.

It is important not to use other sedatives, tranquilizers, or sleeping pills or antihistamines (such as Benadryl) when taking diazepam because of greatly increased side effects.

Oral contraceptives (birth control pills), cimetidine (Tagamet), antifungal agents (such as ketoconazole), fluoxetine (Prozac), propranolol (Inderal), valproate (Depakote), some medicines used to treat HIV/AIDS, and other medicines may increase the levels of diazepam and increase side effects. Ask the doctor.

It is better to limit drinks with caffeine (coffee, tea, soft drinks) because caffeine works in the opposite way from this medicine, and the positive effects might be decreased.

What Could Happen if This Medicine Is Stopped Suddenly?

Many medicines cause problems if stopped suddenly. Diazepam must be decreased slowly (tapered) rather than stopped suddenly. When diazepam is stopped suddenly, there are withdrawal symptoms that are uncomfortable and may even be dangerous, although because diazepam is longer lasting, it causes fewer withdrawal problems than shorter-acting benzodiazepines such as alprazolam (Xanax). Problems are more likely in patients taking high doses of diazepam for 2 months or longer, but even after just a few weeks of taking diazepam it is important to stop it slowly. Withdrawal symptoms may include anxiety, irritability, shaking, sweating, aches and pains, muscle cramps, vomiting, confusion, and trouble sleeping. If large doses taken for a long time are stopped suddenly, seizures (fits, convulsions), hallucinations (hearing voices or seeing things that are not there), or out-of-control behavior may result.

How Long Will This Medicine Be Needed?

Diazepam is usually prescribed for only a few weeks to allow the patient to be calm enough to learn new ways to cope with anxiety and to allow the nervous system to become less excitable. Sometimes antianxiety medicines are used for longer periods to treat panic attacks or anxiety that remains after therapy is completed. Each person is unique, and some people may need these medicines for months or years.

What Else Should I Know About This Medicine?

Because benzodiazepines can be abused (especially by people who abuse alcohol or drugs) and can cause psychological dependence or physical dependence (addiction), they are regulated by special state and federal laws as *controlled substances*. These laws place limitations on telephone prescriptions and refills, and prescriptions expire if they are not filled promptly.

People with sleep apnea (breathing stops while they are asleep) should not take diazepam. Tell the doctor if your child snores very loudly.

Diazepam should be avoided during pregnancy, especially in the first 3 months, because it may cause birth defects in the baby. If taken regularly at the end of pregnancy, diazepam may cause withdrawal symptoms in the baby. Tell the doctor right away if you think that your daughter might be pregnant.

Notes

Use this space to take notes or to write down questions you want to ask the doctor.

_____

_____

_____

_____

_____

_____

_____

_____

_____

_____

_____

_____

From Dulcan MK, Ballard R (editors): _Helping Parents and Teachers Understand Medications for Behavioral and Emotional Problems: A Resource Book of Medication Information Handouts_, Fourth Edition. Washington, DC, American Psychiatric Publishing, 2015

Medication Information for Parents and Teachers

Diphenhydramine—Benadryl

General Information About Medication

Each child and adolescent is different. No one has exactly the same combination of medical and psychological problems. It is a good idea to talk with the doctor or nurse about the reasons a medicine is being used. It is very important to keep all appointments and to be in touch by telephone if you have concerns. It is important to communicate with the doctor, nurse, or therapist. An *advanced practice nurse* (APN) has additional education and training after becoming a registered nurse (RN). Your child's medication may be prescribed by a medical doctor (MD or DO) or an APN. In addition, a *physician assistant* (PA) working with a physician may prescribe certain medications. In this information sheet, "doctor" includes medical doctors as well as APNs and PAs who prescribe medication. Often a nurse (RN) will be part of the team and answer questions and give information.

It is very important that the medicine be taken exactly as the doctor instructs. However, once in a while, everyone forgets to give a medicine on time. It is a good idea to ask the doctor or nurse what to do if this happens. Do not stop or change a medicine without asking the doctor or nurse first.

If the medicine seems to stop working, it may be because it is not being taken regularly. The youth may be "cheeking" or hiding the medicine or forgetting to take it (especially at school). The doses may be too far apart or a different dose or medicine may be needed. Something at school, at home, or in the neighborhood may be upsetting the youth, or he or she may need special help for learning disabilities or tutoring. Please discuss your concerns with the doctor. **Do not just increase the dose.** It is also very important not to decrease the dose or stop the medicine without talking to the doctor first. The problem being treated may come back, or there could be uncomfortable or even dangerous results.

All medicines should be kept in a safe place, out of the reach of children, and should be supervised by an adult. If someone takes too much of a medicine, call the doctor, the poison control center, or a hospital emergency room.

Each medicine has a "generic" or chemical name. Just like laundry detergents or paper towels, some medicines are sold by more than one company under different brand names. The same medicine may be available under a generic name and several brand names. The generic medications are usually less expensive than the brand name ones. The generic medications have the same chemical formula, but they may or may not be exactly the same strength as the brand-name medications. Also, some brands of pills contain dye or other things that can cause allergic reactions. It is a good idea to talk to the doctor and the pharmacist about whether it is important to use a specific brand of medicine.

Any medicine can cause an allergic reaction. Examples are hives, itching, rashes, swelling, and trouble breathing. Even a tiny amount of a medicine can cause a reaction in patients who are allergic to that medicine. Be *sure* to talk to the doctor before restarting a medicine that has caused an allergic reaction and tell the doctor about any reactions to medicine that your child has had before.

Taking more than one medicine at the same time may cause more side effects or cause one of the medicines to not work as well. Always ask the doctor, nurse, or pharmacist before adding another medicine, either prescription or bought without a prescription in a store or on the Internet. Be sure

167

that each doctor knows about *all* of the medicines your child is taking. **Also tell the doctor about any vitamins, herbal medicines, or supplements your child may be taking.** Some of these may have side effects alone or when taken with this medication. It is a very good idea to keep a list with you of the names and doses of all medicines that your child is taking.

Everyone taking medicine should have a physical examination at least once a year.

If you think that your child may be using drugs or alcohol, please tell the doctor right away.

Pregnancy requires special care in the use of medicine. Some medicines can cause birth defects if taken by a pregnant mother. **Please tell the doctor immediately if you suspect the teenager is at risk of becoming pregnant.** The doctor may wish to discuss sexual behavior and/or birth control with your daughter.

Printed information like this applies to children and adolescents in general. If you have questions about the medicine, or if you notice changes or anything unusual, please ask the doctor or nurse. As scientific research advances, knowledge increases and advice changes. Even experts do not always agree. Many medicines have not been "approved" by the U.S. Food and Drug Administration (FDA) for use in children or use for particular problems. For this reason, use of the medicine for a problem or age group often is not listed in the *Physicians' Desk Reference*. This does not necessarily mean that the medicine is dangerous or does not work, only that the company that makes the medicine has not received permission to advertise the medicine for use in children. Companies often do not apply for this permission because it is expensive to do the tests needed to apply for approval for use in children. Once a medication is approved by the FDA for any purpose, a doctor is allowed to prescribe it according to research and clinical experience.

Note to Teachers

It is a good idea to talk with the parent(s) about the reason(s) that a medication is being used. If the parent(s) sign consent to release information, it is often helpful for you to talk with the doctor. If the parent(s) give permission, the doctor may ask you to fill out rating forms about your experience with the student's behavior, feelings, academic performance, and medication side effects. This information is very useful in selecting and monitoring medication treatment. If you have observations that you think are important, do not hesitate to share these with the student's parent(s) and treating clinicians (with parental consent).

It is very important that the medicine be taken exactly as the doctor instructs. However, everyone forgets to give a medicine on time once in a while. It is a good idea to ask the parent(s) in advance what to do if this happens. Do not stop or change the time you are giving a medicine at school without parental permission. If a medication is to be taken with food, but lunchtime or snack time changes, be sure to notify the parent(s) so appropriate adjustments can be made.

All medicines should be kept in a secure place and should be supervised by an adult. If someone takes too much of a medicine, follow your school procedure for an urgent medical problem.

Taking medicine is a private matter and is best managed discreetly and confidentially. It is important to be sensitive to the student's feelings about taking medicine.

If you suspect that the student is using drugs or alcohol, please tell the parent(s) or a school counselor right away.

Please tell the parent(s) or school nurse if you suspect medication side effects.

Modifications of the classroom environment or assignments may be useful in addition to medication. The student may need to be evaluated for additional help or a 504 plan or an Individualized Education Plan for learning problems or emotional or behavioral issues.

Any expression of suicidal thoughts or feelings or self-harm by a child or adolescent is a signal of distress and should be taken seriously. These behaviors should not be dismissed as "attention seeking." School procedures for safety issues should be followed.

What Is Diphenhydramine (Benadryl)?

Diphenhydramine is called an *antihistamine*. These medicines were developed to treat allergies. It is sometimes used to treat anxiety (nervousness), insomnia (difficulty falling asleep), or the side effects of certain other medicines (such as antipsychotics).

Diphenhydramine comes in many different forms—including tablet, capsule, chewable tablet, orally disintegrating tablet (dissolves in the mouth), suspension (liquid), and as one ingredient in many combination over-the-counter medicines for colds and allergies. The medicine also comes in a skin cream or spray and an injection (shot).

How Can This Medicine Help?

Diphenhydramine may decrease nervousness. When used for anxiety, it works best when used for a short time along with psychotherapy. Diphenhydramine can help with insomnia when used for a short time along with a behavioral program, such as regular soothing routines at bedtime and increased exercise in the daytime. It can reduce some of the movement side effects of the antipsychotic medicines, such as severe restlessness, agitation, and pacing *(akathisia)*; muscle spasms *(dystonia)*; muscle stiffness *(cogwheeling rigidity)*; or trembling. Sometimes these are called *parkinsonian* or *extrapyramidal* symptoms. Diphenhydramine can be given regularly to prevent or treat these problems. If there is a sudden, severe muscle spasm, diphenhydramine may be given as a pill or, if needed, as a shot that works within 15 minutes.

How Does This Medicine Work?

Diphenhydramine can help decrease anxiety and help falling asleep because of its *sedative* effect—that is, it makes people a little sleepy so that they feel less nervous and also fall asleep more easily.

Diphenhydramine works in a different way to counteract the effects of the antipsychotic medicines in parts of the brain that control muscle action (and cause stiffness or restlessness), but without decreasing the positive effects of the antipsychotic medicines on thinking and other psychiatric symptoms.

How Long Does This Medicine Last?

Diphenhydramine lasts for 4–7 hours. When used with an antipsychotic medicine, it is usually taken three or four times a day.

How Will the Doctor Monitor This Medicine?

The doctor will review your child's medical history and physical examination before starting diphenhydramine. Be sure to tell the doctor if your child or anyone in the family has a history of asthma or of heart rhythm problems, palpitations, or fainting. The doctor or nurse may measure your child's height, weight, pulse, and blood pressure before starting the medicine. An examination such as the AIMS (Abnormal Involuntary Movement Scale) test may be used to check your child's tongue, legs, and arms for unusual movements that could be helped by the medicine.

After the medicine is started, the doctor will want to have regular appointments with you and your child to see how the medicine is working, to see if a dose change is needed, to watch for side effects, to see if diphenhydramine is still needed, and to see if any other treatment is needed. The doctor or nurse may check your child's height, weight, pulse, and blood pressure.

What Side Effects Can This Medicine Have?

Any medicine can have side effects, including an allergy to the medicine. Because each patient is different, the doctor will monitor the youth closely, especially when the medicine is started. The doctor will work with you to increase the positive effects and decrease the negative effects of the medicine. Please tell the doctor if any of the listed side effects appear or if you think that the medicine is causing any other problems. Not all of the rare or unusual side effects are listed.

Side effects are most common after starting the medicine or after a dose increase. Many side effects can be avoided or lessened by starting with a very low dose and increasing it slowly—ask the doctor.

Allergic Reaction

Tell the doctor in a day or two (if possible, before the next dose of medicine):

- Hives
- Itching
- Rash

Stop the medicine and get *immediate* medical care:

- Trouble breathing or chest tightness
- Swelling of lips, tongue, or throat

Common Side Effects

Tell the doctor within a week or two:

- Daytime sleepiness—Do not allow your child to drive, ride a bicycle or motorcycle, or operate machinery if this happens.
- Decreased attention, memory, or learning in school
- Dry mouth—Have your child try using sugar-free gum or candy.
- Headache
- Blurred vision
- Constipation—Encourage your child to drink more fluids and eat high-fiber foods; if necessary, the doctor may recommend a fiber medicine such as Benefiber or a stool softener such as Colace or mineral oil.
- Trouble passing urine
- Dizziness or light-headedness—This side effect is worse when the child stands up quickly, especially when getting out of bed in the morning; try having the child stand up slowly.
- Loss of appetite, nausea, or upset stomach

Less Common Side Effects

Call the doctor within a day or two:

- Poor coordination
- Motor tics (fast, repeated movements)
- Unusual muscle movements
- Irritability, overactivity
- Waking up after sleeping for a short time and being unable to get back to sleep
- Exposure to sunlight may cause severe sunburn, skin rash, redness, or itching; avoid direct exposure to sunlight or use sunscreen

Very Rare, but Serious, Side Effects

Call the doctor immediately:

- Worsening of asthma or trouble breathing
- Seizure (fit, convulsion)
- Uncontrollable behavior
- Hallucinations (seeing things that are not really there)
- Severe muscle stiffness
- Irregular heartbeat (pulse), fainting, palpitations

Some Interactions With Other Medicines or Food

Please note that the following are only the most likely interactions with other medicines or food.

If other medicines that can cause sleepiness are taken with diphenhydramine, severe sleepiness can result.

What Could Happen if This Medicine Is Stopped Suddenly?

Stopping these medicines suddenly does not usually cause problems, but diarrhea or feeling sick may result if diphenhydramine has been taken for a long time. The problem being treated may come back. Always ask the doctor whether a medicine can be stopped suddenly or must be decreased slowly (tapered).

How Long Will This Medicine Be Needed?

When used for nervousness or sleep, diphenhydramine is usually prescribed for a very short time to allow the patient to be calm enough to learn new ways to cope. If the person needs treatment for a longer time, another medicine is usually prescribed.

When being used to reduce the motor side effects of an antipsychotic medicine, sometimes the diphenhydramine will be needed as long as the person is on the antipsychotic medicine, but sometimes it can be carefully tapered (decreased) and stopped if the person has gotten used to the antipsychotic medicine and there are no longer motor side effects.

What Else Should I Know About This Medicine?

People who take diphenhydramine must not drink alcohol. Severe sleepiness or even loss of consciousness may result.

Diphenhydramine may be confused with desipramine. Benadryl may be confused with Caladryl. Be sure to check the medicine when you get it from the pharmacist.

Notes

Use this space to take notes or to write down questions you want to ask the doctor.

_____

_____

_____

_____

_____

_____

_____

_____

_____

_____

_____

_____

_____

_____

concerning drug dosages, schedules, routes of administration, and side effects is accurate as of the time of publication and consistent with standards set by the U.S. Food and Drug Administration and the general medical community and accepted child psychiatric practice. The information on this medication sheet does not cover all the possible uses, precautions, side effects, or interactions of this drug. For a complete listing of side effects, see the manufacturer's package insert, which can be obtained from your physician or pharmacist. As medical research and practice advance, therapeutic standards may change. For this reason and because human and mechanical errors sometimes occur, we recommend that readers follow the advice of a physician who is directly involved in their care or the care of a member of their family.

From Dulcan MK, Ballard R (editors): *Helping Parents and Teachers Understand Medications for Behavioral and Emotional Problems: A Resource Book of Medication Information Handouts*, Fourth Edition. Washington, DC, American Psychiatric Publishing, 2015

Duloxetine—Cymbalta

General Information About Medication

Each child and adolescent is different. No one has exactly the same combination of medical and psychological problems. It is a good idea to talk with the doctor or nurse about the reasons a medicine is being used. It is very important to keep all appointments and to be in touch by telephone if you have concerns. It is important to communicate with the doctor, nurse, or therapist. An *advanced practice nurse* (APN) has additional education and training after becoming a registered nurse (RN). Your child's medication may be prescribed by a medical doctor (MD or DO) or an APN. In addition, a *physician assistant* (PA) working with a physician may prescribe certain medications. In this information sheet, "doctor" includes medical doctors as well as APNs and PAs who prescribe medication. Often a nurse (RN) will be part of the team and answer questions and give information.

It is very important that the medicine be taken exactly as the doctor instructs. However, once in a while, everyone forgets to give a medicine on time. It is a good idea to ask the doctor or nurse what to do if this happens. Do not stop or change a medicine without asking the doctor or nurse first.

If the medicine seems to stop working, it may be because it is not being taken regularly. The youth may be "cheeking" or hiding the medicine or forgetting to take it (especially at school). The doses may be too far apart or a different dose or medicine may be needed. Something at school, at home, or in the neighborhood may be upsetting the youth, or he or she may need special help for learning disabilities or tutoring. Please discuss your concerns with the doctor. **Do not just increase the dose.** It is also very important not to decrease the dose or stop the medicine without talking to the doctor first. The problem being treated may come back, or there could be uncomfortable or even dangerous results.

All medicines should be kept in a safe place, out of the reach of children, and should be supervised by an adult. If someone takes too much of a medicine, call the doctor, the poison control center, or a hospital emergency room.

Each medicine has a "generic" or chemical name. Just like laundry detergents or paper towels, some medicines are sold by more than one company under different brand names. The same medicine may be available under a generic name and several brand names. The generic medications are usually less expensive than the brand name ones. The generic medications have the same chemical formula, but they may or may not be exactly the same strength as the brand-name medications. Also, some brands of pills contain dye or other things that can cause allergic reactions. It is a good idea to talk to the doctor and the pharmacist about whether it is important to use a specific brand of medicine.

Any medicine can cause an allergic reaction. Examples are hives, itching, rashes, swelling, and trouble breathing. Even a tiny amount of a medicine can cause a reaction in patients who are allergic to that medicine. Be *sure* to talk to the doctor before restarting a medicine that has caused an allergic reaction and tell the doctor about any reactions to medicine that your child has had before.

Taking more than one medicine at the same time may cause more side effects or cause one of the medicines to not work as well. Always ask the doctor, nurse, or pharmacist before adding another

175

medicine, either prescription or bought without a prescription in a store or on the Internet. **Be sure that each doctor knows about** *all* **of the medicines your child is taking. Also tell the doctor about any vitamins, herbal medicines, or supplements your child may be taking.** Some of these may have side effects alone or when taken with this medication. It is a very good idea to keep a list with you of the names and doses of all medicines that your child is taking.

Everyone taking medicine should have a physical examination at least once a year.

If you think that your child may be using drugs or alcohol, please tell the doctor right away.

Pregnancy requires special care in the use of medicine. Some medicines can cause birth defects if taken by a pregnant mother. **Please tell the doctor immediately if you suspect the teenager is at risk of becoming pregnant.** The doctor may wish to discuss sexual behavior and/or birth control with your daughter.

Printed information like this applies to children and adolescents in general. If you have questions about the medicine, or if you notice changes or anything unusual, please ask the doctor or nurse. As scientific research advances, knowledge increases and advice changes. Even experts do not always agree. Many medicines have not been "approved" by the U.S. Food and Drug Administration (FDA) for use in children or use for particular problems. For this reason, use of the medicine for a problem or age group often is not listed in the *Physicians' Desk Reference*. This does not necessarily mean that the medicine is dangerous or does not work, only that the company that makes the medicine has not received permission to advertise the medicine for use in children. Companies often do not apply for this permission because it is expensive to do the tests needed to apply for approval for use in children. Once a medication is approved by the FDA for any purpose, a doctor is allowed to prescribe it according to research and clinical experience.

Note to Teachers

It is a good idea to talk with the parent(s) about the reason(s) that a medication is being used. If the parent(s) sign consent to release information, it is often helpful for you to talk with the doctor. If the parent(s) give permission, the doctor may ask you to fill out rating forms about your experience with the student's behavior, feelings, academic performance, and medication side effects. This information is very useful in selecting and monitoring medication treatment. If you have observations that you think are important, do not hesitate to share these with the student's parent(s) and treating clinicians (with parental consent).

It is very important that the medicine be taken exactly as the doctor instructs. However, everyone forgets to give a medicine on time once in a while. It is a good idea to ask the parent(s) in advance what to do if this happens. Do not stop or change the time you are giving a medicine at school without parental permission. If a medication is to be taken with food, but lunchtime or snack time changes, be sure to notify the parent(s) so appropriate adjustments can be made.

All medicines should be kept in a secure place and should be supervised by an adult. If someone takes too much of a medicine, follow your school procedure for an urgent medical problem.

Taking medicine is a private matter and is best managed discreetly and confidentially. It is important to be sensitive to the student's feelings about taking medicine.

If you suspect that the student is using drugs or alcohol, please tell the parent(s) or a school counselor right away.

Please tell the parent(s) or school nurse if you suspect medication side effects.

Modifications of the classroom environment or assignments may be useful in addition to medication. The student may need to be evaluated for additional help or a 504 plan or an Individualized Education Plan for learning problems or emotional or behavioral issues.

Any expression of suicidal thoughts or feelings or self-harm by a child or adolescent is a signal of distress and should be taken seriously. These behaviors should not be dismissed as "attention seeking." School procedures for safety issues should be followed.

What Is Duloxetine (Cymbalta)?

Duloxetine is an *antidepressant*. It is known as a *serotonin-norepinephrine reuptake inhibitor* (SNRI). It comes in brand name Cymbalta and generic delayed-release capsules. Compared with the *selective serotonin reuptake inhibitors* (SSRIs), less is known about duloxetine's safety and effectiveness in children and adolescents.

How Can This Medicine Help?

Duloxetine is used to treat depression and generalized anxiety disorder. Less is known about whether it helps obsessive-compulsive disorder (OCD), posttraumatic stress disorder (PTSD), panic disorder, or separation anxiety disorder. It is also used to treat chronic muscle or bone pain or diabetic nerve pain in adults.

How Does This Medicine Work?

Duloxetine increases the amount of two neurotransmitters—*serotonin* and *norepinephrine*—in parts of the brain. *Neurotransmitters* are the chemicals used by brain cells to communicate. People with depression and anxiety may have low levels of serotonin and norepinephrine in certain parts of the brain. Duloxetine helps by increasing the action of these neurotransmitters to more normal levels.

How Long Does This Medicine Last?

Duloxetine is taken once or twice a day.

How Will the Doctor Monitor This Medicine?

The doctor will review your child's medical history and physical examination before starting duloxetine. Be sure to tell the doctor if your child or anyone in the family has had liver problems. The doctor may order some blood or urine tests to be sure your child does not have a hidden medical condition that would make it unsafe to use this medicine. Extra care is needed when using duloxetine in youth with seizures (epilepsy), liver or kidney problems, or diabetes. The doctor or nurse may measure your child's pulse, blood pressure, and weight before starting the medicine.

Be sure to tell the doctor if your child or anyone in the family has bipolar illness (manic-depressive illness) or has tried to kill himself or herself.

After the medicine is started, the doctor will want to have regular appointments with you and your child to see how the medicine is working, to see if a dose change is needed, to watch for side effects, to see if duloxetine is still needed, and to see if any other treatment is needed. The doctor or nurse may check your child's height, weight, pulse, and blood pressure. Duloxetine may cause small increases in blood pressure. No blood tests are usually required while taking duloxetine.

Before using medicine and at times afterward, the doctor may ask your child to fill out a rating scale about depression and anxiety, to help see how your child is doing.

What Side Effects Can This Medicine Have?

Any medicine can have side effects, including an allergy to the medicine. Because each patient is different, the doctor will monitor the youth closely, especially when the medicine is started. The doctor will work with you to increase the positive effects and decrease the negative effects of the medicine. Please tell the doctor if any of the listed side effects appear or if you think that the medicine is causing any other problems. Not all of the rare or unusual side effects are listed.

Side effects are most common after starting the medicine or after a dose increase. Many side effects can be avoided or lessened by starting with a very low dose and increasing it slowly—ask the doctor.

Allergic Reaction

Tell the doctor in a day or two (if possible, before the next dose of medicine):

- Hives
- Itching
- Rash

Stop the medicine and get *immediate* medical care:

- Trouble breathing or chest tightness
- Swelling of lips, tongue, or throat
- Severe skin rash or skin blisters

Common Side Effects

Tell the doctor within a week or two:

- Nausea, upset stomach, vomiting
- Headaches
- Decreased appetite
- Dry mouth—Have your child try using sugar-free gum or candy.
- Constipation—Encourage your child to drink more fluids and eat high-fiber foods; if necessary, the doctor may recommend a fiber medicine such as Benefiber or a stool softener such as Colace or mineral oil.
- Insomnia (trouble sleeping)
- Daytime sleepiness or tiredness—Do not allow your child to drive, ride a bicycle or motorcycle, or operate machinery if this happens.
- Dizziness—This side effect is worse when the child stands up quickly, especially when getting out of bed in the morning; try having the child stand up slowly.
- Excessive sweating
- Rapid heartbeat (palpitations)
- Weight gain

Less Common, but More Serious, Side Effects

Call the doctor within a day or two:

- Significant suicidal thoughts or self-injurious behavior
- Increased activity, rapid speech, feeling "speeded up," decreased need for sleep, being very excited or irritable (cranky)
- Abnormal bleeding, such as easy bruising, nosebleeds, or bleeding with surgery
- Yellowing of skin or eyes, dark urine, pale bowel movements, abdominal pain or fullness, unexplained flu-like symptoms, itchy skin—These side effects are extremely rare but could be signs of liver damage.

Serious Side Effects

Call the doctor *immediately* or go to the nearest emergency room:

- Seizure (fit, convulsion)
- Stiffness, high fever, confusion, tremors (shaking)
- Overheating or heatstroke—Prevent by decreasing activity in hot weather, staying out of the sun, and drinking water.

Serotonin Syndrome

A very serious side effect called *serotonin syndrome* can happen when certain kinds of medicines (including SSRI antidepressants, clomipramine, and other medicines, such as triptans for migraine headaches, buspirone, linezolid, tramadol, or St. John's wort) are taken by the same person. Very rarely, serotonin syndrome can happen at high doses of just one medicine. The early signs are restlessness, confusion, shaking, skin turning red, sweating, muscle stiffness, sweating, and jerking of muscles. If you see these symptoms, stop the medicine and send or take the youth to an emergency room right away.

Some Interactions With Other Medicines or Food

Please note that the following are only the most likely interactions with other medicines or food.

Duloxetine may be taken with or without food.

Duloxetine interacts with many other medicines, including some antibiotics and other psychiatric medicines. It is especially important to tell the doctor and pharmacist about all of the medicines your child is taking or has taken in the past few months, including over-the-counter and herbal medicines. Sometimes one medicine can increase or decrease the blood level of another medicine, so that different doses are needed. Ciprofloxacin (Cipro) and cimetidine (Tagamet) both increase the level of duloxetine. When switching from fluvoxamine, paroxetine, or fluoxetine to duloxetine, lower than usual doses of duloxetine are needed, because those other antidepressants increase the levels of duloxetine. The herbal medicine St. John's wort also increases serotonin and can cause serious side effects if taken with duloxetine. Taking duloxetine with aspirin, nonsteroidal anti-inflammatory drugs (NSAIDs; medications including ibuprofen or naproxen), or anticoagulant medications (including warfarin) increases risk of abnormal bleeding.

It can be *very dangerous* to take duloxetine at the same time as or even within a month of taking another type of medicine called a *monoamine oxidase inhibitor* (MAOI), such as selegiline (Eldepryl), phenelzine (Nardil), tranylcypromine (Parnate), or isocarboxazid (Marplan).

Duloxetine can be taken with or without food.

Caffeine may increase side effects.

What Could Happen if This Medicine Is Stopped Suddenly?

If duloxetine is stopped suddenly, there may be uncomfortable withdrawal feelings, including dizziness, headache, irritability, and nightmares. Do not stop this medicine suddenly, and tell the doctor if these symptoms happen as the medicine is being tapered (dose decreased).

How Long Will This Medicine Be Needed?

Duloxetine may take up to 1–2 months to reach its full effect. If your child has a good response to duloxetine, it is a good idea to continue the medicine for at least 6 months. Ask the doctor about this.

What Else Should I Know About This Medicine?

In youth who have bipolar disorder or who may be at risk for bipolar disorder, any antidepressant medicine may increase the risk of hypomania or mania (excitement, agitation, increased activity, decreased sleep).

Smoking may lower the levels of duloxetine, making it not work as well.

In hot weather, make sure your child drinks enough water or other liquids and does not get overheated.

Sometimes, after a person has improved while taking duloxetine, he or she loses interest in school or friends or just stops trying. Please tell your child's doctor if this happens—it may be a side effect of the medicine. A lower dose or a different medicine may be needed.

Store the medicine away from sunlight, heat, moisture, and humidity.

Duloxetine capsules should not be crushed, chewed, sprinkled on food, or mixed with juice but should be swallowed whole.

Black Box Antidepressant Warning

In 2004, an advisory committee to the FDA decided that there might be an increased risk of suicidal behavior for some youth taking medicines called *antidepressants*. In the research studies that the committee reviewed, about 3%–4% of youth with depression who took an antidepressant medicine—and 1%–2% of youth with depression who took a placebo (pill without active medicine)—talked about suicidal thoughts (thinking about killing themselves or wishing they were dead) or did something to harm themselves. This means that almost twice as many youth who were taking an antidepressant to treat their depression talked about suicide or had suicidal behavior compared with youth with depression who were taking inactive medicine. There were *no* completed suicides in any of these research studies, which included more than 4,000 children and adolescents. For youth being treated for anxiety, there was no difference in suicidal talking or behavior between those taking antidepressant medication and those taking placebo.

The FDA told drug companies to add a *black box warning* label to all antidepressant medicines. Because of this label, a doctor (or advanced practice nurse) prescribing one of these medicines has to warn youth and their families that there might be more suicidal thoughts and actions in youth taking these medicines.

On the other hand, in places where more youth are taking the newer antidepressant medicines, the number of adolescents who commit suicide has gotten smaller. Also, thinking about or attempting suicide is more common in surveys of teenagers in the community than it is in depressed youth treated in research studies with antidepressant medicine.

If a youth is being treated with this medicine and is doing well, then no changes are needed as a result of this warning. Increased suicidal talk or action is most likely to happen in the first few months of treatment with a medicine. If your child has recently started this medicine or is about to start, then you and your doctor (or advanced practice nurse) should watch for any changes in behavior. People who are depressed often have suicidal thoughts or actions. It is hard to know whether suicidal thoughts or actions in depressed people are caused by the depression itself or by the medicine. Also, as their depression is getting better, some people talk more about the suicidal thoughts that they had before but did not talk about. As young people get better from depression, they might be at higher risk of doing something about suicidal thoughts that they have had for some time, because they have more energy.

What Should A Parent Do?

1. Be honest with your child about possible risks and benefits of medicine.

2. Talk to your child about whether he or she is having any suicidal thoughts, and tell your child to come to you if he or she is having such thoughts.

3. You, your child, and your child's doctor or nurse should develop a safety plan. Pick adults whom your child can tell if he or she is thinking about suicide.

4. Be sure to tell your child's doctor, nurse, or therapist if you suspect that your child is using alcohol or drugs or if something has happened that might make your child feel worse, such as a family separation, breaking up with a boyfriend or girlfriend, someone close dying or attempting suicide, physical or sexual abuse, or failure in school.

5. Be sure that there are no guns in the home and that all medicines (including over-the-counter medicines like Tylenol) are closely supervised by an adult and kept in a safe place.

6. Watch for new or worse thoughts of suicide, self-harm, depression, anxiety (nerves), feeling very agitated or restless, being angry or aggressive, having more trouble sleeping, or anything else that you see for the first time, seems worse, or worries your child or you. If these appear, contact a mental health professional **right away.** Do not just stop or change the dose of the medicine on your own. If the problems are serious, and you cannot reach one of your clinicians, call a 24-hour psychiatry emergency telephone number or take your child to an emergency room.

Youth taking antidepressant medicine should be watched carefully by their parent(s), clinician(s) (doctor, advanced practice nurse, nurse, therapist), and other concerned adults for the first weeks of treatment. It is a good idea to have regular contact with the doctor, APN, nurse, or therapist for the first months to check for feelings of depression or sadness, thoughts of killing or harming himself or herself, and any problems with the medication. If you have questions, be sure to ask the doctor, APN, nurse, or therapist.

For more information, see http://www.parentsmedguide.org/.

Notes

Use this space to take notes or to write down questions you want to ask the doctor.

_____

_____

_____

_____

_____

_____

_____

_____

_____

_____

_____

_____

Escitalopram—Lexapro

General Information About Medication

Each child and adolescent is different. No one has exactly the same combination of medical and psychological problems. It is a good idea to talk with the doctor or nurse about the reasons a medicine is being used. It is very important to keep all appointments and to be in touch by telephone if you have concerns. It is important to communicate with the doctor, nurse, or therapist. An *advanced practice nurse* (APN) has additional education and training after becoming a registered nurse (RN). Your child's medication may be prescribed by a medical doctor (MD or DO) or an APN. In addition, a *physician assistant* (PA) working with a physician may prescribe certain medications. In this information sheet, "doctor" includes medical doctors as well as APNs and PAs who prescribe medication. Often a nurse (RN) will be part of the team and answer questions and give information.

It is very important that the medicine be taken exactly as the doctor instructs. However, once in a while, everyone forgets to give a medicine on time. It is a good idea to ask the doctor or nurse what to do if this happens. Do not stop or change a medicine without asking the doctor or nurse first.

If the medicine seems to stop working, it may be because it is not being taken regularly. The youth may be "cheeking" or hiding the medicine or forgetting to take it (especially at school). The doses may be too far apart or a different dose or medicine may be needed. Something at school, at home, or in the neighborhood may be upsetting the youth, or he or she may need special help for learning disabilities or tutoring. Please discuss your concerns with the doctor. **Do not just increase the dose.** It is also very important not to decrease the dose or stop the medicine without talking to the doctor first. The problem being treated may come back, or there could be uncomfortable or even dangerous results.

All medicines should be kept in a safe place, out of the reach of children, and should be supervised by an adult. If someone takes too much of a medicine, call the doctor, the poison control center, or a hospital emergency room.

Each medicine has a "generic" or chemical name. Just like laundry detergents or paper towels, some medicines are sold by more than one company under different brand names. The same medicine may be available under a generic name and several brand names. The generic medications are usually less expensive than the brand name ones. The generic medications have the same chemical formula, but they may or may not be exactly the same strength as the brand-name medications. Also, some brands of pills contain dye or other things that can cause allergic reactions. It is a good idea to talk to the doctor and the pharmacist about whether it is important to use a specific brand of medicine.

Any medicine can cause an allergic reaction. Examples are hives, itching, rashes, swelling, and trouble breathing. Even a tiny amount of a medicine can cause a reaction in patients who are allergic to that medicine. Be *sure* to talk to the doctor before restarting a medicine that has caused an allergic reaction and tell the doctor about any reactions to medicine that your child has had before.

Taking more than one medicine at the same time may cause more side effects or cause one of the medicines to not work as well. Always ask the doctor, nurse, or pharmacist before adding another

medicine, either prescription or bought without a prescription in a store or on the Internet. **Be sure that each doctor knows about *all* of the medicines your child is taking. Also tell the doctor about any vitamins, herbal medicines, or supplements your child may be taking.** Some of these may have side effects alone or when taken with this medication. It is a very good idea to keep a list with you of the names and doses of all medicines that your child is taking.

Everyone taking medicine should have a physical examination at least once a year.

If you think that your child may be using drugs or alcohol, please tell the doctor right away.

Pregnancy requires special care in the use of medicine. Some medicines can cause birth defects if taken by a pregnant mother. **Please tell the doctor immediately if you suspect the teenager is at risk of becoming pregnant.** The doctor may wish to discuss sexual behavior and/or birth control with your daughter.

Printed information like this applies to children and adolescents in general. If you have questions about the medicine, or if you notice changes or anything unusual, please ask the doctor or nurse. As scientific research advances, knowledge increases and advice changes. Even experts do not always agree. Many medicines have not been "approved" by the U.S. Food and Drug Administration (FDA) for use in children or use for particular problems. For this reason, use of the medicine for a problem or age group often is not listed in the *Physicians' Desk Reference.* This does not necessarily mean that the medicine is dangerous or does not work, only that the company that makes the medicine has not received permission to advertise the medicine for use in children. Companies often do not apply for this permission because it is expensive to do the tests needed to apply for approval for use in children. Once a medication is approved by the FDA for any purpose, a doctor is allowed to prescribe it according to research and clinical experience.

Note to Teachers

It is a good idea to talk with the parent(s) about the reason(s) that a medication is being used. If the parent(s) sign consent to release information, it is often helpful for you to talk with the doctor. If the parent(s) give permission, the doctor may ask you to fill out rating forms about your experience with the student's behavior, feelings, academic performance, and medication side effects. This information is very useful in selecting and monitoring medication treatment. If you have observations that you think are important, do not hesitate to share these with the student's parent(s) and treating clinicians (with parental consent).

It is very important that the medicine be taken exactly as the doctor instructs. However, everyone forgets to give a medicine on time once in a while. It is a good idea to ask the parent(s) in advance what to do if this happens. Do not stop or change the time you are giving a medicine at school without parental permission. If a medication is to be taken with food, but lunchtime or snack time changes, be sure to notify the parent(s) so appropriate adjustments can be made.

All medicines should be kept in a secure place and should be supervised by an adult. If someone takes too much of a medicine, follow your school procedure for an urgent medical problem.

Taking medicine is a private matter and is best managed discreetly and confidentially. It is important to be sensitive to the student's feelings about taking medicine.

If you suspect that the student is using drugs or alcohol, please tell the parent(s) or a school counselor right away.

Please tell the parent(s) or school nurse if you suspect medication side effects.

Modifications of the classroom environment or assignments may be useful in addition to medication. The student may need to be evaluated for additional help or a 504 plan or an Individualized Education Plan for learning problems or emotional or behavioral issues.

Any expression of suicidal thoughts or feelings or self-harm by a child or adolescent is a signal of distress and should be taken seriously. These behaviors should not be dismissed as "attention seeking." School procedures for safety issues should be followed.

What Is Escitalopram (Lexapro)?

Escitalopram is an antidepressant known as a *selective serotonin reuptake inhibitor* (SSRI). It comes in generic and brand name Lexapro tablets and liquid.

How Can This Medicine Help?

Escitalopram is used to treat depression and anxiety disorders such as obsessive-compulsive disorder (OCD), posttraumatic stress disorder (PTSD), panic disorder, separation anxiety disorder, selective mutism, social anxiety disorder, and generalized anxiety disorder.

How Does This Medicine Work?

Escitalopram increases the amount of a *neurotransmitter* called *serotonin* in certain parts of the brain. People with emotional and behavioral problems, such as depression and anxiety, may have low levels of serotonin in certain parts of the brain. SSRIs such as escitalopram help by increasing the action of brain serotonin to more normal levels.

How Long Does This Medicine Last?

Escitalopram can be taken only once a day for most people.

How Will the Doctor Monitor This Medicine?

The doctor will review your child's medical history and physical examination before starting escitalopram. The doctor may order some blood or urine tests to be sure your child does not have a hidden medical condition that would make it unsafe to use this medicine. Extra care is needed when using SSRIs in youth with seizures (epilepsy); heart, liver, or kidney problems; or diabetes. The doctor or nurse may measure your child's pulse, blood pressure, and weight before starting the medicine.

Be sure to tell the doctor if your child or anyone in the family has bipolar disorder or has tried to kill himself or herself.

After the medicine is started, the doctor will want to have regular appointments with you and your child to see how the medicine is working, to see if a dose change is needed, to watch for side effects, to see if escitalopram is still needed, and to see if any other treatment is needed. The doctor or nurse may check your child's height, weight, pulse, and blood pressure.

Before using medicine and at times afterward, the doctor may ask your child to fill out a rating scale about depression or anxiety to help see how your child is doing.

What Side Effects Can This Medicine Have?

Any medicine can have side effects, including an allergy to the medicine. Because each patient is different, the doctor will monitor the youth closely, especially when the medicine is started. The doctor will work with you to increase the positive effects and decrease the negative effects of the medicine. Please tell the doctor if any of the listed side effects appear or if you think that the medicine is causing any other problems. Not all of the rare or unusual side effects are listed.

Side effects are most common after starting the medicine or after a dose increase. Many side effects can be avoided or lessened by starting with a very low dose and increasing it slowly—ask the doctor.

Allergic Reaction

Tell the doctor in a day or two (if possible, before the next dose of medicine):

- Hives
- Itching
- Rash

Stop the medicine and get *immediate* medical care:

- Trouble breathing or chest tightness
- Swelling of lips, tongue, or throat

Common Side Effects

Tell the doctor within a week or two, or sooner if the problems are getting worse:

- Nausea, upset stomach, vomiting
- Diarrhea or excessive gas
- Dry mouth—Have your child try using sugar-free gum or candy.
- Constipation—Encourage your child to drink more fluids and eat high-fiber foods; if necessary, the doctor may recommend a fiber medicine such as Benefiber or a stool softener such as Colace or mineral oil.
- Headache
- Anxiety or nervousness
- Insomnia (trouble sleeping)
- Restlessness, increased activity level
- Daytime sleepiness or tiredness—Do not allow your child to drive, ride a bicycle or motorcycle, or operate machinery if this side effect is present.
- Dizziness—This side effect is worse when the child stands up quickly, especially when getting out of bed in the morning; try having the child stand up slowly.
- Tremor (shakiness)
- Excessive sweating
- Apathy, lack of interest in school or friends—This may happen after an initial good response to treatment.
- Decreased sexual interest, trouble with sexual functioning
- Weight gain
- Weight loss

Less Common, but More Serious, Side Effects

Call the doctor within a day or two:

- Significant suicidal thoughts or self-injurious behavior
- Increased activity, rapid speech, feeling "speeded up," decreased need for sleep, being very excited or irritable (cranky), agitation, acting out of character
- Bleeding, such as bruising or nosebleeds, or bleeding with surgery

Serious Side Effects

Call the doctor *immediately* or go to the nearest emergency room:

- Seizure (fit, convulsion)
- Stiffness, high fever, confusion, tremors (shaking)
- Overheating or heatstroke—Prevent by decreasing activity in hot weather, staying out of the sun, and drinking water.

Serotonin Syndrome

A very serious side effect called *serotonin syndrome* can happen when certain kinds of medicines (including SSRI antidepressants, clomipramine, and other medicines, such as triptans for migraine headaches, buspirone, linezolid, tramadol, or St. John's wort) are taken by the same person. Very rarely, serotonin syndrome can happen at high doses of just one medicine. The early signs are restlessness, confusion, shaking, skin turning red, sweating, muscle stiffness, sweating, and jerking of muscles. If you see these symptoms, stop the medicine and send or take the youth to an emergency room right away.

Some Interactions With Other Medicines or Food

Please note that the following are only the most likely interactions with other medicines or food.

Escitalopram interacts with many other prescription and over the counter medicines, including some antibiotics and other psychiatric medicines. It is especially important to tell the doctor and pharmacist about all of the medicines your child is taking or has taken in the past few months, including over-the-counter and herbal medicines. Sometimes one medicine can increase or decrease the blood level of another medicine, so that different doses are needed. Erythromycin and similar antibiotics, as well as antifungal agents such as ketoconazole, may increase levels of escitalopram and increase side effects. Escitalopram may increase the heart side effects of pimozide (Orap), so those two medicines should not be taken by the same person. Tryptophan or the herbal medicine St. John's Wort also increases serotonin and can cause serious side effects if taken with escitalopram. Taking escitalopram with aspirin, nonsteroidal anti-inflammatory drugs (NSAIDs) (medications including ibuprofen or naproxen), or anticoagulant medications (including warfarin) increases risk of abnormal bleeding.

It can be *very dangerous* to take an SSRI at the same time as or even within a month of taking another type of medicine called a *monoamine oxidase inhibitor* (MAOI), such as selegiline (Eldepryl), phenelzine (Nardil), tranylcypromine (Parnate), or isocarboxazid (Marplan).

Escitalopram can be taken with or without food.

Caffeine may increase side effects of escitalopram.

What Could Happen if This Medicine Is Stopped Suddenly?

No known serious medical effects occur if escitalopram is stopped suddenly, but there may be uncomfortable feelings, which should be avoided if possible. Your child might have trouble sleeping, nervousness, irritability, dizziness, and flu-like symptoms. Ask the doctor before stopping escitalopram or if these symptoms happen while the dose is being decreased.

How Long Will This Medicine Be Needed?

Escitalopram may take up to 1–2 months to reach its full effect. If your child has a good response to escitalopram, it is a good idea to continue the medicine for at least 6–12 months. It is important to review this with your doctor.

What Else Should I Know About This Medicine?

In youth who have bipolar disorder or who may be at risk for bipolar disorder, any antidepressant medicine may increase the risk of hypomania or mania (excitement, agitation, increased activity, decreased sleep).

In hot weather, make sure your child drinks enough water or other liquids and does not get overheated.

Sometimes, after a person has improved while taking escitalopram, he or she loses interest in school or friends or just stops trying. Please tell your child's doctor if this happens—it may be a side effect of the medicine. A lower dose or a different medicine may be needed.

Store the medicine away from sunlight, heat, moisture, and humidity.

Black Box Antidepressant Warning

In 2004, an advisory committee to the FDA decided that there might be an increased risk of suicidal behavior for some youth taking medicines called *antidepressants*. In the research studies that the committee reviewed, about 3%–4% of youth with depression who took an antidepressant medicine—and 1%–2% of youth with depression who took a placebo (pill without active medicine)—talked about suicidal thoughts (thinking about killing themselves or wishing they were dead) or did something to harm themselves. This means that almost twice as many youth who were taking an antidepressant to treat their depression talked about suicide or had suicidal behavior compared with youth with depression who were taking inactive medicine. There were *no* completed suicides in any of these research studies, which included more than 4,000 children and adolescents. For youth being treated for anxiety, there was no difference in suicidal talking or behavior between those taking antidepressant medication and those taking placebo.

The FDA told drug companies to add a *black box warning* label to all antidepressant medicines. Because of this label, a doctor (or advanced practice nurse) prescribing one of these medicines has to warn youth and their families that there might be more suicidal thoughts and actions in youth taking these medicines.

On the other hand, in places where more youth are taking the newer antidepressant medicines, the number of adolescents who commit suicide has gotten smaller. Also, thinking about or attempting suicide is more common in surveys of teenagers in the community than it is in depressed youth treated in research studies with antidepressant medicine.

If a youth is being treated with this medicine and is doing well, then no changes are needed as a result of this warning. Increased suicidal talk or action is most likely to happen in the first few months of treatment with a medicine. If your child has recently started this medicine or is about to start, then you and your doctor (or advanced practice nurse) should watch for any changes in behavior. People who are depressed often have suicidal thoughts or actions. It is hard to know whether suicidal thoughts or actions in depressed people are caused by the depression itself or by the medicine. Also, as their depression is getting better, some people talk more about the suicidal thoughts that they had before but did not talk about. As young people get better from depression, they might be at higher risk of doing something about suicidal thoughts that they have had for some time, because they have more energy.

What Should a Parent Do?

1. Be honest with your child about possible risks and benefits of medicine.
2. Talk to your child about whether he or she is having any suicidal thoughts, and tell your child to come to you if he or she is having such thoughts.
3. You, your child, and your child's doctor or nurse should develop a safety plan. Pick adults whom your child can tell if he or she is thinking about suicide.
4. Be sure to tell your child's doctor, nurse, or therapist if you suspect that your child is using alcohol or drugs or if something has happened that might make your child feel worse, such as a family separation, breaking up with a boyfriend or girlfriend, someone close dying or attempting suicide, physical or sexual abuse, or failure in school.
5. Be sure that there are no guns in the home and that all medicines (including over-the-counter medicines like Tylenol) are closely supervised by an adult and kept in a safe place.
6. Watch for new or worse thoughts of suicide, self-harm, depression, anxiety (nerves), feeling very agitated or restless, being angry or aggressive, having more trouble sleeping, or anything else that you see for the first time, seems worse, or worries your child or you. If these appear, contact a mental health professional **right away.** Do not just stop or change the dose of the medicine on your own. If the problems are serious, and you cannot reach one of your clinicians, call a 24-hour psychiatry emergency telephone number or take your child to an emergency room.

Youth taking antidepressant medicine should be watched carefully by their parent(s), clinician(s) (doctor, advanced practice nurse, nurse, therapist), and other concerned adults for the first weeks of treatment. It is a good idea to have regular contact with the doctor, APN, nurse, or therapist for the first months to check for feelings of depression or sadness, thoughts of killing or harming himself or herself, and any problems with the medication. If you have questions, be sure to ask the doctor, APN, nurse, or therapist.

For more information, see http://www.parentsmedguide.org/.

Notes

Use this space to take notes or to write down questions you want to ask the doctor.

_____

_____

_____

_____

_____

_____

_____

_____

_____

_____

_____

_____

_____

_____

Medication Information for Parents and Teachers

Fluoxetine—Prozac, Symbyax

General Information About Medication

Each child and adolescent is different. No one has exactly the same combination of medical and psychological problems. It is a good idea to talk with the doctor or nurse about the reasons a medicine is being used. It is very important to keep all appointments and to be in touch by telephone if you have concerns. It is important to communicate with the doctor, nurse, or therapist. An *advanced practice nurse* (APN) has additional education and training after becoming a registered nurse (RN). Your child's medication may be prescribed by a medical doctor (MD or DO) or an APN. In addition, a *physician assistant* (PA) working with a physician may prescribe certain medications. In this information sheet, "doctor" includes medical doctors as well as APNs and PAs who prescribe medication. Often a nurse (RN) will be part of the team and answer questions and give information.

It is very important that the medicine be taken exactly as the doctor instructs. However, once in a while, everyone forgets to give a medicine on time. It is a good idea to ask the doctor or nurse what to do if this happens. Do not stop or change a medicine without asking the doctor or nurse first.

If the medicine seems to stop working, it may be because it is not being taken regularly. The youth may be "cheeking" or hiding the medicine or forgetting to take it (especially at school). The doses may be too far apart or a different dose or medicine may be needed. Something at school, at home, or in the neighborhood may be upsetting the youth, or he or she may need special help for learning disabilities or tutoring. Please discuss your concerns with the doctor. **Do not just increase the dose.** It is also very important not to decrease the dose or stop the medicine without talking to the doctor first. The problem being treated may come back, or there could be uncomfortable or even dangerous results.

All medicines should be kept in a safe place, out of the reach of children, and should be supervised by an adult. If someone takes too much of a medicine, call the doctor, the poison control center, or a hospital emergency room.

Each medicine has a "generic" or chemical name. Just like laundry detergents or paper towels, some medicines are sold by more than one company under different brand names. The same medicine may be available under a generic name and several brand names. The generic medications are usually less expensive than the brand name ones. The generic medications have the same chemical formula, but they may or may not be exactly the same strength as the brand-name medications. Also, some brands of pills contain dye or other things that can cause allergic reactions. It is a good idea to talk to the doctor and the pharmacist about whether it is important to use a specific brand of medicine.

Any medicine can cause an allergic reaction. Examples are hives, itching, rashes, swelling, and trouble breathing. Even a tiny amount of a medicine can cause a reaction in patients who are allergic to that medicine. Be *sure* to talk to the doctor before restarting a medicine that has caused an allergic reaction and tell the doctor about any reactions to medicine that your child has had before.

Taking more than one medicine at the same time may cause more side effects or cause one of the medicines to not work as well. Always ask the doctor, nurse, or pharmacist before adding another

191

medicine, either prescription or bought without a prescription in a store or on the Internet. **Be sure that each doctor knows about *all* of the medicines your child is taking. Also tell the doctor about any vitamins, herbal medicines, or supplements your child may be taking.** Some of these may have side effects alone or when taken with this medication. It is a very good idea to keep a list with you of the names and doses of all medicines that your child is taking.

Everyone taking medicine should have a physical examination at least once a year.

If you think that your child may be using drugs or alcohol, please tell the doctor right away.

Pregnancy requires special care in the use of medicine. Some medicines can cause birth defects if taken by a pregnant mother. **Please tell the doctor immediately if you suspect the teenager is at risk of becoming pregnant.** The doctor may wish to discuss sexual behavior and/or birth control with your daughter.

Printed information like this applies to children and adolescents in general. If you have questions about the medicine, or if you notice changes or anything unusual, please ask the doctor or nurse. As scientific research advances, knowledge increases and advice changes. Even experts do not always agree. Many medicines have not been "approved" by the U.S. Food and Drug Administration (FDA) for use in children or use for particular problems. For this reason, use of the medicine for a problem or age group often is not listed in the *Physicians' Desk Reference.* This does not necessarily mean that the medicine is dangerous or does not work, only that the company that makes the medicine has not received permission to advertise the medicine for use in children. Companies often do not apply for this permission because it is expensive to do the tests needed to apply for approval for use in children. Once a medication is approved by the FDA for any purpose, a doctor is allowed to prescribe it according to research and clinical experience.

Note to Teachers

It is a good idea to talk with the parent(s) about the reason(s) that a medication is being used. If the parent(s) sign consent to release information, it is often helpful for you to talk with the doctor. If the parent(s) give permission, the doctor may ask you to fill out rating forms about your experience with the student's behavior, feelings, academic performance, and medication side effects. This information is very useful in selecting and monitoring medication treatment. If you have observations that you think are important, do not hesitate to share these with the student's parent(s) and treating clinicians (with parental consent).

It is very important that the medicine be taken exactly as the doctor instructs. However, everyone forgets to give a medicine on time once in a while. It is a good idea to ask the parent(s) in advance what to do if this happens. Do not stop or change the time you are giving a medicine at school without parental permission. If a medication is to be taken with food, but lunchtime or snack time changes, be sure to notify the parent(s) so appropriate adjustments can be made.

All medicines should be kept in a secure place and should be supervised by an adult. If someone takes too much of a medicine, follow your school procedure for an urgent medical problem.

Taking medicine is a private matter and is best managed discreetly and confidentially. It is important to be sensitive to the student's feelings about taking medicine.

If you suspect that the student is using drugs or alcohol, please tell the parent(s) or a school counselor right away.

Please tell the parent(s) or school nurse if you suspect medication side effects.

Modifications of the classroom environment or assignments may be useful in addition to medication. The student may need to be evaluated for additional help or a 504 plan or an Individualized Education Plan for learning problems or emotional or behavioral issues.

Any expression of suicidal thoughts or feelings or self-harm by a child or adolescent is a signal of distress and should be taken seriously. These behaviors should not be dismissed as "attention seeking." School procedures for safety issues should be followed.

What Is Fluoxetine (Prozac)?

Fluoxetine is an antidepressant known as a *selective serotonin reuptake inhibitor* (SSRI). It comes in generic and brand name Prozac capsules, once-weekly extended release forms (Prozac Weekly), and generic liquid form. For very small doses or for children who cannot swallow pills, the pill form can be dissolved in cranberry or orange juice and kept in the refrigerator. Fluoxetine is also sold under the brand name Sarafem (or generic tablet) for premenstrual dysphoric disorder. There is a capsule that combines fluoxetine and olanzapine that comes in brand name Symbyax and generic.

How Can This Medicine Help?

Fluoxetine is used to treat depression and anxiety disorders such as obsessive-compulsive disorder (OCD), posttraumatic stress disorder (PTSD), panic disorder, separation anxiety disorder, selective mutism, social anxiety disorder, and generalized anxiety disorder. Symbyax is used to treat depression in people with bipolar disorder.

How Does This Medicine Work?

Fluoxetine increases the amount of a *neurotransmitter* called *serotonin* in certain parts of the brain. People with emotional and behavioral problems, such as depression and anxiety, may have low levels of serotonin in certain parts of the brain. SSRIs such as fluoxetine help by increasing the action of brain serotonin to more normal levels.

How Long Does This Medicine Last?

Fluoxetine lasts a very long time. It has some action in the body for as long as 4 weeks after it is stopped. It is usually taken once a day.

How Will the Doctor Monitor This Medicine?

The doctor will review your child's medical history and physical examination before starting fluoxetine. The doctor may order some blood or urine tests to be sure your child does not have a hidden medical condition that would make it unsafe to use this medicine. Extra care is needed when using SSRIs in youth with seizures (epilepsy); heart, liver, or kidney problems; or diabetes. The doctor or nurse may measure your child's pulse, blood pressure, and weight before starting the medicine.

Be sure to tell the doctor if your child or anyone in the family has bipolar disorder or has tried to kill himself or herself.

After the medicine is started, the doctor will want to have regular appointments with you and your child to see how the medicine is working, to see if a dose change is needed, to watch for side effects, to see if fluoxetine is still needed, and to see if any other treatment is needed. The doctor or nurse may check your child's height, weight, pulse, and blood pressure.

Before using medicine and at times afterward, the doctor may ask your child to fill out a rating scale about depression or anxiety to help see how your child is doing.

What Side Effects Can This Medicine Have?

Any medicine can have side effects, including an allergy to the medicine. Because each patient is different, the doctor will monitor the youth closely, especially when the medicine is started. The doctor will work with you to increase the positive effects and decrease the negative effects of the medicine. Please tell the doctor if any of the listed side effects appear or if you think that the medicine is causing any other problems. Not all of the rare or unusual side effects are listed.

Side effects are most common after starting the medicine or after a dose increase. Many side effects can be avoided or lessened by starting with a very low dose and increasing it slowly—ask the doctor.

For the fluoxetine-olanzapine combination Symbyax, see also the information sheet for olanzapine.

Allergic Reaction

Tell the doctor in a day or two (if possible, before the next dose of medicine):

- Hives
- Itching
- Rash

Stop the medicine and get *immediate* medical care:

- Trouble breathing or chest tightness
- Swelling of lips, tongue, or throat

Common Side Effects

Tell the doctor within a week or two, or sooner if the problems are getting worse:

- Nausea, upset stomach, vomiting
- Diarrhea or excessive gas
- Dry mouth—Have your child try using sugar-free gum or candy.
- Constipation—Encourage your child to drink more fluids and eat high-fiber foods; if necessary, the doctor may recommend a fiber medicine such as Benefiber or a stool softener such as Colace or mineral oil.
- Headache
- Anxiety or nervousness
- Insomnia (trouble sleeping)
- Restlessness, increased activity level
- Daytime sleepiness or tiredness—Do not allow your child to drive, ride a bicycle or motorcycle, or operate machinery if this side effect is present.
- Dizziness—This side effect is worse when the child stands up quickly, especially when getting out of bed in the morning; try having the child stand up slowly.
- Tremor (shakiness)

- Excessive sweating
- Apathy, lack of interest in school or friends—This may happen after an initial good response to treatment.
- Decreased sexual interest, trouble with sexual functioning
- Weight gain
- Weight loss

Less Common, but More Serious, Side Effects

Call the doctor within a day or two:

- Significant suicidal thoughts or self-injurious behavior
- Increased activity, rapid speech, feeling "speeded up," decreased need for sleep, being very excited or irritable (cranky), agitation, acting out of character
- Bleeding, such as bruising or nosebleeds, or bleeding with surgery

Serious Side Effects

Call the doctor *immediately* or go to the nearest emergency room:

- Seizure (fit, convulsion)
- Stiffness, high fever, confusion, tremors (shaking)
- Overheating or heatstroke—Prevent by decreasing activity in hot weather, staying out of the sun, and drinking water.

Serotonin Syndrome

A very serious side effect called *serotonin syndrome* can happen when certain kinds of medicines (including SSRI antidepressants, clomipramine, and other medicines, such as triptans for migraine headaches, buspirone, linezolid, tramadol, or St. John's wort) are taken by the same person. Very rarely, serotonin syndrome can happen at high doses of just one medicine. The early signs are restlessness, confusion, shaking, skin turning red, sweating, muscle stiffness, sweating, and jerking of muscles. If you see these symptoms, stop the medicine and send or take the youth to an emergency room right away.

Some Interactions With Other Medicines or Food

Please note that the following are only the most likely interactions with other medicines or food.

Fluoxetine interacts with many other prescription and over the counter medicines, including some antibiotics and other psychiatric medicines. It is especially important to tell the doctor and pharmacist about all of the medicines your child is taking or has taken in the past few months, including over-the-counter and herbal medicines. Sometimes one medicine can increase or decrease the blood level of another medicine, so that different doses are needed. Erythromycin and similar antibiotics, as well as antifungal agents such as ketoconazole, may increase levels of fluoxetine and increase side effects. Fluoxetine may increase the heart side effects of pimozide (Orap), so those two medicines should not be taken by the same person. Tryptophan or the herbal medicine St. John's wort also increases serotonin and can cause serious side effects if taken with fluoxetine. Taking fluoxetine with aspirin, nonsteroidal anti-inflammatory drugs (NSAIDs) (medications including ibuprofen or naproxen), or anticoagulant medications (including warfarin) increases risk of abnormal bleeding.

It can be *very dangerous* to take an SSRI at the same time as or even within a month of taking another type of medicine called a *monoamine oxidase inhibitor* (MAOI), such as selegiline (Eldepryl), phenelzine (Nardil), tranylcypromine (Parnate), or isocarboxazid (Marplan).

Fluoxetine can be taken with or without food.

Caffeine may increase side effects of fluoxetine.

What Could Happen if This Medicine Is Stopped Suddenly?

No known serious medical effects occur if fluoxetine is stopped suddenly, but there may be uncomfortable feelings, which should be avoided if possible. Your child might have trouble sleeping, nervousness, irritability, dizziness, and flu-like symptoms. Ask the doctor before stopping fluoxetine or if these symptoms happen while the dose is being decreased.

How Long Will This Medicine Be Needed?

Fluoxetine may take up to 1–2 months to reach its full effect. If your child has a good response to fluoxetine, it is a good idea to continue the medicine for at least 6–12 months. It is important to review this with your doctor.

What Else Should I Know About This Medicine?

In youth who have bipolar disorder or who may be at risk for bipolar disorder, any antidepressant medicine may increase the risk of hypomania or mania (excitement, agitation, increased activity, decreased sleep).

In hot weather, make sure your child drinks enough water or other liquids and does not get overheated.

Sometimes, after a person has improved while taking fluoxetine, he or she loses interest in school or friends or just stops trying. Please tell your child's doctor if this happens—it may be a side effect of the medicine. A lower dose or a different medicine may be needed.

Store the medicine away from sunlight, heat, moisture, and humidity.

Fluoxetine (Prozac) and fluvoxamine (Luvox) are sometimes confused. Be sure to check the medicine when you get it from the pharmacy.

Black Box Antidepressant Warning

In 2004, an advisory committee to the FDA decided that there might be an increased risk of suicidal behavior for some youth taking medicines called *antidepressants*. In the research studies that the committee reviewed, about 3%–4% of youth with depression who took an antidepressant medicine—and 1%–2% of youth with depression who took a placebo (pill without active medicine)—talked about suicidal thoughts (thinking about killing themselves or wishing they were dead) or did something to harm themselves. This means that almost twice as many youth who were taking an antidepressant to treat their depression talked about suicide or had suicidal behavior compared with youth with depression who were taking inactive medicine. There were *no* completed suicides in any of these research studies, which included more than 4,000 children and adolescents. For youth being treated for anxiety, there was no difference in suicidal talking or behavior between those taking antidepressant medication and those taking placebo.

The FDA told drug companies to add a *black box warning* label to all antidepressant medicines. Because of this label, a doctor (or advanced practice nurse) prescribing one of these medicines has to warn youth and their families that there might be more suicidal thoughts and actions in youth taking these medicines.

On the other hand, in places where more youth are taking the newer antidepressant medicines, the number of adolescents who commit suicide has gotten smaller. Also, thinking about or attempting suicide is more common in surveys of teenagers in the community than it is in depressed youth treated in research studies with antidepressant medicine.

If a youth is being treated with this medicine and is doing well, then no changes are needed as a result of this warning. Increased suicidal talk or action is most likely to happen in the first few months of treatment with a medicine. If your child has recently started this medicine or is about to start, then you and your doctor (or advanced practice nurse) should watch for any changes in behavior. People who are depressed often have suicidal thoughts or actions. It is hard to know whether suicidal thoughts or actions in depressed people are caused by the depression itself or by the medicine. Also, as their depression is getting better, some people talk more about the suicidal thoughts that they had before but did not talk about. As young people get better from depression, they might be at higher risk of doing something about suicidal thoughts that they have had for some time, because they have more energy.

What Should a Parent Do?

1. Be honest with your child about possible risks and benefits of medicine.

2. Talk to your child about whether he or she is having any suicidal thoughts, and tell your child to come to you if he or she is having such thoughts.

3. You, your child, and your child's doctor or nurse should develop a safety plan. Pick adults whom your child can tell if he or she is thinking about suicide.

4. Be sure to tell your child's doctor, nurse, or therapist if you suspect that your child is using alcohol or drugs or if something has happened that might make your child feel worse, such as a family separation, breaking up with a boyfriend or girlfriend, someone close dying or attempting suicide, physical or sexual abuse, or failure in school.

5. Be sure that there are no guns in the home and that all medicines (including over-the-counter medicines like Tylenol) are closely supervised by an adult and kept in a safe place.

6. Watch for new or worse thoughts of suicide, self-harm, depression, anxiety (nerves), feeling very agitated or restless, being angry or aggressive, having more trouble sleeping, or anything else that you see for the first time, seems worse, or worries your child or you. If these appear, contact a mental health professional **right away.** Do not just stop or change the dose of the medicine on your own. If the problems are serious, and you cannot reach one of your clinicians, call a 24-hour psychiatry emergency telephone number or take your child to an emergency room.

Youth taking antidepressant medicine should be watched carefully by their parent(s), clinician(s) (doctor, advanced practice nurse, nurse, therapist), and other concerned adults for the first weeks of treatment. It is a good idea to have regular contact with the doctor, APN, nurse, or therapist for the first months to check for feelings of depression or sadness, thoughts of killing or harming himself or herself, and any problems with the medication. If you have questions, be sure to ask the doctor, APN, nurse, or therapist.

For more information, see http://www.parentsmedguide.org/.

Notes

Use this space to take notes or to write down questions you want to ask the doctor.

_____

_____

_____

_____

_____

_____

_____

_____

_____

_____

_____

_____

From Dulcan MK, Ballard R (editors): _Helping Parents and Teachers Understand Medications for Behavioral and Emotional Problems: A Resource Book of Medication Information Handouts_, Fourth Edition. Washington, DC, American Psychiatric Publishing, 2015

Medication Information for Parents and Teachers

Fluphenazine

General Information About Medication

Each child and adolescent is different. No one has exactly the same combination of medical and psychological problems. It is a good idea to talk with the doctor or nurse about the reasons a medicine is being used. It is very important to keep all appointments and to be in touch by telephone if you have concerns. It is important to communicate with the doctor, nurse, or therapist. An *advanced practice nurse* (APN) has additional education and training after becoming a registered nurse (RN). Your child's medication may be prescribed by a medical doctor (MD or DO) or an APN. In addition, a *physician assistant* (PA) working with a physician may prescribe certain medications. In this information sheet, "doctor" includes medical doctors as well as APNs and PAs who prescribe medication. Often a nurse (RN) will be part of the team and answer questions and give information.

It is very important that the medicine be taken exactly as the doctor instructs. However, once in a while, everyone forgets to give a medicine on time. It is a good idea to ask the doctor or nurse what to do if this happens. Do not stop or change a medicine without asking the doctor or nurse first.

If the medicine seems to stop working, it may be because it is not being taken regularly. The youth may be "cheeking" or hiding the medicine or forgetting to take it (especially at school). The doses may be too far apart or a different dose or medicine may be needed. Something at school, at home, or in the neighborhood may be upsetting the youth, or he or she may need special help for learning disabilities or tutoring. Please discuss your concerns with the doctor. **Do not just increase the dose.** It is also very important not to decrease the dose or stop the medicine without talking to the doctor first. The problem being treated may come back, or there could be uncomfortable or even dangerous results.

All medicines should be kept in a safe place, out of the reach of children, and should be supervised by an adult. If someone takes too much of a medicine, call the doctor, the poison control center, or a hospital emergency room.

Each medicine has a "generic" or chemical name. Just like laundry detergents or paper towels, some medicines are sold by more than one company under different brand names. The same medicine may be available under a generic name and several brand names. The generic medications are usually less expensive than the brand name ones. The generic medications have the same chemical formula, but they may or may not be exactly the same strength as the brand-name medications. Also, some brands of pills contain dye or other things that can cause allergic reactions. It is a good idea to talk to the doctor and the pharmacist about whether it is important to use a specific brand of medicine.

Any medicine can cause an allergic reaction. Examples are hives, itching, rashes, swelling, and trouble breathing. Even a tiny amount of a medicine can cause a reaction in patients who are allergic to that medicine. Be *sure* to talk to the doctor before restarting a medicine that has caused an allergic reaction and tell the doctor about any reactions to medicine that your child has had before.

Taking more than one medicine at the same time may cause more side effects or cause one of the medicines to not work as well. Always ask the doctor, nurse, or pharmacist before adding another

199

medicine, either prescription or bought without a prescription in a store or on the Internet. **Be sure that each doctor knows about *all* of the medicines your child is taking. Also tell the doctor about any vitamins, herbal medicines, or supplements your child may be taking.** Some of these may have side effects alone or when taken with this medication. It is a very good idea to keep a list with you of the names and doses of all medicines that your child is taking.

Everyone taking medicine should have a physical examination at least once a year.

If you think that your child may be using drugs or alcohol, please tell the doctor right away.

Pregnancy requires special care in the use of medicine. Some medicines can cause birth defects if taken by a pregnant mother. **Please tell the doctor immediately if you suspect the teenager is at risk of becoming pregnant.** The doctor may wish to discuss sexual behavior and/or birth control with your daughter.

Printed information like this applies to children and adolescents in general. If you have questions about the medicine, or if you notice changes or anything unusual, please ask the doctor or nurse. As scientific research advances, knowledge increases and advice changes. Even experts do not always agree. Many medicines have not been "approved" by the U.S. Food and Drug Administration (FDA) for use in children or use for particular problems. For this reason, use of the medicine for a problem or age group often is not listed in the *Physicians' Desk Reference*. This does not necessarily mean that the medicine is dangerous or does not work, only that the company that makes the medicine has not received permission to advertise the medicine for use in children. Companies often do not apply for this permission because it is expensive to do the tests needed to apply for approval for use in children. Once a medication is approved by the FDA for any purpose, a doctor is allowed to prescribe it according to research and clinical experience.

Note to Teachers

It is a good idea to talk with the parent(s) about the reason(s) that a medication is being used. If the parent(s) sign consent to release information, it is often helpful for you to talk with the doctor. If the parent(s) give permission, the doctor may ask you to fill out rating forms about your experience with the student's behavior, feelings, academic performance, and medication side effects. This information is very useful in selecting and monitoring medication treatment. If you have observations that you think are important, do not hesitate to share these with the student's parent(s) and treating clinicians (with parental consent).

It is very important that the medicine be taken exactly as the doctor instructs. However, everyone forgets to give a medicine on time once in a while. It is a good idea to ask the parent(s) in advance what to do if this happens. Do not stop or change the time you are giving a medicine at school without parental permission. If a medication is to be taken with food, but lunchtime or snack time changes, be sure to notify the parent(s) so appropriate adjustments can be made.

All medicines should be kept in a secure place and should be supervised by an adult. If someone takes too much of a medicine, follow your school procedure for an urgent medical problem.

Taking medicine is a private matter and is best managed discreetly and confidentially. It is important to be sensitive to the student's feelings about taking medicine.

If you suspect that the student is using drugs or alcohol, please tell the parent(s) or a school counselor right away.

Please tell the parent(s) or school nurse if you suspect medication side effects.

Modifications of the classroom environment or assignments may be useful in addition to medication. The student may need to be evaluated for additional help or a 504 plan or an Individualized Education Plan for learning problems or emotional or behavioral issues.

Any expression of suicidal thoughts or feelings or self-harm by a child or adolescent is a signal of distress and should be taken seriously. These behaviors should not be dismissed as "attention seeking." School procedures for safety issues should be followed.

What Is Fluphenazine?

Fluphenazine is sometimes called a *typical, conventional,* or *first-generation antipsychotic* medicine. It is also called a *neuroleptic* or *phenothiazine.* It used to be called a *major tranquilizer.* It used to come in brand name Prolixin. Now it comes in generic tablets, liquid, and two kinds of shots (injections): immediate-acting and very long-acting (fluphenazine decanoate).

How Can This Medicine Help?

Fluphenazine is used to treat psychosis, such as in schizophrenia, mania, or very severe depression. It can reduce hallucinations (hearing voices or seeing things that are not there) and delusions (troubling beliefs that other people do not share). It can help the patient be less upset and agitated. It can improve the patient's ability to think clearly.

Sometimes fluphenazine is used to decrease severe aggression or very serious behavioral problems in young people with conduct disorder, intellectual disability, or autism spectrum disorder.

This medicine is very powerful and should be used to treat very serious problems or symptoms that other medicines do not help. Be patient; the positive effects of this medicine may not appear for 2–3 weeks.

How Does This Medicine Work?

Cells in the brain (neurons) communicate using chemicals called *neurotransmitters.* Too much or too little of these substances in certain parts of the brain can cause problems. Fluphenazine reduces the activity of one of these neurotransmitters, *dopamine.* Blocking the effect of dopamine in certain parts of the brain reduces what have been called *positive symptoms* of psychosis: delusions; hallucinations; disorganized and unusual thinking, speaking, and behavior; excessive activity (agitation); and lack of activity (catatonia). Blocking dopamine can also reduce tics. Reducing dopamine action in other parts of the brain may lead to the side effects of this medicine.

How Long Does This Medicine Last?

Fluphenazine usually may be taken only once a day, unless divided doses are used to lessen side effects. An injection of fluphenazine decanoate lasts for 2–3 weeks.

How Will the Doctor Monitor This Medicine?

The doctor will review your child's medical history and physical examination before starting fluphenazine. The doctor may order some blood or urine tests to be sure your child does not have a hidden medical condition. The doctor or nurse may measure your child's pulse and blood pressure before starting fluphenazine.

Before your child starts taking fluphenazine and every so often afterward, a test such as the AIMS (Abnormal Involuntary Movement Scale) may be used to check your child's tongue, legs, and arms for unusual movements that could be caused by the medicine.

After the medicine is started, the doctor will want to have regular appointments with you and your child to see how the medicine is working, to see if a dose change is needed, to watch for side effects, to see if fluphenazine is still needed, and to see if any other treatment is needed. The doctor or nurse may check your child's height, weight, pulse, and blood pressure, and watch for abnormal movements.

What Side Effects Can This Medicine Have?

Any medicine can have side effects, including an allergy to the medicine. Because each patient is different, the doctor will monitor the youth closely, especially when the medicine is started. The doctor will work with you to increase the positive effects and decrease the negative effects of the medicine. Please tell the doctor if any of the listed side effects appear or if you think that the medicine is causing any other problems. Not all of the rare or unusual side effects are listed.

Side effects are most common after starting the medicine or after a dose increase. Many side effects can be avoided or lessened by starting with a very low dose and increasing it slowly—ask the doctor.

Allergic Reaction

Tell the doctor in a day or two (if possible, before the next dose of medicine):

- Hives
- Itching
- Rash

Stop the medicine and get *immediate* medical care:

- Trouble breathing or chest tightness
- Swelling of lips, tongue, or throat

Common, but Not Usually Serious, Side Effects

Discuss the following side effects with your child's doctor within a week or two. They often can be helped by lowering the dose of medicine, changing the times medicine is taken, or adding another medicine.

- Dry mouth—Have your child try using sugar-free gum or candy.
- Constipation—Encourage your child to drink more fluids and eat high-fiber foods; if necessary, a fiber medicine such as Benefiber or a stool softener such as Colace or mineral oil may be used.
- Mild trouble urinating
- Blurred vision
- Weight gain—Seek nutritional counseling; provide your child with low-calorie snacks and encourage regular exercise.
- Sadness, irritability, nervousness, clinginess, not wanting to go to school
- Restlessness or inability to sit still
- Shaking of hands and fingers

Less Common, but Not Usually Serious, Side Effects

Discuss the following side effects with your child's doctor within a week or two. They often can be helped by lowering the dose of medicine, changing the times medicine is taken, or adding another medicine.

- Daytime sleepiness or tiredness—Do not allow your child to drive, ride a bicycle or motorcycle, or operate machinery if this happens. This problem may be lessened by taking the medicine at bedtime.
- Dizziness—This side effect is worse when the child stands up quickly, especially when getting out of bed in the morning; try having the child stand up slowly.
- Decreased or slowed movement and decreased facial expressions
- Drooling
- Decreased sexual interest or ability
- Changes in menstrual cycle
- Increase in breast size or discharge from the breasts (in both boys and girls)—This may go away with time.

Less Common, but Potentially Serious, Side Effects

Call the doctor or go to an emergency room *right away:*

- Stiffness of the tongue, jaw, neck, back, or legs
- Overheating or heatstroke—Prevent by decreasing activity in hot weather, staying out of the sun, and drinking water.
- Seizure (fit, convulsion)—This is more likely in people with a history of seizures or head injury.
- Severe confusion

Serious, but Rare, Side Effects

- Extreme stiffness or lack of movement, very high fever, mental confusion, irregular pulse rate, or eye pain—**This is a medical emergency. Go to an emergency room** *right away.*
- Sudden stiffness and inability to breathe or swallow—**Go to an emergency room or call 911.** Tell the paramedics, nurses, and doctors that the patient is taking fluphenazine. Other medicines can be used to treat this problem fast.
- Increased thirst, frequent urination, lethargy, tiredness, dizziness—These could be signs of diabetes (especially if your child is overweight or there is a family history of diabetes). **Talk to a doctor within a day.**

What Else Should I Know About Side Effects?

Most side effects lessen over time. If they are troublesome, talk with your child's doctor. Some side effects can be decreased by taking a smaller dose of medicine, by stopping the medicine, by changing to another medicine, or by adding another medicine.

One side effect that may not go away is *tardive dyskinesia* (or TD). Patients with tardive dyskinesia have involuntary movements of the body, especially the mouth and tongue. The patient may look as though he or she is making faces over and over again. Jerky movements of the arms, legs, or body may occur. There may be fine, wormlike, or sudden repeated movements of the tongue, or the person may appear to be chewing something or smacking or puckering his or her lips. The fingers may look as though they are rolling something. If you notice any unusual movements, be sure to tell the doctor. The doctor may use the AIMS test to look for these movements.

The medicine may increase the level of *prolactin*, a natural hormone made in the part of the brain called the *pituitary*. This may cause side effects such as breast tenderness or swelling or production of milk, in both boys and girls. It also may interfere with sexual functioning in teenage boys and with regular menstrual cycles (periods) in teenage girls. A blood test can measure the level of prolactin. If these side effects do not go away and are troublesome, talk with your child's doctor about substituting another medicine for fluphenazine.

Heart problems are more common if other medicines are being taken also. Be sure to tell your child's doctors and your pharmacist about all medications your child is taking.

Neuroleptic malignant syndrome is a very rare side effect that can lead to death. The symptoms are severe muscle stiffness, high fever, increased heart rate and blood pressure, irregular heartbeat (pulse), and sweating. It may lead to unconsciousness. If you suspect this, **call 911 or go to an emergency room right away.**

Some Interactions With Other Medicines or Food

Please note that the following are only the most likely interactions with other medicines or food.

Fluphenazine may be taken with or without food. If the medicine causes stomach upset, taking it with food may help.

Fluoxetine (Prozac) or paroxetine (Paxil) may increase the levels of fluphenazine, increasing the risk of side effects.

It is better to limit drinks with caffeine (coffee, tea, soft drinks) because caffeine works in the opposite way from this medicine, and the positive effects might be decreased.

What Could Happen if This Medicine Is Stopped Suddenly?

Involuntary movements, or *withdrawal dyskinesias*, may appear within 1–4 weeks of lowering the dose or stopping the medicine. Usually these go away, but they can last for days to months. If fluphenazine is stopped suddenly, emotional problems such as irritability, nervousness, or moodiness; behavior problems; or physical problems such as stomachache, loss of appetite, nausea, vomiting, diarrhea, sweating, indigestion, trouble sleeping, trembling, or shaking may appear. These problems usually last only a few days to a few weeks. If they happen, tell your child's doctor. The medicine dose may need to be lowered more slowly (tapered). Always check with the doctor before stopping a medicine.

How Long Will This Medicine Be Needed?

How long your child will need to be on fluphenazine depends partly on the reason that it was prescribed. Some problems last for only a few months, whereas others last much longer. Sometimes fluphenazine is used for only a short time until other medicines or behavioral treatments start to work. Some people need to take fluphenazine for years. It is especially important with medicines as powerful as this one to ask the doctor whether it is still needed. Every few months, you should discuss with your child's doctor the reasons for using fluphenazine and whether it is time for a trial of lowering the dose.

What Else Should I Know About This Medicine?

There are many older and newer medicines that are used for the same kinds of problems. If your child is having bad side effects or the medicine does not seem to be working, ask the doctor if another medicine in this group might work as well or better and have fewer side effects for your child.

Be sure to tell the doctor if there is anyone in your family who died suddenly or had a heart problem.

Sometimes this medicine can cause a *dystonic reaction*. This is a sudden stiffening of the muscles, most often in the jaw, neck, tongue, face, or shoulders. If this happens, and your child is not having trouble breathing, you may give a dose of diphenhydramine (Benadryl). Follow the dose instructions on the package for your child's age. This should relax the muscles in a few minutes. Then call your doctor to tell him or her what happened. If the muscles do not relax, take your child to the emergency department.

Notes

Use this space to take notes or to write down questions you want to ask the doctor.

_____

_____

_____

_____

_____

_____

_____

_____

_____

From Dulcan MK, Ballard R (editors): *Helping Parents and Teachers Understand Medications for Behavioral and Emotional Problems: A Resource Book of Medication Information Handouts,* Fourth Edition. Washington, DC, American Psychiatric Publishing, 2015

Medication Information for Parents and Teachers

Fluvoxamine—Luvox CR

General Information About Medication

Each child and adolescent is different. No one has exactly the same combination of medical and psychological problems. It is a good idea to talk with the doctor or nurse about the reasons a medicine is being used. It is very important to keep all appointments and to be in touch by telephone if you have concerns. It is important to communicate with the doctor, nurse, or therapist. An *advanced practice nurse* (APN) has additional education and training after becoming a registered nurse (RN). Your child's medication may be prescribed by a medical doctor (MD or DO) or an APN. In addition, a *physician assistant* (PA) working with a physician may prescribe certain medications. In this information sheet, "doctor" includes medical doctors as well as APNs and PAs who prescribe medication. Often a nurse (RN) will be part of the team and answer questions and give information.

It is very important that the medicine be taken exactly as the doctor instructs. However, once in a while, everyone forgets to give a medicine on time. It is a good idea to ask the doctor or nurse what to do if this happens. Do not stop or change a medicine without asking the doctor or nurse first.

If the medicine seems to stop working, it may be because it is not being taken regularly. The youth may be "cheeking" or hiding the medicine or forgetting to take it (especially at school). The doses may be too far apart or a different dose or medicine may be needed. Something at school, at home, or in the neighborhood may be upsetting the youth, or he or she may need special help for learning disabilities or tutoring. Please discuss your concerns with the doctor. **Do not just increase the dose.** It is also very important not to decrease the dose or stop the medicine without talking to the doctor first. The problem being treated may come back, or there could be uncomfortable or even dangerous results.

All medicines should be kept in a safe place, out of the reach of children, and should be supervised by an adult. If someone takes too much of a medicine, call the doctor, the poison control center, or a hospital emergency room.

Each medicine has a "generic" or chemical name. Just like laundry detergents or paper towels, some medicines are sold by more than one company under different brand names. The same medicine may be available under a generic name and several brand names. The generic medications are usually less expensive than the brand name ones. The generic medications have the same chemical formula, but they may or may not be exactly the same strength as the brand-name medications. Also, some brands of pills contain dye or other things that can cause allergic reactions. It is a good idea to talk to the doctor and the pharmacist about whether it is important to use a specific brand of medicine.

Any medicine can cause an allergic reaction. Examples are hives, itching, rashes, swelling, and trouble breathing. Even a tiny amount of a medicine can cause a reaction in patients who are allergic to that medicine. Be *sure* to talk to the doctor before restarting a medicine that has caused an allergic reaction and tell the doctor about any reactions to medicine that your child has had before.

Taking more than one medicine at the same time may cause more side effects or cause one of the medicines to not work as well. Always ask the doctor, nurse, or pharmacist before adding another

medicine, either prescription or bought without a prescription in a store or on the Internet. **Be sure that each doctor knows about** *all* **of the medicines your child is taking. Also tell the doctor about any vitamins, herbal medicines, or supplements your child may be taking.** Some of these may have side effects alone or when taken with this medication. It is a very good idea to keep a list with you of the names and doses of all medicines that your child is taking.

Everyone taking medicine should have a physical examination at least once a year.

If you think that your child may be using drugs or alcohol, please tell the doctor right away.

Pregnancy requires special care in the use of medicine. Some medicines can cause birth defects if taken by a pregnant mother. **Please tell the doctor immediately if you suspect the teenager is at risk of becoming pregnant.** The doctor may wish to discuss sexual behavior and/or birth control with your daughter.

Printed information like this applies to children and adolescents in general. If you have questions about the medicine, or if you notice changes or anything unusual, please ask the doctor or nurse. As scientific research advances, knowledge increases and advice changes. Even experts do not always agree. Many medicines have not been "approved" by the U.S. Food and Drug Administration (FDA) for use in children or use for particular problems. For this reason, use of the medicine for a problem or age group often is not listed in the *Physicians' Desk Reference*. This does not necessarily mean that the medicine is dangerous or does not work, only that the company that makes the medicine has not received permission to advertise the medicine for use in children. Companies often do not apply for this permission because it is expensive to do the tests needed to apply for approval for use in children. Once a medication is approved by the FDA for any purpose, a doctor is allowed to prescribe it according to research and clinical experience.

Note to Teachers

It is a good idea to talk with the parent(s) about the reason(s) that a medication is being used. If the parent(s) sign consent to release information, it is often helpful for you to talk with the doctor. If the parent(s) give permission, the doctor may ask you to fill out rating forms about your experience with the student's behavior, feelings, academic performance, and medication side effects. This information is very useful in selecting and monitoring medication treatment. If you have observations that you think are important, do not hesitate to share these with the student's parent(s) and treating clinicians (with parental consent).

It is very important that the medicine be taken exactly as the doctor instructs. However, everyone forgets to give a medicine on time once in a while. It is a good idea to ask the parent(s) in advance what to do if this happens. Do not stop or change the time you are giving a medicine at school without parental permission. If a medication is to be taken with food, but lunchtime or snack time changes, be sure to notify the parent(s) so appropriate adjustments can be made.

All medicines should be kept in a secure place and should be supervised by an adult. If someone takes too much of a medicine, follow your school procedure for an urgent medical problem.

Taking medicine is a private matter and is best managed discreetly and confidentially. It is important to be sensitive to the student's feelings about taking medicine.

If you suspect that the student is using drugs or alcohol, please tell the parent(s) or a school counselor right away.

Please tell the parent(s) or school nurse if you suspect medication side effects.

Modifications of the classroom environment or assignments may be useful in addition to medication. The student may need to be evaluated for additional help or a 504 plan or an Individualized Education Plan for learning problems or emotional or behavioral issues.

Any expression of suicidal thoughts or feelings or self-harm by a child or adolescent is a signal of distress and should be taken seriously. These behaviors should not be dismissed as "attention seeking." School procedures for safety issues should be followed.

What Is Fluvoxamine (Luvox CR)?

Fluvoxamine is an antidepressant known as a *selective serotonin reuptake inhibitor* (SSRI). It comes in generic tablets and brand name Luvox CR and generic extended-release capsules (developed for use in adults). It used to come in brand name Luvox.

How Can This Medicine Help?

Fluvoxamine is used to treat depression and anxiety disorders such as obsessive-compulsive disorder (OCD), posttraumatic stress disorder (PTSD), panic disorder, separation anxiety disorder, selective mutism, social anxiety disorder, and generalized anxiety disorder.

How Does This Medicine Work?

Fluvoxamine increases the amount of a *neurotransmitter* called *serotonin* in certain parts of the brain. People with emotional and behavioral problems, such as depression and anxiety, may have low levels of serotonin in certain parts of the brain. SSRIs such as fluvoxamine help by increasing the action of brain serotonin to more normal levels.

How Long Does This Medicine Last?

Fluvoxamine can be taken only once a day, although at higher doses it should be divided into two daily doses to lessen side effects.

How Will the Doctor Monitor This Medicine?

The doctor will review your child's medical history and physical examination before starting fluvoxamine. The doctor may order some blood or urine tests to be sure your child does not have a hidden medical condition that would make it unsafe to use this medicine. Extra care is needed when using SSRIs in youth with seizures (epilepsy); heart, liver, or kidney problems; or diabetes. The doctor or nurse may measure your child's pulse, blood pressure, and weight before starting the medicine.

Be sure to tell the doctor if your child or anyone in the family has bipolar disorder or has tried to kill himself or herself.

After the medicine is started, the doctor will want to have regular appointments with you and your child to see how the medicine is working, to see if a dose change is needed, to watch for side effects, to see if fluvoxamine is still needed, and to see if any other treatment is needed. The doctor or nurse may check your child's height, weight, pulse, and blood pressure.

Before using medicine and at times afterward, the doctor may ask your child to fill out a rating scale about depression or anxiety to help see how your child is doing.

What Side Effects Can This Medicine Have?

Any medicine can have side effects, including an allergy to the medicine. Because each patient is different, the doctor will monitor the youth closely, especially when the medicine is started. The doctor will work with you to increase the positive effects and decrease the negative effects of the medicine. Please tell the doctor if any of the listed side effects appear or if you think that the medicine is causing any other problems. Not all of the rare or unusual side effects are listed.

Side effects are most common after starting the medicine or after a dose increase. Many side effects can be avoided or lessened by starting with a very low dose and increasing it slowly—ask the doctor.

Allergic Reaction

Tell the doctor in a day or two (if possible, before the next dose of medicine):

- Hives
- Itching
- Rash

Stop the medicine and get *immediate* medical care:

- Trouble breathing or chest tightness
- Swelling of lips, tongue, or throat

Common Side Effects

Tell the doctor within a week or two, or sooner if the problems are getting worse:

- Nausea, upset stomach, vomiting
- Diarrhea or excessive gas
- Dry mouth—Have your child try using sugar-free gum or candy.
- Constipation—Encourage your child to drink more fluids and eat high-fiber foods; if necessary, the doctor may recommend a fiber medicine such as Benefiber or a stool softener such as Colace or mineral oil.
- Headache
- Anxiety or nervousness
- Insomnia (trouble sleeping)
- Restlessness, increased activity level
- Daytime sleepiness or tiredness—Do not allow your child to drive, ride a bicycle or motorcycle, or operate machinery if this side effect is present.
- Dizziness—This side effect is worse when the child stands up quickly, especially when getting out of bed in the morning; try having the child stand up slowly.
- Tremor (shakiness)
- Excessive sweating
- Apathy, lack of interest in school or friends—This may happen after an initial good response to treatment.
- Decreased sexual interest, trouble with sexual functioning
- Weight gain
- Weight loss

Less Common, but More Serious, Side Effects

Call the doctor within a day or two:

- Significant suicidal thoughts or self-injurious behavior
- Increased activity, rapid speech, feeling "speeded up," decreased need for sleep, being very excited or irritable (cranky), agitation, acting out of character
- Bleeding, such as bruising or nosebleeds, or bleeding with surgery

Serious Side Effects

Call the doctor *immediately* or go to the nearest emergency room:

- Seizure (fit, convulsion)
- Stiffness, high fever, confusion, tremors (shaking)
- Overheating or heatstroke—Prevent by decreasing activity in hot weather, staying out of the sun, and drinking water.

Serotonin Syndrome

A very serious side effect called *serotonin syndrome* can happen when certain kinds of medicines (including SSRI antidepressants, clomipramine, and other medicines, such as triptans for migraine headaches, buspirone, linezolid, tramadol, or St. John's wort) are taken by the same person. Very rarely, serotonin syndrome can happen at high doses of just one medicine. The early signs are restlessness, confusion, shaking, skin turning red, sweating, muscle stiffness, sweating, and jerking of muscles. If you see these symptoms, stop the medicine and send or take the youth to an emergency room right away.

Some Interactions With Other Medicines or Food

Please note that the following are only the most likely interactions with other medicines or food.

Fluvoxamine interacts with many other prescription and over the counter medicines, including some antibiotics and other psychiatric medicines. It is especially important to tell the doctor and pharmacist about all of the medicines your child is taking or has taken in the past few months, including over-the-counter and herbal medicines. Sometimes one medicine can increase or decrease the blood level of another medicine, so that different doses are needed. Erythromycin and similar antibiotics, as well as antifungal agents such as ketoconazole, may increase levels of fluvoxamine and increase side effects. Fluvoxamine may increase the heart side effects of pimozide (Orap), so those two medicines should not be taken by the same person. Tryptophan and the herbal medicine St. John's wort also increase serotonin and can cause serious side effects if taken with fluvoxamine. Taking fluvoxamine with aspirin, nonsteroidal anti-inflammatory drugs (NSAIDs) (medications including ibuprofen or naproxen), or anticoagulant medications (including warfarin) increases risk of abnormal bleeding. Taking fluvoxamine with clozapine may increase levels of clozapine and increase side effects, especially sedation or seizures.

It can be *very dangerous* to take an SSRI at the same time as or even within a month of taking another type of medicine called a *monoamine oxidase inhibitor* (MAOI), such as selegiline (Eldepryl), phenelzine (Nardil), tranylcypromine (Parnate), or isocarboxazid (Marplan).

Fluvoxamine can be taken with or without food.

Caffeine may increase side effects.

What Could Happen if This Medicine Is Stopped Suddenly?

No known serious medical effects occur if fluvoxamine is stopped suddenly, but there may be uncomfortable feelings, which should be avoided if possible. Your child might have trouble sleeping, nervousness, irritability, dizziness, and flu-like symptoms. Ask the doctor before stopping fluvoxamine or if these symptoms happen while the dose is being decreased.

How Long Will This Medicine Be Needed?

Fluvoxamine may take up to 1–2 months to reach its full effect. If your child has a good response to fluvoxamine, it is a good idea to continue the medicine for at least 6–12 months. It is important to review this with your doctor.

What Else Should I Know About This Medicine?

In youth who have bipolar disorder or who may be at risk for bipolar disorder, any antidepressant medicine may increase the risk of hypomania or mania (excitement, agitation, increased activity, decreased sleep).

In hot weather, make sure your child drinks enough water or other liquids and does not get overheated.

Sometimes, after a person has improved while taking fluvoxamine, he or she loses interest in school or friends or just stops trying. Please tell your child's doctor if this happens—it may be a side effect of the medicine. A lower dose or a different medicine may be needed.

Store the medicine away from sunlight, heat, moisture, and humidity.

Fluoxetine (Prozac) and fluvoxamine (Luvox) are sometimes confused. Be sure to check the medicine when you get it from the pharmacy.

Black Box Antidepressant Warning

In 2004, an advisory committee to the FDA decided that there might be an increased risk of suicidal behavior for some youth taking medicines called *antidepressants*. In the research studies that the committee reviewed, about 3%–4% of youth with depression who took an antidepressant medicine—and 1%–2% of youth with depression who took a placebo (pill without active medicine)—talked about suicidal thoughts (thinking about killing themselves or wishing they were dead) or did something to harm themselves. This means that almost twice as many youth who were taking an antidepressant to treat their depression talked about suicide or had suicidal behavior compared with youth with depression who were taking inactive medicine. There were *no* completed suicides in any of these research studies, which included more than 4,000 children and adolescents. For youth being treated for anxiety, there was no difference in suicidal talking or behavior between those taking antidepressant medication and those taking placebo.

The FDA told drug companies to add a *black box warning* label to all antidepressant medicines. Because of this label, a doctor (or advanced practice nurse) prescribing one of these medicines has to warn youth and their families that there might be more suicidal thoughts and actions in youth taking these medicines.

On the other hand, in places where more youth are taking the newer antidepressant medicines, the number of adolescents who commit suicide has gotten smaller. Also, thinking about or attempting suicide is more common in surveys of teenagers in the community than it is in depressed youth treated in research studies with antidepressant medicine.

If a youth is being treated with this medicine and is doing well, then no changes are needed as a result of this warning. Increased suicidal talk or action is most likely to happen in the first few months of treatment with a medicine. If your child has recently started this medicine or is about to start, then you and your doctor (or advanced practice nurse) should watch for any changes in behavior. People who are depressed often have suicidal thoughts or actions. It is hard to know whether suicidal thoughts or actions in depressed people are caused by the depression itself or by the medicine. Also, as their depression is getting better, some people talk more about the suicidal thoughts that they had before but did not talk about. As young people get better from depression, they might be at higher risk of doing something about suicidal thoughts that they have had for some time, because they have more energy.

What Should a Parent Do?

1. Be honest with your child about possible risks and benefits of medicine.
2. Talk to your child about whether he or she is having any suicidal thoughts, and tell your child to come to you if he or she is having such thoughts.
3. You, your child, and your child's doctor or nurse should develop a safety plan. Pick adults whom your child can tell if he or she is thinking about suicide.
4. Be sure to tell your child's doctor, nurse, or therapist if you suspect that your child is using alcohol or drugs or if something has happened that might make your child feel worse, such as a family separation, breaking up with a boyfriend or girlfriend, someone close dying or attempting suicide, physical or sexual abuse, or failure in school.
5. Be sure that there are no guns in the home and that all medicines (including over-the-counter medicines like Tylenol) are closely supervised by an adult and kept in a safe place.
6. Watch for new or worse thoughts of suicide, self-harm, depression, anxiety (nerves), feeling very agitated or restless, being angry or aggressive, having more trouble sleeping, or anything else that you see for the first time, seems worse, or worries your child or you. If these appear, contact a mental health professional **right away.** Do not just stop or change the dose of the medicine on your own. If the problems are serious, and you cannot reach one of your clinicians, call a 24-hour psychiatry emergency telephone number or take your child to an emergency room.

Youth taking antidepressant medicine should be watched carefully by their parent(s), clinician(s) (doctor, advanced practice nurse, nurse, therapist), and other concerned adults for the first weeks of treatment. It is a good idea to have regular contact with the doctor, APN, nurse, or therapist for the first months to check for feelings of depression or sadness, thoughts of killing or harming himself or herself, and any problems with the medication. If you have questions, be sure to ask the doctor, APN, nurse, or therapist.

For more information, see http://www.parentsmedguide.org/.

Notes

Use this space to take notes or to write down questions you want to ask the doctor.

_____

_____

_____

_____

_____

_____

_____

_____

_____

_____

Gabapentin—Neurontin, Gralise, Gralise Starter

General Information About Medication

Each child and adolescent is different. No one has exactly the same combination of medical and psychological problems. It is a good idea to talk with the doctor or nurse about the reasons a medicine is being used. It is very important to keep all appointments and to be in touch by telephone if you have concerns. It is important to communicate with the doctor, nurse, or therapist. An *advanced practice nurse* (APN) has additional education and training after becoming a registered nurse (RN). Your child's medication may be prescribed by a medical doctor (MD or DO) or an APN. In addition, a *physician assistant* (PA) working with a physician may prescribe certain medications. In this information sheet, "doctor" includes medical doctors as well as APNs and PAs who prescribe medication. Often a nurse (RN) will be part of the team and answer questions and give information.

It is very important that the medicine be taken exactly as the doctor instructs. However, once in a while, everyone forgets to give a medicine on time. It is a good idea to ask the doctor or nurse what to do if this happens. Do not stop or change a medicine without asking the doctor or nurse first.

If the medicine seems to stop working, it may be because it is not being taken regularly. The youth may be "cheeking" or hiding the medicine or forgetting to take it (especially at school). The doses may be too far apart or a different dose or medicine may be needed. Something at school, at home, or in the neighborhood may be upsetting the youth, or he or she may need special help for learning disabilities or tutoring. Please discuss your concerns with the doctor. **Do not just increase the dose.** It is also very important not to decrease the dose or stop the medicine without talking to the doctor first. The problem being treated may come back, or there could be uncomfortable or even dangerous results.

All medicines should be kept in a safe place, out of the reach of children, and should be supervised by an adult. If someone takes too much of a medicine, call the doctor, the poison control center, or a hospital emergency room.

Each medicine has a "generic" or chemical name. Just like laundry detergents or paper towels, some medicines are sold by more than one company under different brand names. The same medicine may be available under a generic name and several brand names. The generic medications are usually less expensive than the brand name ones. The generic medications have the same chemical formula, but they may or may not be exactly the same strength as the brand-name medications. Also, some brands of pills contain dye or other things that can cause allergic reactions. It is a good idea to talk to the doctor and the pharmacist about whether it is important to use a specific brand of medicine.

Any medicine can cause an allergic reaction. Examples are hives, itching, rashes, swelling, and trouble breathing. Even a tiny amount of a medicine can cause a reaction in patients who are allergic to that medicine. Be *sure* to talk to the doctor before restarting a medicine that has caused an allergic reaction and tell the doctor about any reactions to medicine that your child has had before.

Taking more than one medicine at the same time may cause more side effects or cause one of the medicines to not work as well. Always ask the doctor, nurse, or pharmacist before adding another

medicine, either prescription or bought without a prescription in a store or on the Internet. **Be sure that each doctor knows about** *all* **of the medicines your child is taking. Also tell the doctor about any vitamins, herbal medicines, or supplements your child may be taking.** Some of these may have side effects alone or when taken with this medication. It is a very good idea to keep a list with you of the names and doses of all medicines that your child is taking.

Everyone taking medicine should have a physical examination at least once a year.

If you think that your child may be using drugs or alcohol, please tell the doctor right away.

Pregnancy requires special care in the use of medicine. Some medicines can cause birth defects if taken by a pregnant mother. **Please tell the doctor immediately if you suspect the teenager is at risk of becoming pregnant.** The doctor may wish to discuss sexual behavior and/or birth control with your daughter.

Printed information like this applies to children and adolescents in general. If you have questions about the medicine, or if you notice changes or anything unusual, please ask the doctor or nurse. As scientific research advances, knowledge increases and advice changes. Even experts do not always agree. Many medicines have not been "approved" by the U.S. Food and Drug Administration (FDA) for use in children or use for particular problems. For this reason, use of the medicine for a problem or age group often is not listed in the *Physicians' Desk Reference*. This does not necessarily mean that the medicine is dangerous or does not work, only that the company that makes the medicine has not received permission to advertise the medicine for use in children. Companies often do not apply for this permission because it is expensive to do the tests needed to apply for approval for use in children. Once a medication is approved by the FDA for any purpose, a doctor is allowed to prescribe it according to research and clinical experience.

Note to Teachers

It is a good idea to talk with the parent(s) about the reason(s) that a medication is being used. If the parent(s) sign consent to release information, it is often helpful for you to talk with the doctor. If the parent(s) give permission, the doctor may ask you to fill out rating forms about your experience with the student's behavior, feelings, academic performance, and medication side effects. This information is very useful in selecting and monitoring medication treatment. If you have observations that you think are important, do not hesitate to share these with the student's parent(s) and treating clinicians (with parental consent).

It is very important that the medicine be taken exactly as the doctor instructs. However, everyone forgets to give a medicine on time once in a while. It is a good idea to ask the parent(s) in advance what to do if this happens. Do not stop or change the time you are giving a medicine at school without parental permission. If a medication is to be taken with food, but lunchtime or snack time changes, be sure to notify the parent(s) so appropriate adjustments can be made.

All medicines should be kept in a secure place and should be supervised by an adult. If someone takes too much of a medicine, follow your school procedure for an urgent medical problem.

Taking medicine is a private matter and is best managed discreetly and confidentially. It is important to be sensitive to the student's feelings about taking medicine.

If you suspect that the student is using drugs or alcohol, please tell the parent(s) or a school counselor right away.

Please tell the parent(s) or school nurse if you suspect medication side effects.

Modifications of the classroom environment or assignments may be useful in addition to medication. The student may need to be evaluated for additional help or a 504 plan or an Individualized Education Plan for learning problems or emotional or behavioral issues.

Any expression of suicidal thoughts or feelings or self-harm by a child or adolescent is a signal of distress and should be taken seriously. These behaviors should not be dismissed as "attention seeking." School procedures for safety issues should be followed.

What Is Gabapentin (Neurontin, Gralise)?

Gabapentin was first used to treat seizures (fits, convulsions), so it is sometimes called an *anticonvulsant* or an *antiepileptic.* Now it is also used for behavioral problems or bipolar disorder whether or not the patient has seizures. It also may be used when the patient has a history of severe mood changes, sometimes called *mood swings.* When used in psychiatry, this medicine is more commonly called a *mood stabilizer.* It may also be used to treat chronic nerve pain or *restless leg syndrome,* when it interferes with sleep.

It comes in brand name Neurontin and generic tablets, capsules, and liquid and extended-release Gralise tablets.

How Can This Medicine Help?

Gabapentin can reduce aggression, anger, severe mood swings, and neuropathic pain (chronic severe pain from nerve problems).

How Does This Medicine Work?

Gabapentin is thought to work by stabilizing a part of the brain cell (the cell membrane or envelope) and by changing the concentrations of certain *neurotransmitters* (chemicals in the brain) such as *GABA* and *serotonin.*

How Long Does This Medicine Last?

Gabapentin needs to be taken two or three times a day. Extended-release Gralise can be taken once a day.

How Will the Doctor Monitor This Medicine?

The doctor will review your child's medical history and physical examination before starting gabapentin. The doctor may order some blood tests to be sure your child does not have a hidden kidney condition that would make it unsafe to use this medicine. The doctor or nurse may measure your child's pulse and blood pressure before starting gabapentin.

After the medicine is started, the doctor will want to have regular appointments with you and your child to see how the medicine is working, to see if a dose change is needed, to watch for side effects, to see if gabapentin is still needed, and to see if any other treatment is needed. The doctor or nurse may check your child's height, weight, pulse, and blood pressure.

What Side Effects Can This Medicine Have?

Any medicine can have side effects, including an allergy to the medicine. Because each patient is different, the doctor will monitor the youth closely, especially when the medicine is started. The doctor will work with you

to increase the positive effects and decrease the negative effects of the medicine. Please tell the doctor if any of the listed side effects appear or if you think that the medicine is causing any other problems. Not all of the rare or unusual side effects are listed.

Side effects are most common after starting the medicine or after a dose increase. Many side effects can be avoided or lessened by starting with a very low dose and increasing it slowly—ask the doctor.

Allergic Reaction

Tell the doctor in a day or two (if possible, before the next dose of medicine):

- Hives
- Itching
- Rash

Stop the medicine and get *immediate* medical care:

- Trouble breathing or chest tightness
- Swelling of lips, tongue, or throat

General Side Effects

These side effects are more common when first starting the medicine. Tell the doctor within a week or two:

- Daytime sleepiness or tiredness—Do not allow your child to drive, ride a bicycle or motorcycle, or operate machinery if this happens.
- Dizziness
- Unsteadiness
- Rapid, involuntary movements of the eyes
- Tremor
- Double vision
- Fatigue
- Muscle pain

Side Effects on Thinking, Behavior, and Emotions

Tell the doctor within a week:

- Worsening of behavioral problems
- Temper tantrums, increased irritability, anger and/or aggression
- Problems with concentration or doing schoolwork

Tell the doctor right away:

- Increased suicidal thoughts or behaviors or new or worse depression or anxiety

Some Interactions With Other Medicines or Food

Please note that the following are only the most likely interactions with other medicines or food.

Caffeine may increase side effects.

Taking gabapentin with another medicine may cause more side effects. Be sure that each doctor knows about *all* of the medicines being taken.

Antacids decrease the levels of gabapentin so that it does not work as well. Do not give antacids within 2 hours before or after gabapentin.

What Could Happen if This Medicine Is Stopped Suddenly?

Stopping gabapentin suddenly could lead to an increase in seizures or convulsions if your child is being treated for epilepsy (seizures).

How Long Will This Medicine Be Needed?

The length of time a person needs to take gabapentin depends on what problem is being treated. For example, someone with an impulse control disorder usually takes the medicine only until behavioral therapy begins to work. Someone with bipolar disorder may need to take the medicine for many years. Please ask the doctor about the length of treatment needed.

What Else Should I Know About This Medicine?

Taking gabapentin with food may decrease stomach upset.

Keep the medicine in a safe place under close supervision. Keep the pill container tightly closed and in a dry place, away from bathrooms, showers, and humidifiers.

Children with kidney problems may have more serious side effects from this medicine.

Notes

Use this space to take notes or to write down questions you want to ask the doctor.

_____

_____

_____

_____

_____

_____

_____

_____

Medication Information for Parents and Teachers

Guanfacine—Tenex, Intuniv

General Information About Medication

Each child and adolescent is different. No one has exactly the same combination of medical and psychological problems. It is a good idea to talk with the doctor or nurse about the reasons a medicine is being used. It is very important to keep all appointments and to be in touch by telephone if you have concerns. It is important to communicate with the doctor, nurse, or therapist. An *advanced practice nurse* (APN) has additional education and training after becoming a registered nurse (RN). Your child's medication may be prescribed by a medical doctor (MD or DO) or an APN. In addition, a *physician assistant* (PA) working with a physician may prescribe certain medications. In this information sheet, "doctor" includes medical doctors as well as APNs and PAs who prescribe medication. Often a nurse (RN) will be part of the team and answer questions and give information.

It is very important that the medicine be taken exactly as the doctor instructs. However, once in a while, everyone forgets to give a medicine on time. It is a good idea to ask the doctor or nurse what to do if this happens. Do not stop or change a medicine without asking the doctor or nurse first.

If the medicine seems to stop working, it may be because it is not being taken regularly. The youth may be "cheeking" or hiding the medicine or forgetting to take it (especially at school). The doses may be too far apart or a different dose or medicine may be needed. Something at school, at home, or in the neighborhood may be upsetting the youth, or he or she may need special help for learning disabilities or tutoring. Please discuss your concerns with the doctor. **Do not just increase the dose.** It is also very important not to decrease the dose or stop the medicine without talking to the doctor first. The problem being treated may come back, or there could be uncomfortable or even dangerous results.

All medicines should be kept in a safe place, out of the reach of children, and should be supervised by an adult. If someone takes too much of a medicine, call the doctor, the poison control center, or a hospital emergency room.

Each medicine has a "generic" or chemical name. Just like laundry detergents or paper towels, some medicines are sold by more than one company under different brand names. The same medicine may be available under a generic name and several brand names. The generic medications are usually less expensive than the brand name ones. The generic medications have the same chemical formula, but they may or may not be exactly the same strength as the brand-name medications. Also, some brands of pills contain dye or other things that can cause allergic reactions. It is a good idea to talk to the doctor and the pharmacist about whether it is important to use a specific brand of medicine.

Any medicine can cause an allergic reaction. Examples are hives, itching, rashes, swelling, and trouble breathing. Even a tiny amount of a medicine can cause a reaction in patients who are allergic to that medicine. Be *sure* to talk to the doctor before restarting a medicine that has caused an allergic reaction and tell the doctor about any reactions to medicine that your child has had before.

Taking more than one medicine at the same time may cause more side effects or cause one of the medicines to not work as well. Always ask the doctor, nurse, or pharmacist before adding another

medicine, either prescription or bought without a prescription in a store or on the Internet. **Be sure that each doctor knows about** *all* **of the medicines your child is taking. Also tell the doctor about any vitamins, herbal medicines, or supplements your child may be taking.** Some of these may have side effects alone or when taken with this medication. It is a very good idea to keep a list with you of the names and doses of all medicines that your child is taking.

Everyone taking medicine should have a physical examination at least once a year.

If you think that your child may be using drugs or alcohol, please tell the doctor right away.

Pregnancy requires special care in the use of medicine. Some medicines can cause birth defects if taken by a pregnant mother. **Please tell the doctor immediately if you suspect the teenager is at risk of becoming pregnant.** The doctor may wish to discuss sexual behavior and/or birth control with your daughter.

Printed information like this applies to children and adolescents in general. If you have questions about the medicine, or if you notice changes or anything unusual, please ask the doctor or nurse. As scientific research advances, knowledge increases and advice changes. Even experts do not always agree. Many medicines have not been "approved" by the U.S. Food and Drug Administration (FDA) for use in children or use for particular problems. For this reason, use of the medicine for a problem or age group often is not listed in the *Physicians' Desk Reference*. This does not necessarily mean that the medicine is dangerous or does not work, only that the company that makes the medicine has not received permission to advertise the medicine for use in children. Companies often do not apply for this permission because it is expensive to do the tests needed to apply for approval for use in children. Once a medication is approved by the FDA for any purpose, a doctor is allowed to prescribe it according to research and clinical experience.

Note to Teachers

It is a good idea to talk with the parent(s) about the reason(s) that a medication is being used. If the parent(s) sign consent to release information, it is often helpful for you to talk with the doctor. If the parent(s) give permission, the doctor may ask you to fill out rating forms about your experience with the student's behavior, feelings, academic performance, and medication side effects. This information is very useful in selecting and monitoring medication treatment. If you have observations that you think are important, do not hesitate to share these with the student's parent(s) and treating clinicians (with parental consent).

It is very important that the medicine be taken exactly as the doctor instructs. However, everyone forgets to give a medicine on time once in a while. It is a good idea to ask the parent(s) in advance what to do if this happens. Do not stop or change the time you are giving a medicine at school without parental permission. If a medication is to be taken with food, but lunchtime or snack time changes, be sure to notify the parent(s) so appropriate adjustments can be made.

All medicines should be kept in a secure place and should be supervised by an adult. If someone takes too much of a medicine, follow your school procedure for an urgent medical problem.

Taking medicine is a private matter and is best managed discreetly and confidentially. It is important to be sensitive to the student's feelings about taking medicine.

If you suspect that the student is using drugs or alcohol, please tell the parent(s) or a school counselor right away.

Please tell the parent(s) or school nurse if you suspect medication side effects.

Modifications of the classroom environment or assignments may be useful in addition to medication. The student may need to be evaluated for additional help or a 504 plan or an Individualized Education Plan for learning problems or emotional or behavioral issues.

Any expression of suicidal thoughts or feelings or self-harm by a child or adolescent is a signal of distress and should be taken seriously. These behaviors should not be dismissed as "attention seeking." School procedures for safety issues should be followed.

What Is Guanfacine (Tenex, Intuniv)?

Guanfacine was first used to treat high blood pressure, so it is sometimes called an *antihypertensive*. Now it is also used to treat symptoms of attention-deficit/hyperactivity disorder (ADHD), Tourette's disorder, chronic tics (fast, repeated movements), and aggression. It comes in brand name Tenex and generic tablets and Intuniv. Intuniv is an extended-release version of guanfacine that is used to treat symptoms of ADHD. It can be used by itself or with stimulant medications also used to treat symptoms of ADHD.

How Can This Medicine Help?

Guanfacine can decrease symptoms of hyperactivity, impulsivity, anxiety, irritability, temper tantrums, explosive anger, and tics. It can increase patience and frustration tolerance as well as improve self-control and cooperation with adults. Guanfacine may be used together with a stimulant medication (methylphenidate or amphetamine) for ADHD or with an atypical or pimozide (Orap) for Tourette's disorder. The positive effects usually do not start for 2 weeks after a stable dose is reached. The full benefit may not be seen for 2–4 months.

How Does This Medicine Work?

Guanfacine works by decreasing the level of excitement in parts of the brain. It is sometimes called an *alpha-adrenergic agonist*. It affects the levels of *norepinephrine*, one of the *neurotransmitters*—a chemical that the brain makes for nerve cells to communicate with each other. This effect helps people with tic disorders to stop moving or making noises when they do not want to and helps people with ADHD to slow down and think before doing something. It calms parts of the brain that are too excited in people with severe anxiety. This medicine is chemically different from sedatives or tranquilizers, even though it may make your child sleepy when he or she first starts taking it.

How Long Does This Medicine Last?

Although guanfacine lasts 24 hours in the body after a dose, when children take it for problems with emotions or behavior the short-acting form must be taken three times a day. The extended-release version, Intuniv, is taken once a day.

How Will the Doctor Monitor This Medicine?

The doctor will review your child's medical history and physical examination before starting guanfacine. The doctor may order some blood or urine tests to be sure your child does not have a hidden medical condition. Be sure to tell the doctor if your child or anyone in the family has high blood pressure, heart disease, fainting, diabetes, or kidney disease. If Intuniv is being considered, tell the doctor if your child cannot swallow pills. The doctor also may want to obtain an ECG (electrocardiogram or heart rhythm test) before starting the medicine. The doctor or nurse will measure your child's height, weight, pulse, and blood pressure before starting guanfacine.

After the medicine is started, the doctor will want to have regular appointments with you and your child to see how the medicine is working, to see if a dose change is needed, to watch for side effects, to see if guanfacine is still needed, and to see if any other treatment is needed. The doctor or nurse will check your child's height, weight, pulse, and blood pressure.

What Side Effects Can This Medicine Have?

Any medicine can have side effects, including an allergy to the medicine. Because each patient is different, the doctor will monitor the youth closely, especially when the medicine is started. The doctor will work with you to increase the positive effects and decrease the negative effects of the medicine. Please tell the doctor if any of the listed side effects appear or if you think that the medicine is causing any other problems. Not all of the rare or unusual side effects are listed.

Side effects are most common after starting the medicine or after a dose increase. Many side effects can be avoided or lessened by starting with a very low dose and increasing it slowly—ask the doctor.

Allergic Reaction

Tell the doctor in a day or two (if possible, before the next dose of medicine):

- Hives
- Itching
- Rash

Stop the medicine and get *immediate* medical care:

- Trouble breathing or chest tightness
- Swelling of lips, tongue, or throat

Common, but Usually Mild, Side Effects

The following side effects are more common at first or as the dose is increased. If they do not go away after a week or two, ask the doctor about lowering the dose.

- Daytime sleepiness, especially when bored or not doing anything (usually worst in the first 2–4 weeks)—Do not allow your child to drive, ride a bicycle or motorcycle, or operate machinery if this happens.
- Fatigue or tiredness
- Low blood pressure (rarely a serious problem)
- Dizziness or light-headedness—This side effect is worse when the child stands up quickly, especially when getting out of bed in the morning; try having the child stand up slowly.
- Headache
- Stomachache

If one of the following side effects appears, call the doctor within a day or two:

- Slow pulse rate (heartbeat)
- Insomnia (trouble sleeping)—This may be caused by the medicine wearing off during the night.
- Ringing in the ears

Less Common Side Effects

Call the doctor within a day or two:

- Depression or increased irritability
- Confusion
- Bed-wetting
- Muscle cramps
- Itching
- Runny nose

Less Common, but Serious, Side Effects

Call the doctor *immediately:*

- Severe or increased dizziness or light-headedness
- Fainting

Very Rare, but Serious, Side Effects

Call the doctor *immediately:*

- Irregular heartbeat
- Trouble breathing
- Decreased frequency of passing urine; puffy swelling of the body (especially the legs and feet); sudden headaches with nausea and vomiting—These could be signs of kidney failure.

Side Effects Reported in Adults but Rare in Children

Tell the doctor within a week:

- Dry mouth—Have your child try using sugar-free gum or candy.
- Constipation—Encourage your child to drink more fluids and eat high-fiber foods; if necessary, the doctor may recommend a fiber medicine such as Benefiber or a stool softener such as Colace or mineral oil.
- Low blood pressure
- Weakness
- Nightmares
- Increased blood sugar (mainly in persons with diabetes)
- Sensation of cold or pain in fingers or toes
- Weight gain

Some Interactions With Other Medicines or Food

Please note that the following are only the most likely interactions with other medicines or food.

Increased sleepiness will occur in combination with medications for anxiety (sedatives or tranquilizers), sleep (hypnotics), allergy or colds (antihistamines), psychosis, or seizures (anticonvulsants).

If guanfacine is taken with valproate, the valproate levels may get too high. If taking rifampin, guanfacine levels may be decreased and your doctor may consider increasing the dose. If taking ketoconazole, guanfacine levels may be elevated and your doctor may recommend decreasing the dose of guanfacine.

What Could Happen if This Medicine Is Stopped Suddenly?

Withdrawal effects are rare, but the following could happen:

- Very high blood pressure, even if blood pressure was normal before starting the medicine *(rebound hypertension):* This occurs 2–4 days after withdrawal.
- Temporary worsening of behavioral problems or tics
- Nervousness or anxiety
- Rapid or irregular heartbeat
- Chest pain
- Headache
- Stomach cramps, nausea, vomiting
- Trouble sleeping

Because of these effects, it is important not to stop guanfacine suddenly but to decrease it slowly (taper) as directed by the doctor. It is also important not to miss a dose of guanfacine, because withdrawal symptoms such as heart or blood pressure problems may occur. **Be sure not to let the prescription run out!**

How Long Will This Medicine Be Needed?

There is no way to know how long a person will need to take guanfacine. The parent(s), the doctor, and the school will work together to determine what is right for each patient. Some people need the medicine for a few years; some people may need it longer.

What Else Should I Know About This Medicine?

If a child is sleepy from the guanfacine, something active or interesting to do will help the child to stay awake. Sleeping extra hours will not help. Sleepiness usually decreases as the child gets used to the medicine. If the youth is still sleepy in the daytime after 4 weeks on the same dose, a lower dose or a different medicine may be needed.

Intuniv must be taken whole and swallowed. It should not be chewed, crushed, or broken. Intuniv should not be taken with a high-fat meal, as this can increase blood levels of Intuniv and side effects.

If your child is taking either the short-acting or the extended-release form of guanfacine (Intuniv), your doctor will tell you how to gradually increase to the right dose. If your child stops taking the medication for several days, you should not restart right away at the same dose because your child may become very sleepy or have very low blood pressure. Talk with your doctor about the best way to restart the medication.

Tenex may be confused with Xanax. Intuniv may be confused with Invega. Be sure to check the medicine when you get it from the pharmacy.

Notes

Use this space to take notes or to write down questions you want to ask the doctor.

_____

_____

_____

_____

_____

_____

_____

_____

_____

_____

_____

_____

_____

_____

From Dulcan MK, Ballard R (editors): *Helping Parents and Teachers Understand Medications for Behavioral and Emotional Problems: A Resource Book of Medication Information Handouts,* Fourth Edition. Washington, DC, American Psychiatric Publishing, 2015

Haloperidol—Haldol

General Information About Medication

Each child and adolescent is different. No one has exactly the same combination of medical and psychological problems. It is a good idea to talk with the doctor or nurse about the reasons a medicine is being used. It is very important to keep all appointments and to be in touch by telephone if you have concerns. It is important to communicate with the doctor, nurse, or therapist. An *advanced practice nurse* (APN) has additional education and training after becoming a registered nurse (RN). Your child's medication may be prescribed by a medical doctor (MD or DO) or an APN. In addition, a *physician assistant* (PA) working with a physician may prescribe certain medications. In this information sheet, "doctor" includes medical doctors as well as APNs and PAs who prescribe medication. Often a nurse (RN) will be part of the team and answer questions and give information.

It is very important that the medicine be taken exactly as the doctor instructs. However, once in a while, everyone forgets to give a medicine on time. It is a good idea to ask the doctor or nurse what to do if this happens. Do not stop or change a medicine without asking the doctor or nurse first.

If the medicine seems to stop working, it may be because it is not being taken regularly. The youth may be "cheeking" or hiding the medicine or forgetting to take it (especially at school). The doses may be too far apart or a different dose or medicine may be needed. Something at school, at home, or in the neighborhood may be upsetting the youth, or he or she may need special help for learning disabilities or tutoring. Please discuss your concerns with the doctor. **Do not just increase the dose.** It is also very important not to decrease the dose or stop the medicine without talking to the doctor first. The problem being treated may come back, or there could be uncomfortable or even dangerous results.

All medicines should be kept in a safe place, out of the reach of children, and should be supervised by an adult. If someone takes too much of a medicine, call the doctor, the poison control center, or a hospital emergency room.

Each medicine has a "generic" or chemical name. Just like laundry detergents or paper towels, some medicines are sold by more than one company under different brand names. The same medicine may be available under a generic name and several brand names. The generic medications are usually less expensive than the brand name ones. The generic medications have the same chemical formula, but they may or may not be exactly the same strength as the brand-name medications. Also, some brands of pills contain dye or other things that can cause allergic reactions. It is a good idea to talk to the doctor and the pharmacist about whether it is important to use a specific brand of medicine.

Any medicine can cause an allergic reaction. Examples are hives, itching, rashes, swelling, and trouble breathing. Even a tiny amount of a medicine can cause a reaction in patients who are allergic to that medicine. Be *sure* to talk to the doctor before restarting a medicine that has caused an allergic reaction and tell the doctor about any reactions to medicine that your child has had before.

Taking more than one medicine at the same time may cause more side effects or cause one of the medicines to not work as well. Always ask the doctor, nurse, or pharmacist before adding another

medicine, either prescription or bought without a prescription in a store or on the Internet. **Be sure that each doctor knows about *all* of the medicines your child is taking. Also tell the doctor about any vitamins, herbal medicines, or supplements your child may be taking.** Some of these may have side effects alone or when taken with this medication. It is a very good idea to keep a list with you of the names and doses of all medicines that your child is taking.

Everyone taking medicine should have a physical examination at least once a year.

If you think that your child may be using drugs or alcohol, please tell the doctor right away.

Pregnancy requires special care in the use of medicine. Some medicines can cause birth defects if taken by a pregnant mother. **Please tell the doctor immediately if you suspect the teenager is at risk of becoming pregnant.** The doctor may wish to discuss sexual behavior and/or birth control with your daughter.

Printed information like this applies to children and adolescents in general. If you have questions about the medicine, or if you notice changes or anything unusual, please ask the doctor or nurse. As scientific research advances, knowledge increases and advice changes. Even experts do not always agree. Many medicines have not been "approved" by the U.S. Food and Drug Administration (FDA) for use in children or use for particular problems. For this reason, use of the medicine for a problem or age group often is not listed in the *Physicians' Desk Reference.* This does not necessarily mean that the medicine is dangerous or does not work, only that the company that makes the medicine has not received permission to advertise the medicine for use in children. Companies often do not apply for this permission because it is expensive to do the tests needed to apply for approval for use in children. Once a medication is approved by the FDA for any purpose, a doctor is allowed to prescribe it according to research and clinical experience.

Note to Teachers

It is a good idea to talk with the parent(s) about the reason(s) that a medication is being used. If the parent(s) sign consent to release information, it is often helpful for you to talk with the doctor. If the parent(s) give permission, the doctor may ask you to fill out rating forms about your experience with the student's behavior, feelings, academic performance, and medication side effects. This information is very useful in selecting and monitoring medication treatment. If you have observations that you think are important, do not hesitate to share these with the student's parent(s) and treating clinicians (with parental consent).

It is very important that the medicine be taken exactly as the doctor instructs. However, everyone forgets to give a medicine on time once in a while. It is a good idea to ask the parent(s) in advance what to do if this happens. Do not stop or change the time you are giving a medicine at school without parental permission. If a medication is to be taken with food, but lunchtime or snack time changes, be sure to notify the parent(s) so appropriate adjustments can be made.

All medicines should be kept in a secure place and should be supervised by an adult. If someone takes too much of a medicine, follow your school procedure for an urgent medical problem.

Taking medicine is a private matter and is best managed discreetly and confidentially. It is important to be sensitive to the student's feelings about taking medicine.

If you suspect that the student is using drugs or alcohol, please tell the parent(s) or a school counselor right away.

Please tell the parent(s) or school nurse if you suspect medication side effects.

Modifications of the classroom environment or assignments may be useful in addition to medication. The student may need to be evaluated for additional help or a 504 plan or an Individualized Education Plan for learning problems or emotional or behavioral issues.

Any expression of suicidal thoughts or feelings or self-harm by a child or adolescent is a signal of distress and should be taken seriously. These behaviors should not be dismissed as "attention seeking." School procedures for safety issues should be followed.

What Is Haloperidol (Haldol)?

Haloperidol is sometimes called a *typical, conventional,* or *first-generation antipsychotic* medicine. It is also called a *neuroleptic.* It used to be called a *major tranquilizer.* It comes in generic tablets and liquid and two kinds of shots (injections) in both brand name Haldol and generic: immediate-acting and very long-acting (haloperidol decanoate).

How Can This Medicine Help?

Haloperidol is used to treat psychosis, such as in schizophrenia, mania, or very severe depression. It can reduce hallucinations (hearing voices or seeing things that are not there) and delusions (troubling beliefs that other people do not share). It can help the patient be less upset and agitated. It can improve the patient's ability to think clearly.

Sometimes haloperidol is used to decrease severe aggression or very serious behavioral problems in young people with conduct disorder, intellectual disability, or autism spectrum disorder.

Haloperidol is occasionally used to reduce motor and vocal tics (fast, repeated movements or sounds) and behavioral problems in people with Tourette's disorder.

This medicine is very powerful and should be used to treat very serious problems or symptoms that other medicines do not help. Be patient; the positive effects of this medicine may not appear for 2–3 weeks.

How Does This Medicine Work?

Cells in the brain (neurons) communicate using chemicals called *neurotransmitters.* Too much or too little of these substances in certain parts of the brain can cause problems. Haloperidol reduces the activity of one of these neurotransmitters, *dopamine.* Blocking the effect of dopamine in certain parts of the brain reduces what have been called *positive symptoms* of psychosis: delusions; hallucinations; disorganized and unusual thinking, speaking, and behavior; excessive activity (agitation); and lack of activity (catatonia). Blocking dopamine can also reduce tics. Reducing dopamine action in other parts of the brain may lead to the side effects of this medicine.

How Long Does This Medicine Last?

Haloperidol usually may be taken only once a day, unless divided doses are used to lessen side effects. An injection of haloperidol decanoate lasts for 3–4 weeks.

How Will the Doctor Monitor This Medicine?

The doctor will review your child's medical history and physical examination before starting haloperidol. The doctor may order some blood or urine tests to be sure your child does not have a hidden medical condition. The doctor or nurse may measure your child's pulse and blood pressure before starting haloperidol.

Be sure to tell the doctor if anyone in the family is hearing impaired or has had heart problems or died suddenly.

Before your child starts taking haloperidol and every so often afterward, a test such as the AIMS (Abnormal Involuntary Movement Scale) may be used to check your child's tongue, legs, and arms for unusual movements that could be caused by the medicine.

After the medicine is started, the doctor will want to have regular appointments with you and your child to see how the medicine is working, to see if a dose change is needed, to watch for side effects, to see if haloperidol is still needed, and to see if any other treatment is needed. The doctor or nurse may check your child's height, weight, pulse, and blood pressure, and watch for abnormal movements.

What Side Effects Can This Medicine Have?

Any medicine can have side effects, including an allergy to the medicine. Because each patient is different, the doctor will monitor the youth closely, especially when the medicine is started. The doctor will work with you to increase the positive effects and decrease the negative effects of the medicine. Please tell the doctor if any of the listed side effects appear or if you think that the medicine is causing any other problems. Not all of the rare or unusual side effects are listed.

Side effects are most common after starting the medicine or after a dose increase. Many side effects can be avoided or lessened by starting with a very low dose and increasing it slowly—ask the doctor.

Allergic Reaction

Tell the doctor in a day or two (if possible, before the next dose of medicine):

- Hives
- Itching
- Rash

Stop the medicine and get *immediate* medical care:

- Trouble breathing or chest tightness
- Swelling of lips, tongue, or throat

Common, but Not Usually Serious, Side Effects

Discuss the following side effects with your child's doctor within a week or two. They often can be helped by lowering the dose of medicine, changing the times medicine is taken, or adding another medicine.

- Dry mouth—Have your child try using sugar-free gum or candy.
- Constipation—Encourage your child to drink more fluids and eat high-fiber foods; if necessary, the doctor may recommend a fiber medicine such as Benefiber or a stool softener such as Colace or mineral oil.
- Mild trouble urinating
- Blurred vision
- Weight gain—Seek nutritional counseling; provide your child with low-calorie snacks and encourage regular exercise.
- Sadness, irritability, nervousness, clinginess, not wanting to go to school
- Restlessness or inability to sit still
- Shaking of hands and fingers

Less Common, but Not Usually Serious, Side Effects

Discuss the following side effects with your child's doctor within a week or two. They often can be helped by lowering the dose of medicine, changing the times medicine is taken, or adding another medicine.

- Daytime sleepiness or tiredness—Do not allow your child to drive, ride a bicycle or motorcycle, or operate machinery if this happens. This problem may be lessened by taking the medicine at bedtime.
- Dizziness—This side effect is worse when the child stands up quickly, especially when getting out of bed in the morning; try having the child stand up slowly.
- Decreased or slowed movement and decreased facial expressions
- Drooling
- Decreased sexual interest or ability
- Changes in menstrual cycle
- Increase in breast size or discharge from the breasts (in both boys and girls)—This may go away with time.

Less Common, but Potentially Serious, Side Effects

Call the doctor or go to an emergency room *right away:*

- Stiffness of the tongue, jaw, neck, back, or legs
- Overheating or heatstroke—Prevent by decreasing activity in hot weather, staying out of the sun, and drinking water.
- Seizure (fit, convulsion)—This is more likely in people with a history of seizures or head injury.
- Severe confusion

Rare, but Serious, Side Effects

- Extreme stiffness or lack of movement, very high fever, mental confusion, irregular pulse rate, or eye pain—**This is a medical emergency. Go to an emergency room *right away.***
- Sudden stiffness and inability to breathe or swallow—**Go to an emergency room or call 911.** Tell the paramedics, nurses, and doctors that the patient is taking haloperidol. Other medicines can be used to treat this problem fast.
- Increased thirst, frequent urination, lethargy, tiredness, dizziness—These could be signs of diabetes (especially if your child is overweight or there is a family history of diabetes). **Talk to a doctor within a day.**

What Else Should I Know About Side Effects?

Most side effects lessen over time. If they are troublesome, talk with your child's doctor. Some side effects can be decreased by taking a smaller dose of medicine, by stopping the medicine, by changing to another medicine, or by adding another medicine.

One side effect that may not go away is *tardive dyskinesia* (or TD). Patients with tardive dyskinesia have involuntary movements of the body, especially the mouth and tongue. The patient may look as though he or she is making faces over and over again. Jerky movements of the arms, legs, or body may occur. There may be fine, wormlike, or sudden repeated movements of the tongue, or the person may appear to be chewing something or smacking or puckering his or her lips. The fingers may look as though they are rolling something. If you notice any unusual movements, be sure to tell the doctor. The doctor may use the AIMS test to look for these movements.

The medicine may increase the level of *prolactin*, a natural hormone made in the part of the brain called the *pituitary*. This may cause side effects such as breast tenderness or swelling or production of milk, in both boys and girls. It also may interfere with sexual functioning in teenage boys and with regular menstrual cycles (periods) in teenage girls. A blood test can measure the level of prolactin. If these side effects do not go away and are troublesome, talk with your child's doctor about substituting another medicine for haloperidol.

Heart problems are more common if other medicines are being taken as well. Be sure to tell all your child's doctors and your pharmacist about all medications your child is taking.

Neuroleptic malignant syndrome is a very rare side effect that can lead to death. The symptoms are severe muscle stiffness, high fever, increased heart rate and blood pressure, irregular heartbeat (pulse), and sweating. It may lead to unconsciousness. If you suspect this, **call 911 or go to an emergency room right away.**

Some Interactions With Other Medicines or Food

Please note that the following are only the most likely interactions with other medicines or food.

Haloperidol may be taken with or without food. If the medicine causes stomach upset, taking it with food may help.

Carbamazepine (Tegretol) may decrease levels of haloperidol so that it does not work as well.

Fluoxetine (Prozac) may increase the levels of haloperidol, increasing the risk of side effects.

It is better to limit drinks with caffeine (coffee, tea, soft drinks) because caffeine works in the opposite way from this medicine, and the positive effects might be decreased.

What Could Happen if This Medicine Is Stopped Suddenly?

Involuntary movements, or *withdrawal dyskinesias*, may appear within 1–4 weeks of lowering the dose or stopping the medicine. Usually these go away, but they can last for days to months. If haloperidol is stopped suddenly, emotional problems such as irritability, nervousness, or moodiness; behavior problems; or physical problems such as stomachache, loss of appetite, nausea, vomiting, diarrhea, sweating, indigestion, trouble sleeping, trembling, or shaking may appear. These problems usually last only a few days to a few weeks. If they happen, tell your child's doctor. The medicine dose may need to be lowered more slowly (tapered). Always check with the doctor before stopping a medicine.

How Long Will This Medicine Be Needed?

How long your child will need to be on haloperidol depends partly on the reason that it was prescribed. Some problems last for only a few months, whereas others last much longer. Sometimes haloperidol is used for only a short time until other medicines or behavioral treatments start to work. Some people need to take haloperidol for years. It is especially important with medicines as powerful as this one to ask the doctor whether it is still needed. Every few months, you should discuss with your child's doctor the reasons for using haloperidol and whether it is time for a trial of lowering the dose.

What Else Should I Know About This Medicine?

There are many other medicines that are used for the same kinds of problems. If your child is having bad side effects or the medicine does not seem to be working, ask the doctor if another medicine in this group might work as well or better and have fewer side effects for your child.

Be sure to tell the doctor if there is anyone in your family who died suddenly or had a heart problem.

Sometimes this medicine can cause a *dystonic reaction*. This is a sudden stiffening of the muscles, most often in the jaw, neck, tongue, face, or shoulders. If this happens, and your child is not having trouble breathing, you may give a dose of diphenhydramine (Benadryl). Follow the dose instructions on the package for your child's age. This should relax the muscles in a few minutes. Then call your doctor to tell him or her what happened. If the muscles do not relax, take your child to the emergency department.

Notes

Use this space to take notes or to write down questions you want to ask the doctor.

_____

_____

_____

_____

_____

_____

_____

_____

_____

_____

_____

community and accepted child psychiatric practice. The information on this medication sheet does not cover all the possible uses, precautions, side effects, or interactions of this drug. For a complete listing of side effects, see the manufacturer's package insert, which can be obtained from your physician or pharmacist. As medical research and practice advance, therapeutic standards may change. For this reason and because human and mechanical errors sometimes occur, we recommend that readers follow the advice of a physician who is directly involved in their care or the care of a member of their family.

From Dulcan MK, Ballard R (editors): *Helping Parents and Teachers Understand Medications for Behavioral and Emotional Problems: A Resource Book of Medication Information Handouts*, Fourth Edition. Washington, DC, American Psychiatric Publishing, 2015

Medication Information for Parents and Teachers

Hydroxyzine—Vistaril

General Information About Medication

Each child and adolescent is different. No one has exactly the same combination of medical and psychological problems. It is a good idea to talk with the doctor or nurse about the reasons a medicine is being used. It is very important to keep all appointments and to be in touch by telephone if you have concerns. It is important to communicate with the doctor, nurse, or therapist. An *advanced practice nurse* (APN) has additional education and training after becoming a registered nurse (RN). Your child's medication may be prescribed by a medical doctor (MD or DO) or an APN. In addition, a *physician assistant* (PA) working with a physician may prescribe certain medications. In this information sheet, "doctor" includes medical doctors as well as APNs and PAs who prescribe medication. Often a nurse (RN) will be part of the team and answer questions and give information.

It is very important that the medicine be taken exactly as the doctor instructs. However, once in a while, everyone forgets to give a medicine on time. It is a good idea to ask the doctor or nurse what to do if this happens. Do not stop or change a medicine without asking the doctor or nurse first.

If the medicine seems to stop working, it may be because it is not being taken regularly. The youth may be "cheeking" or hiding the medicine or forgetting to take it (especially at school). The doses may be too far apart or a different dose or medicine may be needed. Something at school, at home, or in the neighborhood may be upsetting the youth, or he or she may need special help for learning disabilities or tutoring. Please discuss your concerns with the doctor. **Do not just increase the dose.** It is also very important not to decrease the dose or stop the medicine without talking to the doctor first. The problem being treated may come back, or there could be uncomfortable or even dangerous results.

All medicines should be kept in a safe place, out of the reach of children, and should be supervised by an adult. If someone takes too much of a medicine, call the doctor, the poison control center, or a hospital emergency room.

Each medicine has a "generic" or chemical name. Just like laundry detergents or paper towels, some medicines are sold by more than one company under different brand names. The same medicine may be available under a generic name and several brand names. The generic medications are usually less expensive than the brand name ones. The generic medications have the same chemical formula, but they may or may not be exactly the same strength as the brand-name medications. Also, some brands of pills contain dye or other things that can cause allergic reactions. It is a good idea to talk to the doctor and the pharmacist about whether it is important to use a specific brand of medicine.

Any medicine can cause an allergic reaction. Examples are hives, itching, rashes, swelling, and trouble breathing. Even a tiny amount of a medicine can cause a reaction in patients who are allergic to that medicine. Be *sure* to talk to the doctor before restarting a medicine that has caused an allergic reaction and tell the doctor about any reactions to medicine that your child has had before.

Taking more than one medicine at the same time may cause more side effects or cause one of the medicines to not work as well. Always ask the doctor, nurse, or pharmacist before adding another

237

medicine, either prescription or bought without a prescription in a store or on the Internet. Be sure that each doctor knows about *all* of the medicines your child is taking. Also tell the doctor about any vitamins, herbal medicines, or supplements your child may be taking. Some of these may have side effects alone or when taken with this medication. It is a very good idea to keep a list with you of the names and doses of all medicines that your child is taking.

Everyone taking medicine should have a physical examination at least once a year.

If you think that your child may be using drugs or alcohol, please tell the doctor right away.

Pregnancy requires special care in the use of medicine. Some medicines can cause birth defects if taken by a pregnant mother. **Please tell the doctor immediately if you suspect the teenager is at risk of becoming pregnant.** The doctor may wish to discuss sexual behavior and/or birth control with your daughter.

Printed information like this applies to children and adolescents in general. If you have questions about the medicine, or if you notice changes or anything unusual, please ask the doctor or nurse. As scientific research advances, knowledge increases and advice changes. Even experts do not always agree. Many medicines have not been "approved" by the U.S. Food and Drug Administration (FDA) for use in children or use for particular problems. For this reason, use of the medicine for a problem or age group often is not listed in the *Physicians' Desk Reference*. This does not necessarily mean that the medicine is dangerous or does not work, only that the company that makes the medicine has not received permission to advertise the medicine for use in children. Companies often do not apply for this permission because it is expensive to do the tests needed to apply for approval for use in children. Once a medication is approved by the FDA for any purpose, a doctor is allowed to prescribe it according to research and clinical experience.

Note to Teachers

It is a good idea to talk with the parent(s) about the reason(s) that a medication is being used. If the parent(s) sign consent to release information, it is often helpful for you to talk with the doctor. If the parent(s) give permission, the doctor may ask you to fill out rating forms about your experience with the student's behavior, feelings, academic performance, and medication side effects. This information is very useful in selecting and monitoring medication treatment. If you have observations that you think are important, do not hesitate to share these with the student's parent(s) and treating clinicians (with parental consent).

It is very important that the medicine be taken exactly as the doctor instructs. However, everyone forgets to give a medicine on time once in a while. It is a good idea to ask the parent(s) in advance what to do if this happens. Do not stop or change the time you are giving a medicine at school without parental permission. If a medication is to be taken with food, but lunchtime or snack time changes, be sure to notify the parent(s) so appropriate adjustments can be made.

All medicines should be kept in a secure place and should be supervised by an adult. If someone takes too much of a medicine, follow your school procedure for an urgent medical problem.

Taking medicine is a private matter and is best managed discreetly and confidentially. It is important to be sensitive to the student's feelings about taking medicine.

If you suspect that the student is using drugs or alcohol, please tell the parent(s) or a school counselor right away.

Please tell the parent(s) or school nurse if you suspect medication side effects.

Modifications of the classroom environment or assignments may be useful in addition to medication. The student may need to be evaluated for additional help or a 504 plan or an Individualized Education Plan for learning problems or emotional or behavioral issues.

Any expression of suicidal thoughts or feelings or self-harm by a child or adolescent is a signal of distress and should be taken seriously. These behaviors should not be dismissed as "attention seeking." School procedures for safety issues should be followed.

What Is Hydroxyzine (Vistaril)?

Hydroxyzine is called an *antihistamine*. Antihistamines were developed to treat allergies. Hydroxyzine is sometimes used to treat anxiety (nervousness) or insomnia (difficulty falling asleep). It may sometimes be used to stop itching or vomiting. It comes in generic capsules, tablets, and syrup and brand name Vistaril capsules. It also comes in an injection (shot).

How Can This Medicine Help?

Hydroxyzine may decrease nervousness. When used for anxiety, it works best when used for a short time along with psychotherapy. Hydroxyzine can help with insomnia when used for a short time along with a behavioral program, such as regular soothing routines at bedtime and increased exercise in the daytime.

How Does This Medicine Work?

Hydroxyzine can help decrease anxiety and help falling asleep because of its *sedative* effect. That is, it makes people a little sleepy so that they feel less nervous and also fall asleep more easily.

How Long Does This Medicine Last?

Hydroxyzine lasts for 4–6 hours.

How Will the Doctor Monitor This Medicine?

The doctor will review your child's medical history and physical examination before starting hydroxyzine. Be sure to tell the doctor if your child or anyone in the family has a history of asthma or of heart rhythm problems, palpitations, or fainting. The doctor or nurse may measure your child's height, weight, pulse, and blood pressure before starting the medicine.

After the medicine is started, the doctor will want to have regular appointments with you and your child to see how the medicine is working, to see if a dose change is needed, to watch for side effects, to see if hydroxyzine is still needed, and to see if any other treatment is needed. The doctor or nurse may check your child's height, weight, pulse, and blood pressure.

What Side Effects Can This Medicine Have?

Any medicine can have side effects, including an allergy to the medicine. Because each patient is different, the doctor will monitor the youth closely, especially when the medicine is started. The doctor will work with you to increase the positive effects and decrease the negative effects of the medicine. Please tell the doctor if any of the listed side effects appear or if you think that the medicine is causing any other problems. Not all of the rare or unusual side effects are listed.

Side effects are most common after starting the medicine or after a dose increase. Many side effects can be avoided or lessened by starting with a very low dose and increasing it slowly—ask the doctor.

Allergic Reaction

Tell the doctor in a day or two (if possible, before the next dose of medicine):

- Hives
- Itching
- Rash

Stop the medicine and get *immediate* medical care:

- Trouble breathing or chest tightness
- Swelling of lips, tongue, or throat

Common Side Effects

Tell the doctor within a week or two:

- Daytime sleepiness—Do not allow your child to drive, ride a bicycle or motorcycle, or operate machinery if this happens.
- Decreased attention, memory, or learning in school
- Dry mouth—Have your child try using sugar-free gum or candy.
- Headache
- Blurred vision
- Constipation—Encourage your child to drink more fluids and eat high-fiber foods; if necessary, the doctor may recommend a fiber medicine such as Benefiber or a stool softener such as Colace or mineral oil.
- Dizziness or light-headedness—This side effect is worse when the child stands up quickly, especially when getting out of bed in the morning; try having the child stand up slowly.
- Loss of appetite, nausea, or upset stomach

Less Common Side Effects

Call the doctor within a day or two:

- Poor coordination
- Motor tics (fast, repeated movements)
- Unusual muscle movements
- Irritability, increased overactivity
- Waking up after sleeping for a short time and being unable to get back to sleep
- Exposure to sunlight may cause severe sunburn, skin rash, redness, or itching; avoid direct exposure to sunlight or use sunscreen.
- Trouble passing urine

Very Rare, but Serious, Side Effects

Call the doctor *immediately:*

- Worsening of asthma or trouble breathing
- Seizure (fit, convulsion)
- Uncontrollable behavior
- Hallucinations (seeing things that are not really there)
- Severe muscle stiffness
- Irregular heartbeat (pulse), fainting, palpitations

Some Interactions With Other Medicines or Food

Please note that the following are only the most likely interactions with other medicines or food.

If other medicines that can cause sleepiness are taken with hydroxyzine, severe sleepiness can result.

What Could Happen if This Medicine Is Stopped Suddenly?

Stopping these medicines suddenly does not usually cause problems, but diarrhea or feeling sick may result if it has been taken for a long time. The problem being treated may come back. Always ask the doctor whether a medicine can be stopped suddenly or must be decreased slowly (tapered).

How Long Will This Medicine Be Needed?

When used for nervousness or sleep, hydroxyzine is usually prescribed for a very short time to allow the patient to be calm enough to learn new ways to cope. If the person needs treatment for a longer time, another medicine is usually prescribed.

What Else Should I Know About This Medicine?

People who take hydroxyzine must not drink alcohol. Severe sleepiness or even loss of consciousness may result.

Notes

Use this space to take notes or to write down questions you want to ask the doctor.

_____

_____

_____

_____

_____

_____

_____

_____

_____

_____

_____

From Dulcan MK, Ballard R (editors): _Helping Parents and Teachers Understand Medications for Behavioral and Emotional Problems: A Resource Book of Medication Information Handouts_, Fourth Edition. Washington, DC, American Psychiatric Publishing, 2015

Medication Information for Parents and Teachers

Hypnotics—Sleep Medications (Nonbenzodiazepines):
Eszopiclone—Lunesta
Zaleplon—Sonata
Zolpidem—Ambien, Ambien CR, Edluar, Intermezzo, Zolpimist

General Information About Medication

Each child and adolescent is different. No one has exactly the same combination of medical and psychological problems. It is a good idea to talk with the doctor or nurse about the reasons a medicine is being used. It is very important to keep all appointments and to be in touch by telephone if you have concerns. It is important to communicate with the doctor, nurse, or therapist. An *advanced practice nurse* (APN) has additional education and training after becoming a registered nurse (RN). Your child's medication may be prescribed by a medical doctor (MD or DO) or an APN. In addition, a *physician assistant* (PA) working with a physician may prescribe certain medications. In this information sheet, "doctor" includes medical doctors as well as APNs and PAs who prescribe medication. Often a nurse (RN) will be part of the team and answer questions and give information.

It is very important that the medicine be taken exactly as the doctor instructs. However, once in a while, everyone forgets to give a medicine on time. It is a good idea to ask the doctor or nurse what to do if this happens. Do not stop or change a medicine without asking the doctor or nurse first.

If the medicine seems to stop working, it may be because it is not being taken regularly. The youth may be "cheeking" or hiding the medicine or forgetting to take it (especially at school). The doses may be too far apart or a different dose or medicine may be needed. Something at school, at home, or in the neighborhood may be upsetting the youth, or he or she may need special help for learning disabilities or tutoring. Please discuss your concerns with the doctor. **Do not just increase the dose.** It is also very important not to decrease the dose or stop the medicine without talking to the doctor first. The problem being treated may come back, or there could be uncomfortable or even dangerous results.

All medicines should be kept in a safe place, out of the reach of children, and should be supervised by an adult. If someone takes too much of a medicine, call the doctor, the poison control center, or a hospital emergency room.

Each medicine has a "generic" or chemical name. Just like laundry detergents or paper towels, some medicines are sold by more than one company under different brand names. The same medicine may be available under a generic name and several brand names. The generic medications are usually less expensive than the brand name ones. The generic medications have the same chemical formula, but they may or may not be exactly the same strength as the brand-name medications. Also, some brands of pills contain dye or other things

243

that can cause allergic reactions. It is a good idea to talk to the doctor and the pharmacist about whether it is important to use a specific brand of medicine.

Any medicine can cause an allergic reaction. Examples are hives, itching, rashes, swelling, and trouble breathing. Even a tiny amount of a medicine can cause a reaction in patients who are allergic to that medicine. Be *sure* to talk to the doctor before restarting a medicine that has caused an allergic reaction and tell the doctor about any reactions to medicine that your child has had before.

Taking more than one medicine at the same time may cause more side effects or cause one of the medicines to not work as well. Always ask the doctor, nurse, or pharmacist before adding another medicine, either prescription or bought without a prescription in a store or on the Internet. Be sure that each doctor knows about *all* of the medicines your child is taking. Also tell the doctor about any vitamins, herbal medicines, or supplements your child may be taking. Some of these may have side effects alone or when taken with this medication. It is a very good idea to keep a list with you of the names and doses of all medicines that your child is taking.

Everyone taking medicine should have a physical examination at least once a year.

If you think that your child may be using drugs or alcohol, please tell the doctor right away.

Pregnancy requires special care in the use of medicine. Some medicines can cause birth defects if taken by a pregnant mother. **Please tell the doctor immediately if you suspect the teenager is at risk of becoming pregnant.** The doctor may wish to discuss sexual behavior and/or birth control with your daughter.

Printed information like this applies to children and adolescents in general. If you have questions about the medicine, or if you notice changes or anything unusual, please ask the doctor or nurse. As scientific research advances, knowledge increases and advice changes. Even experts do not always agree. Many medicines have not been "approved" by the U.S. Food and Drug Administration (FDA) for use in children or use for particular problems. For this reason, use of the medicine for a problem or age group often is not listed in the *Physicians' Desk Reference*. This does not necessarily mean that the medicine is dangerous or does not work, only that the company that makes the medicine has not received permission to advertise the medicine for use in children. Companies often do not apply for this permission because it is expensive to do the tests needed to apply for approval for use in children. Once a medication is approved by the FDA for any purpose, a doctor is allowed to prescribe it according to research and clinical experience.

Note to Teachers

It is a good idea to talk with the parent(s) about the reason(s) that a medication is being used. If the parent(s) sign consent to release information, it is often helpful for you to talk with the doctor. If the parent(s) give permission, the doctor may ask you to fill out rating forms about your experience with the student's behavior, feelings, academic performance, and medication side effects. This information is very useful in selecting and monitoring medication treatment. If you have observations that you think are important, do not hesitate to share these with the student's parent(s) and treating clinicians (with parental consent).

It is very important that the medicine be taken exactly as the doctor instructs. However, everyone forgets to give a medicine on time once in a while. It is a good idea to ask the parent(s) in advance what to do if this happens. Do not stop or change the time you are giving a medicine at school without parental permission. If a medication is to be taken with food, but lunchtime or snack time changes, be sure to notify the parent(s) so appropriate adjustments can be made.

All medicines should be kept in a secure place and should be supervised by an adult. If someone takes too much of a medicine, follow your school procedure for an urgent medical problem.

Taking medicine is a private matter and is best managed discreetly and confidentially. It is important to be sensitive to the student's feelings about taking medicine.

If you suspect that the student is using drugs or alcohol, please tell the parent(s) or a school counselor right away.

Please tell the parent(s) or school nurse if you suspect medication side effects.

Modifications of the classroom environment or assignments may be useful in addition to medication. The student may need to be evaluated for additional help or a 504 plan or an Individualized Education Plan for learning problems or emotional or behavioral issues.

Any expression of suicidal thoughts or feelings or self-harm by a child or adolescent is a signal of distress and should be taken seriously. These behaviors should not be dismissed as "attention seeking." School procedures for safety issues should be followed.

What Are Eszopiclone (Lunesta), Zaleplon (Sonata), and Zolpidem (Ambien, Ambien CR, Edluar, Intermezzo, Zolpimist)?

Zolpidem, eszopiclone, and zaleplon are *hypnotics* or *sedative-hypnotic* medicines. They are *not* benzodiazepines. Zolpidem comes in generic immediate- and controlled-release tablets, Ambien brand name tablets, Ambien CR (controlled-release) tablets, Edluar and Intermezzo oral disintegrating tablets (placed under the tongue), and Zolpimist liquid.

Eszopiclone comes in generic and brand name Lunesta tablets.

Zaleplon comes in generic and brand name Sonata capsules.

How Can These Medicines Help?

These very similar medicines are used to treat insomnia—problems falling asleep or staying asleep—when used for a short time along with a behavioral program.

How Do These Medicines Work?

Zolpidem, eszopiclone, and zaleplon work in certain parts of the brain to help people fall asleep. They work in a different way than other sleep medicines.

Zolpimist is a cherry-flavored liquid.

When zolpidem ER (Ambien CR) is taken, the outer coating of the pill helps the person to fall asleep, and the slow-release medicine inside the pill helps with staying asleep.

Edluar and Intermezzo oral disintegrating tablets dissolve in the mouth and work quickly.

Intermezzo is used when people wake up in the middle of the night. It helps them get back to sleep.

How Long Do These Medicines Last?

Zolpidem, eszopiclone, and zaleplon are taken right before going to bed because these medicines start working very quickly. They also leave the body very quickly, so they are less likely to cause daytime sleepiness or memory problems than other kinds of sleep medicines.

Intermezzo oral disintegrating tablets are used for middle of the night insomnia and to help people fall back to sleep quickly.

How Will the Doctor Monitor These Medicines?

The doctor will review your child's medical history and physical examination before starting these medicines.

After the medicine is started, the doctor will want to have regular appointments with you and your child to see how the medicine is working, to see if a dose change is needed, to watch for side effects, to see if the medicine is still needed, and to see if any other treatment is needed.

What Side Effects Can These Medicines Have?

Any medicine can have side effects, including an allergy to the medicine. Because each patient is different, the doctor will monitor the youth closely, especially when the medicine is started. The doctor will work with you to increase the positive effects and decrease the negative effects of the medicine. Please tell the doctor if any of the listed side effects appear or if you think that the medicine is causing any other problems. Not all of the rare or unusual side effects are listed.

Side effects are most common after starting the medicine or after a dose increase. Many side effects can be avoided or lessened by starting with a very low dose and increasing it slowly—ask the doctor.

Allergic Reaction

Tell the doctor in a day or two (if possible, before the next dose of medicine):

- Hives
- Itching
- Rash

Stop the medicine and get *immediate* medical care:

- Trouble breathing or chest tightness
- Swelling of lips, tongue, or throat

These medicines are usually very safe when used for short periods as the doctor prescribes.

Common Side Effects

Tell the doctor in a week or two:

- Daytime sleepiness—Do not allow your child to drive a car, ride a bicycle or motorcycle, or operate machinery if this happens.
- Dizziness, feeling "spacey," or decreased coordination
- Low energy or tiredness
- Headache
- Eszopiclone (Lunesta) may cause a bad taste in the mouth

Less Common Side Effects

Tell the doctor within a week or two:

- More trouble sleeping
- Nausea
- Vomiting
- Diarrhea
- Memory loss
- Nervousness (anxiety)
- Dry mouth
- Nightmares

Rare, but Serious, Side Effects

Tell the doctor right away:

- Depression
- Thoughts of suicide or self-harm
- Hallucinations (seeing or hearing things that are not really there)
- Agitation
- Loss of coordination
- Signs of infection—Fever, chills, sore throat

The most common side effect is daytime sleepiness. These medicines can also cause dizziness, feeling "spacey," or decreased coordination. If the medicine is causing any of these problems it is very important not to drive a car, ride a bicycle or motorcycle, or operate machinery.

These medicines can cause decreased concentration and memory. These problems, along with daytime sleepiness, may decrease learning and performance in school.

Some children and adolescents who have taken these medicines have had dreamlike states right before falling asleep in which they see or hear things that are not there. Some of the youth had unusual or bizarre behaviors after taking the medicine but before falling asleep. If this happens, these medicines should be stopped and not used again.

People who take sleeping medicine must not drink alcohol. Severe sleepiness or even loss of consciousness may result.

It is possible to become psychologically and physically dependent on these medicines, but that is not a common problem for patients who see their doctors regularly. It is less common for these medicines than for other types of sleep medicines.

Some Interactions With Other Medicines or Food

Please note that the following are only the most likely interactions with other medicines or food.

Caffeine may cause trouble sleeping and make these medicines less effective. If caffeine is eliminated, less sleeping medicine may be needed, or medicine may not be needed at all.

It is important not to use other sedatives, tranquilizers, or sleeping pills or antihistamines (such as Benadryl) when taking these medicines because of increased daytime sleepiness.

What Could Happen if These Medicines Are Stopped Suddenly?

Many medicines cause problems if stopped suddenly. These medicines must be decreased slowly (tapered) rather than stopped suddenly. When these medications are stopped suddenly, there are withdrawal symptoms that are uncomfortable. Problems are more likely in patients taking high doses of these medicines for 2 months or longer, but even after taking these medicines for just a few weeks, it is important to stop them slowly. Withdrawal symptoms may include anxiety, irritability, shaking, sweating, aches and pains, muscle cramps, vomiting, confusion, and trouble sleeping.

How Long Will These Medicines Be Needed?

These medicines are usually prescribed for only a week or so or for occasional use only as needed. A behavioral program, such as regular soothing routines at bedtime and increased exercise in the daytime, should be used along with the medicine to improve sleep. Finding developmentally appropriate bedtimes and wake times and sticking to them is very important. These strategies should be continued after the medicine is tapered (stopped slowly) or when the medicine is used only occasionally.

What Else Should I Know About These Medicines?

Because these medicines can be abused (especially by people who abuse alcohol or drugs) and can cause psychological dependence or physical dependence (addiction), they are regulated by special state and federal laws as a *controlled substance*. These laws place limitations on telephone prescriptions and refills.

People with *sleep apnea* (breathing stops while they are asleep) should not take sleeping medicine. Tell the doctor if your child snores very loudly, which may be a symptom of sleep apnea.

These medicines work faster if taken on an empty stomach.

Do not cut or crush the Ambien CR tablet—it should be swallowed whole.

Notes

Use this space to take notes or to write down questions you want to ask the doctor.

_____

_____

_____

_____

_____

_____

_____

_____

_____

_____

_____

_____

_____

_____

_____

From Dulcan MK, Ballard R (editors): _Helping Parents and Teachers Understand Medications for Behavioral and Emotional Problems: A Resource Book of Medication Information Handouts_, Fourth Edition. Washington, DC, American Psychiatric Publishing, 2015

Medication Information for Parents and Teachers

Iloperidone—Fanapt

General Information About Medication

Each child and adolescent is different. No one has exactly the same combination of medical and psychological problems. It is a good idea to talk with the doctor or nurse about the reasons a medicine is being used. It is very important to keep all appointments and to be in touch by telephone if you have concerns. It is important to communicate with the doctor, nurse, or therapist. An *advanced practice nurse* (APN) has additional education and training after becoming a registered nurse (RN). Your child's medication may be prescribed by a medical doctor (MD or DO) or an APN. In addition, a *physician assistant* (PA) working with a physician may prescribe certain medications. In this information sheet, "doctor" includes medical doctors as well as APNs and PAs who prescribe medication. Often a nurse (RN) will be part of the team and answer questions and give information.

It is very important that the medicine be taken exactly as the doctor instructs. However, once in a while, everyone forgets to give a medicine on time. It is a good idea to ask the doctor or nurse what to do if this happens. Do not stop or change a medicine without asking the doctor or nurse first.

If the medicine seems to stop working, it may be because it is not being taken regularly. The youth may be "cheeking" or hiding the medicine or forgetting to take it (especially at school). The doses may be too far apart or a different dose or medicine may be needed. Something at school, at home, or in the neighborhood may be upsetting the youth, or he or she may need special help for learning disabilities or tutoring. Please discuss your concerns with the doctor. **Do not just increase the dose.** It is also very important not to decrease the dose or stop the medicine without talking to the doctor first. The problem being treated may come back, or there could be uncomfortable or even dangerous results.

All medicines should be kept in a safe place, out of the reach of children, and should be supervised by an adult. If someone takes too much of a medicine, call the doctor, the poison control center, or a hospital emergency room.

Each medicine has a "generic" or chemical name. Just like laundry detergents or paper towels, some medicines are sold by more than one company under different brand names. The same medicine may be available under a generic name and several brand names. The generic medications are usually less expensive than the brand name ones. The generic medications have the same chemical formula, but they may or may not be exactly the same strength as the brand-name medications. Also, some brands of pills contain dye or other things that can cause allergic reactions. It is a good idea to talk to the doctor and the pharmacist about whether it is important to use a specific brand of medicine.

Any medicine can cause an allergic reaction. Examples are hives, itching, rashes, swelling, and trouble breathing. Even a tiny amount of a medicine can cause a reaction in patients who are allergic to that medicine. Be *sure* to talk to the doctor before restarting a medicine that has caused an allergic reaction and tell the doctor about any reactions to medicine that your child has had before.

Taking more than one medicine at the same time may cause more side effects or cause one of the medicines to not work as well. Always ask the doctor, nurse, or pharmacist before adding another medicine, either prescription or bought without a prescription in a store or on the Internet. Be sure

251

that each doctor knows about *all* of the medicines your child is taking. **Also tell the doctor about any vitamins, herbal medicines, or supplements your child may be taking.** Some of these may have side effects alone or when taken with this medication. It is a very good idea to keep a list with you of the names and doses of all medicines that your child is taking.

Everyone taking medicine should have a physical examination at least once a year.

If you think that your child may be using drugs or alcohol, please tell the doctor right away.

Pregnancy requires special care in the use of medicine. Some medicines can cause birth defects if taken by a pregnant mother. **Please tell the doctor immediately if you suspect the teenager is at risk of becoming pregnant.** The doctor may wish to discuss sexual behavior and/or birth control with your daughter.

Printed information like this applies to children and adolescents in general. If you have questions about the medicine, or if you notice changes or anything unusual, please ask the doctor or nurse. As scientific research advances, knowledge increases and advice changes. Even experts do not always agree. Many medicines have not been "approved" by the U.S. Food and Drug Administration (FDA) for use in children or use for particular problems. For this reason, use of the medicine for a problem or age group often is not listed in the *Physicians' Desk Reference*. This does not necessarily mean that the medicine is dangerous or does not work, only that the company that makes the medicine has not received permission to advertise the medicine for use in children. Companies often do not apply for this permission because it is expensive to do the tests needed to apply for approval for use in children. Once a medication is approved by the FDA for any purpose, a doctor is allowed to prescribe it according to research and clinical experience.

Note to Teachers

It is a good idea to talk with the parent(s) about the reason(s) that a medication is being used. If the parent(s) sign consent to release information, it is often helpful for you to talk with the doctor. If the parent(s) give permission, the doctor may ask you to fill out rating forms about your experience with the student's behavior, feelings, academic performance, and medication side effects. This information is very useful in selecting and monitoring medication treatment. If you have observations that you think are important, do not hesitate to share these with the student's parent(s) and treating clinicians (with parental consent).

It is very important that the medicine be taken exactly as the doctor instructs. However, everyone forgets to give a medicine on time once in a while. It is a good idea to ask the parent(s) in advance what to do if this happens. Do not stop or change the time you are giving a medicine at school without parental permission. If a medication is to be taken with food, but lunchtime or snack time changes, be sure to notify the parent(s) so appropriate adjustments can be made.

All medicines should be kept in a secure place and should be supervised by an adult. If someone takes too much of a medicine, follow your school procedure for an urgent medical problem.

Taking medicine is a private matter and is best managed discreetly and confidentially. It is important to be sensitive to the student's feelings about taking medicine.

If you suspect that the student is using drugs or alcohol, please tell the parent(s) or a school counselor right away.

Please tell the parent(s) or school nurse if you suspect medication side effects.

Modifications of the classroom environment or assignments may be useful in addition to medication. The student may need to be evaluated for additional help or a 504 plan or an Individualized Education Plan for learning problems or emotional or behavioral issues.

Any expression of suicidal thoughts or feelings or self-harm by a child or adolescent is a signal of distress and should be taken seriously. These behaviors should not be dismissed as "attention seeking." School procedures for safety issues should be followed.

What Is Iloperidone (Fanapt)?

This medicine is called an *atypical* or *second-generation antipsychotic*. It is sometimes called an *atypical psychotropic agent*, or simply an *atypical*. It comes in brand name Fanapt tablets.

How Can This Medicine Help?

Iloperidone is used to treat psychosis, such as in schizophrenia, mania, or very severe depression. It can reduce *positive symptoms* such as hallucinations (hearing voices or seeing things that are not there); delusions (troubling beliefs that other people do not share); agitation; and very unusual thinking, speech, and behavior. It is also used to lessen the *negative symptoms* of schizophrenia, such as lack of interest in doing things (apathy), lack of motivation, social withdrawal, and lack of energy.

Iloperidone may be used as a *mood stabilizer* in patients with bipolar disorder or severe mood swings. It can reduce mania and may be able to help maintain a stable mood.

Sometimes iloperidone is used to reduce severe aggression or very serious behavioral problems in young people with conduct disorder, intellectual disability, or autism spectrum disorder. This medicine is very powerful and is used to treat very serious problems or symptoms that other medicines do not help. Be patient; the positive effects of this medicine may not appear for 2–3 weeks.

How Does This Medicine Work?

Cells in the brain communicate using chemicals called *neurotransmitters*. Too much or too little of these substances in parts of the brain can cause problems. Iloperidone works by blocking the action of two of these neurotransmitters—*dopamine and serotonin*—in certain areas of the brain.

How Long Does This Medicine Last?

Iloperidone is usually taken twice a day.

How Will the Doctor Monitor This Medicine?

The doctor will review your child's medical history and physical examination before starting iloperidone. The doctor may order some blood or urine tests to be sure your child does not have a hidden medical condition that would make it unsafe to use this medicine. The doctor or nurse may measure your child's pulse and blood pressure before starting iloperidone. The doctor may order other tests, such as baseline tests for blood sugar and cholesterol or an ECG (electrocardiogram or heart rhythm test).

Be sure to tell the doctor if anyone in the family has diabetes, high blood pressure, high cholesterol, or heart disease.

Before your child starts taking iloperidone and every so often afterward, a test such as the Abnormal Involuntary Movement Scale (AIMS) may be used to check your child's tongue, legs, and arms for unusual movements that could be caused by the medicine.

After the medicine is started, the doctor will want to have regular appointments with you and your child to see how the medicine is working, to see if a dose change is needed, to watch for side effects, to see if iloperidone is still needed, and to see if any other treatment is needed. The doctor or nurse will check your child's height, weight, pulse, and blood pressure and watch for abnormal movements. Sometimes blood tests are needed to watch for diabetes or increased cholesterol.

What Side Effects Can This Medicine Have?

Any medicine can have side effects, including an allergy to the medicine. Because each patient is different, the doctor will monitor the youth closely, especially when the medicine is started. The doctor will work with you to increase the positive effects and decrease the negative effects of the medicine. Please tell the doctor if any of the listed side effects appear or if you think that the medicine is causing any other problems. Not all of the rare or unusual side effects are listed.

Side effects are most common after starting the medicine or after a dose increase. Many side effects can be avoided or lessened by starting with a very low dose and increasing it slowly—ask the doctor.

Allergic Reaction

Tell the doctor in a day or two (if possible, before the next dose of medicine):

- Hives
- Itching
- Rash

Stop the medicine and get *immediate* medical care:

- Trouble breathing or chest tightness
- Swelling of lips, tongue, or throat

Common, but Not Usually Serious, Side Effects

Discuss the following side effects with your child's doctor when convenient. These side effects often can be helped by lowering the dose of medicine, changing the times medicine is taken, or adding another medicine.

- Daytime sleepiness or tiredness—Do not allow your child to drive, ride a bicycle or motorcycle, or operate machinery if this happens. This problem may be lessened by taking the medicine at bedtime.
- Dry mouth—Have your child try using sugar-free gum or candy.
- Constipation—Encourage your child to drink more fluids and eat high-fiber foods; if necessary, the doctor may recommend a fiber medicine such as Benefiber or a stool softener such as Colace or mineral oil.
- Dizziness—This side effect is worse when the child stands up quickly, especially when getting out of bed in the morning; try having the child stand up slowly.
- Increased appetite
- Weight gain—Seek nutritional counseling; provide your child with low-calorie snacks and encourage regular exercise.
- Increased risk of sunburn—Have your child wear sunscreen or protective clothing or stay out of the sun.
- Nausea

- Vomiting
- Insomnia (trouble sleeping)

Less Common, but Not Usually Serious, Side Effects

Discuss the following side effects with your child's doctor when convenient. These side effects often can be helped by lowering the dose of medicine, changing the times medicine is taken, or adding another medicine.

- Drooling
- Increased restlessness or inability to sit still
- Shaking of hands and fingers
- Decreased or slowed movement and decreased facial expressions
- Decreased sexual interest or ability
- Changes in menstrual cycle
- Increase in breast size or discharge from the breasts (in both boys and girls)—This may go away with time.

Less Common, but Potentially Serious, Side Effects

Call the doctor *immediately:*

- Stiffness of the tongue, jaw, neck, back, or legs
- Seizure (fit, convulsion)—This is more common in people with a history of seizures or head injury.
- Increased thirst, frequent urination (having to go to the bathroom often), lethargy, tiredness, dizziness, and blurred vision—These could be signs of diabetes, especially if your child is overweight or there is a family history of diabetes. **Talk to a doctor within a day.**

Very Rare, but Serious, Side Effects

- Extreme stiffness or lack of movement, very high fever, mental confusion, irregular pulse rate, or eye pain—**This is a medical emergency. Go to an emergency room right away.**
- Sudden stiffness and inability to breathe or swallow—**Go to an emergency room or call 911.** Tell the paramedics, nurses, and doctors that the patient is taking iloperidone. Other medicines can be used to treat this problem quickly.

What Else Should I Know About Side Effects?

Most side effects lessen over time. If they are troublesome, talk with your child's doctor. Some side effects can be decreased by taking a smaller dose of medicine, by stopping the medicine, by changing to another medicine, or by adding another medicine.

Many young people who take iloperidone gain weight. The weight gain may be from increased appetite and also from ways that the medicine changes how the body processes food. Iloperidone may also change the way that the body handles glucose (sugar) and cause high levels of blood sugar (*hyperglycemia*). People who take iloperidone, especially those who gain a lot of weight, might be at increased risk of developing *diabetes* and of having increased fats (*lipids—cholesterol and triglycerides*) in their blood. Over time, both diabetes and increased fats in the blood may lead to heart disease, stroke, and other complications. The FDA has put warnings on all atypical agents about the increased risks of hyperglycemia, diabetes, and increased blood cholesterol and triglycerides when taking one of these medicines. It is much easier to prevent weight gain than to lose weight later. When your child first starts taking iloperidone, it is a good idea to be sure that he or she eats a well-balanced diet without "junk food" and with healthy snacks like fruits and vegetables, not sweets or fried foods. He or she should drink water or skim milk, not pop, sodas, soft drinks, or sugary juices. Regular exercise is important for maintaining a healthy weight (and may also help with sleep).

The medicine may increase the level of *prolactin*, a natural hormone made in the part of the brain called the *pituitary*. This may cause side effects such as breast tenderness or swelling or production of milk in both boys and girls. It also may interfere with sexual functioning in teenage boys and with regular menstrual cycles (periods) in teenage girls. A blood test can measure the level of prolactin. If these side effects do not go away and are troublesome, talk with your child's doctor about substituting another medicine for iloperidone.

One very rare side effect that may not go away is *tardive dyskinesia* (or TD). Patients with tardive dyskinesia have involuntary movements (movements that they cannot help making) of the body, especially the mouth and tongue. The patient may look as though he or she is making faces over and over again. Jerky movements of the arms, legs, or body may occur. There may be fine, wormlike, or sudden repeated movements of the tongue, or the person may appear to be chewing something or smacking or puckering his or her lips. The fingers may look as though they are rolling something. If you notice any unusual movements, be sure to tell the doctor. The doctor may use the AIMS test to look for these movements.

Neuroleptic malignant syndrome is a very rare side effect that can lead to death. The symptoms are severe muscle stiffness, high fever, increased heart rate and blood pressure, irregular heartbeat (pulse), and sweating. It may lead to unconsciousness. If you suspect this, **call 911 or go to an emergency room right away.**

Sometimes this medicine can cause a *dystonic reaction*. This is a sudden stiffening of the muscles, most often in the jaw, neck, tongue, face, or shoulders. If this happens, and your child is not having trouble breathing, you may give a dose of diphenhydramine (Benadryl). Follow the dose instructions on the package for your child's age. This should relax the muscles in a few minutes. Then call your doctor to tell him or her what happened. If the muscles do not relax, take your child to the emergency department.

Some Interactions With Other Medicines or Food

Please note that the following are only the most likely interactions with other medicines or food.

Iloperidone should be taken without food.

Paroxetine (Paxil), fluoxetine (Prozac), and other selective serotonin reuptake inhibitor (SSRI) antidepressants can increase the levels of iloperidone and increase the risk of side effects.

Heart problems are more common if other medicines that affect the heart are being taken as well. Be sure to tell all your child's doctors and your pharmacist about all medications your child is taking.

It is better to limit drinks with caffeine (coffee, tea, soft drinks) because caffeine works in the opposite way from this medicine, and the positive effects might be decreased.

What Could Happen if This Medicine Is Stopped Suddenly?

Involuntary movements, or *withdrawal dyskinesias*, may appear within 1–4 weeks of lowering the dose or stopping the medicine. Usually these go away, but they can last for days to months. If iloperidone is stopped suddenly, emotional disturbance (such as irritability, nervousness, moodiness, or oppositional behavior) or physical problems (such as stomachache, loss of appetite, nausea, vomiting, diarrhea, sweating, indigestion, trouble sleeping, trembling, or shaking) may appear. These problems usually last only a few days to a few weeks. If they happen, you should tell your child's doctor. The medicine dose may need to be lowered more slowly (tapered). Always check with the doctor before stopping a medicine.

How Long Will This Medicine Be Needed?

How long your child will need to take this medicine depends partly on the reason that it was prescribed. Some problems last for only a few months, whereas others last much longer. It is important to ask the doctor whether medicine is still needed, especially with medicines as powerful as this one. Every few months, you should discuss with your child's doctor the reasons for using the medicine and whether the medicine may be stopped or the dose lowered.

What Else Should I Know About This Medicine?

There are other medicines that are used for the same kinds of problems. If your child is having bad side effects or the medicine does not seem to be working, ask the doctor if another medicine might work as well or better and have fewer side effects for your child. Each person reacts differently to medicines.

Taking this medicine could make overheating or heatstroke more likely. Have your child decrease activity in hot weather, stay out of the sun, and drink water to prevent this.

Notes

Use this space to take notes or to write down questions you want to ask the doctor.

From Dulcan MK, Ballard R (editors): *Helping Parents and Teachers Understand Medications for Behavioral and Emotional Problems: A Resource Book of Medication Information Handouts*, Fourth Edition. Washington, DC, American Psychiatric Publishing, 2015

Medication Information for Parents and Teachers

Imipramine—Tofranil

General Information About Medication

Each child and adolescent is different. No one has exactly the same combination of medical and psychological problems. It is a good idea to talk with the doctor or nurse about the reasons a medicine is being used. It is very important to keep all appointments and to be in touch by telephone if you have concerns. It is important to communicate with the doctor, nurse, or therapist. An *advanced practice nurse* (APN) has additional education and training after becoming a registered nurse (RN). Your child's medication may be prescribed by a medical doctor (MD or DO) or an APN. In addition, a *physician assistant* (PA) working with a physician may prescribe certain medications. In this information sheet, "doctor" includes medical doctors as well as APNs and PAs who prescribe medication. Often a nurse (RN) will be part of the team and answer questions and give information.

It is very important that the medicine be taken exactly as the doctor instructs. However, once in a while, everyone forgets to give a medicine on time. It is a good idea to ask the doctor or nurse what to do if this happens. Do not stop or change a medicine without asking the doctor or nurse first.

If the medicine seems to stop working, it may be because it is not being taken regularly. The youth may be "cheeking" or hiding the medicine or forgetting to take it (especially at school). The doses may be too far apart or a different dose or medicine may be needed. Something at school, at home, or in the neighborhood may be upsetting the youth, or he or she may need special help for learning disabilities or tutoring. Please discuss your concerns with the doctor. **Do not just increase the dose.** It is also very important not to decrease the dose or stop the medicine without talking to the doctor first. The problem being treated may come back, or there could be uncomfortable or even dangerous results.

All medicines should be kept in a safe place, out of the reach of children, and should be supervised by an adult. If someone takes too much of a medicine, call the doctor, the poison control center, or a hospital emergency room.

Each medicine has a "generic" or chemical name. Just like laundry detergents or paper towels, some medicines are sold by more than one company under different brand names. The same medicine may be available under a generic name and several brand names. The generic medications are usually less expensive than the brand name ones. The generic medications have the same chemical formula, but they may or may not be exactly the same strength as the brand-name medications. Also, some brands of pills contain dye or other things that can cause allergic reactions. It is a good idea to talk to the doctor and the pharmacist about whether it is important to use a specific brand of medicine.

Any medicine can cause an allergic reaction. Examples are hives, itching, rashes, swelling, and trouble breathing. Even a tiny amount of a medicine can cause a reaction in patients who are allergic to that medicine. Be *sure* to talk to the doctor before restarting a medicine that has caused an allergic reaction and tell the doctor about any reactions to medicine that your child has had before.

Taking more than one medicine at the same time may cause more side effects or cause one of the medicines to not work as well. Always ask the doctor, nurse, or pharmacist before adding another

medicine, either prescription or bought without a prescription in a store or on the Internet. **Be sure that each doctor knows about** *all* **of the medicines your child is taking. Also tell the doctor about any vitamins, herbal medicines, or supplements your child may be taking.** Some of these may have side effects alone or when taken with this medication. It is a very good idea to keep a list with you of the names and doses of all medicines that your child is taking.

Everyone taking medicine should have a physical examination at least once a year.

If you think that your child may be using drugs or alcohol, please tell the doctor right away.

Pregnancy requires special care in the use of medicine. Some medicines can cause birth defects if taken by a pregnant mother. **Please tell the doctor immediately if you suspect the teenager is at risk of becoming pregnant.** The doctor may wish to discuss sexual behavior and/or birth control with your daughter.

Printed information like this applies to children and adolescents in general. If you have questions about the medicine, or if you notice changes or anything unusual, please ask the doctor or nurse. As scientific research advances, knowledge increases and advice changes. Even experts do not always agree. Many medicines have not been "approved" by the U.S. Food and Drug Administration (FDA) for use in children or use for particular problems. For this reason, use of the medicine for a problem or age group often is not listed in the *Physicians' Desk Reference*. This does not necessarily mean that the medicine is dangerous or does not work, only that the company that makes the medicine has not received permission to advertise the medicine for use in children. Companies often do not apply for this permission because it is expensive to do the tests needed to apply for approval for use in children. Once a medication is approved by the FDA for any purpose, a doctor is allowed to prescribe it according to research and clinical experience.

Note to Teachers

It is a good idea to talk with the parent(s) about the reason(s) that a medication is being used. If the parent(s) sign consent to release information, it is often helpful for you to talk with the doctor. If the parent(s) give permission, the doctor may ask you to fill out rating forms about your experience with the student's behavior, feelings, academic performance, and medication side effects. This information is very useful in selecting and monitoring medication treatment. If you have observations that you think are important, do not hesitate to share these with the student's parent(s) and treating clinicians (with parental consent).

It is very important that the medicine be taken exactly as the doctor instructs. However, everyone forgets to give a medicine on time once in a while. It is a good idea to ask the parent(s) in advance what to do if this happens. Do not stop or change the time you are giving a medicine at school without parental permission. If a medication is to be taken with food, but lunchtime or snack time changes, be sure to notify the parent(s) so appropriate adjustments can be made.

All medicines should be kept in a secure place and should be supervised by an adult. If someone takes too much of a medicine, follow your school procedure for an urgent medical problem.

Taking medicine is a private matter and is best managed discreetly and confidentially. It is important to be sensitive to the student's feelings about taking medicine.

If you suspect that the student is using drugs or alcohol, please tell the parent(s) or a school counselor right away.

Please tell the parent(s) or school nurse if you suspect medication side effects.

Modifications of the classroom environment or assignments may be useful in addition to medication. The student may need to be evaluated for additional help or a 504 plan or an Individualized Education Plan for learning problems or emotional or behavioral issues.

Any expression of suicidal thoughts or feelings or self-harm by a child or adolescent is a signal of distress and should be taken seriously. These behaviors should not be dismissed as "attention seeking." School procedures for safety issues should be followed.

You may notice the following side effects at school:

Common Side Effects

- Dry mouth—Allow the student to chew sugar-free gum, carry a water bottle, or make extra trips to the water fountain.
- Constipation—Allow the student to drink more fluids or to use the bathroom more often.
- Daytime sleepiness—The student should not drive, ride a bicycle or motorcycle, or operate machinery.
- Dizziness (especially when standing up quickly)—This may happen in the classroom or during physical education. Suggest that the student stand up more slowly.
- Irritability

Occasional Side Effects

- Stuttering
- Increased risk of sunburn (this may be a problem if recess or physical education is outdoors in warm weather)—The student should wear sunscreen or protective clothing or stay out of the sun.

Less Common Side Effects

- Nausea—The student may need to take the medicine after a meal or snack.
- Trouble urinating—The student may need more time in the bathroom.
- Blurred vision—The student may have trouble seeing the blackboard.
- Motor tics (fast, repeated movements) or muscle twitches (jerking movements) of parts of the body
- Increased activity, rapid speech, feeling "speeded up," being very excited or irritable (cranky)
- Skin rash

Rare, but Potentially Serious, Side Effects

Call the parent(s) or follow your school's emergency procedures *immediately*:

- Seizure (fit, convulsion) **(This is a medical emergency.)**
- Very fast or irregular heartbeat **(This is a medical emergency.)**
- Fainting
- Hallucinations (hearing voices or seeing things that are not there)
- Inability to urinate
- Confusion
- Severe change in behavior

What Is Imipramine (Tofranil)?

Imipramine is called a *tricyclic antidepressant*. It was first used to treat depression but is now used to treat enuresis (bed-wetting), attention-deficit/hyperactivity disorder (ADHD), school phobia, separation anxiety, panic disorder, and some sleep disorders (such as night terrors and sleepwalking). It comes in brand name Tofranil and generic tablets and Tofranil-PM and generic sustained-release (long-acting) capsules.

261

How Can This Medicine Help?

Imipramine can decrease symptoms of ADHD, anxiety (nervousness), panic, and night terrors or sleepwalking. The medicine may take several weeks to work. Imipramine can also help control urination and decrease bed-wetting (nocturnal enuresis). When treating enuresis, the medicine works right away.

How Does This Medicine Work?

Tricyclic antidepressants affect *neurotransmitters*—the natural substances that are needed for nerves and certain parts of the brain to work normally. They increase the activity of *serotonin* and *norepinephrine*. Science does not yet know how imipramine helps stop bed-wetting.

How Long Does This Medicine Last?

Although a dose lasts for a whole day in adults and older teenagers, in younger children several doses a day may be needed.

How Will the Doctor Monitor This Medicine?

The doctor will review your child's medical history and physical examination, paying special attention to pulse rate, blood pressure, weight, and height, before starting imipramine. These measurements will be taken when the dose is increased and occasionally as long as the medicine is continued. The doctor may order some blood or urine tests to be sure your child does not have a hidden medical condition that would make it unsafe to use this medicine.

Tricyclic antidepressants can slow the speed at which signals move through the heart. This effect is not dangerous if the heart is normal, which is why an ECG (electrocardiogram or heart rhythm test) is done before starting the medicine. The ECG may be repeated as the dose is increased and occasionally while the medicine is being taken. Changes in the heart from the medicine usually can be seen on the ECG before they become a problem, so your child's doctor will order an ECG every so often. When imipramine is used only at night in very low doses to treat bed-wetting, an ECG may not be needed.

To find possible hidden heart risks, it is especially important to tell the doctor if your child or anyone in the family has a history of fainting, palpitations, or irregular heartbeat or if anyone in the family died suddenly.

Be sure to tell the doctor if your child or anyone in the family has bipolar disorder or has tried to kill himself or herself.

Because imipramine may increase the risk of seizures (fits, convulsions), the doctor will want to know whether your child has ever had a seizure or a head injury and if there is any family history of epilepsy. Your child's doctor may want to order an EEG (electroencephalogram or brain wave test) before starting the medicine.

Experts do not agree on whether blood tests are needed to measure the level of this medicine. Blood levels seem to be most useful when your doctor suspects that the dose of medicine is too high or too low. The most accurate level is obtained by drawing blood first thing in the morning after at least 5 days on the same dose, approximately 12 hours after the evening dose of medicine and before the morning dose.

262

After the medicine is started, the doctor will want to have regular appointments with you and your child to see how the medicine is working, to see if a dose change is needed, to watch for side effects, to see if imipramine is still needed, and to see if any other treatment is needed. The doctor or nurse may check your child's height, weight, pulse, and blood pressure or order tests, such as an ECG or blood level.

Before using medicine and at times afterward, the doctor may ask your child to fill out a rating scale about anxiety, to help see how your child is doing.

What Side Effects Can This Medicine Have?

Any medicine can have side effects, including an allergy to the medicine. Because each patient is different, the doctor will monitor the youth closely, especially when the medicine is started. The doctor will work with you to increase the positive effects and decrease the negative effects of the medicine. Please tell the doctor if any of the listed side effects appear or if you think that the medicine is causing any other problems. Not all of the rare or unusual side effects are listed.

Side effects are most common after starting the medicine or after a dose increase. Many side effects can be avoided or lessened by starting with a very low dose and increasing it slowly—ask the doctor.

Allergic Reaction

Tell the doctor in a day or two (if possible, before the next dose of medicine):

- Hives
- Itching
- Rash (may be caused by an allergy to the medicine or to a dye in the specific brand of pill)

Stop the medicine and get *immediate* medical care:

- Trouble breathing or chest tightness
- Swelling of lips, tongue, or throat

Common Side Effects

Tell the doctor within a week or two:

- Dry mouth—Have your child try using sugar-free gum or candy.
- Constipation—Encourage your child to drink more fluids and eat high-fiber foods; if necessary, the doctor may recommend a fiber medicine such as Benefiber or a stool softener such as Colace or mineral oil.
- Daytime sleepiness—Do not allow your child to drive, ride a bicycle or motorcycle, or operate machinery if this happens.
- Dizziness—This side effect is worse when the child stands up quickly, especially when getting out of bed in the morning; try having the child stand up slowly.
- Weight gain
- Loss of appetite and weight loss
- Irritability
- Acne

Occasional Side Effects

Tell the doctor within a week or two:

- Nightmares
- Stuttering
- Blurred vision
- Increase in breast size, nipple discharge, or both (in girls)
- Increase in breast size (in boys)

Less Common, but More Serious, Side Effects

Call the doctor within a day or two:

- High or low blood pressure
- Nausea
- Trouble urinating
- Motor tics (fast, repeated movements) or muscle twitches (jerking movements)
- Increased activity, rapid speech, feeling "speeded up," decreased need for sleep, being very excited or irritable (cranky)
- Yellowing of skin or eyes, dark urine, pale bowel movements, abdominal pain or fullness, unexplained flu-like symptoms, itchy skin—These side effects are extremely rare but could be signs of liver damage.

Rare, but Potentially Serious, Side Effects

Call the doctor *immediately*:

- Seizure (fit, convulsion)—**Go to an emergency room.**
- Very fast or irregular heartbeat—**Go to an emergency room.**
- Fainting
- Hallucinations (hearing voices or seeing things that are not there)
- Inability to pass urine
- Confusion
- Severe change in behavior

Some Interactions With Other Medicines or Food

Please note that the following are only the most likely interactions with other medicines or food.

Check with your child's doctor before giving your child decongestants or over-the-counter cold medicine.

Taking another antidepressant or Depakote with imipramine may increase the level of imipramine and increase side effects.

Taking carbamazepine (Tegretol) with imipramine may decrease the positive effects of imipramine and increase the side effects of carbamazepine.

It can be *very dangerous* to take imipramine at the same time as or even within a month of taking another type of medicine called a *monoamine oxidase inhibitor* (MAOI), such as selegiline (Eldepryl), phenelzine (Nardil), tranylcypromine (Parnate), or isocarboxazid (Marplan).

The combination of imipramine and linezolid may be dangerous. Taking imipramine and pimozide may cause side effects in the heart. Ask the doctor.

Caffeine may worsen side effects on the heart or symptoms of anxiety. It is best not to drink coffee, tea, or soft drinks with caffeine while taking this medicine.

What Could Happen if This Medicine Is Stopped Suddenly?

Stopping the medicine suddenly or skipping a dose is not dangerous but can be very uncomfortable. Your child may feel like he or she has the flu—with a headache, muscle aches, stomachache, and upset stomach. Behavioral problems, sadness, nervousness, or trouble sleeping also may occur. If these feelings appear every day, the medicine may need to be given more often during each day.

How Long Will This Medicine Be Needed?

There is no way to know how long a person will need to take this medicine. Parents work together with the doctor to determine what is right for each child. For bed-wetting, the medicine may be used for 6–12 months and may be stopped if the child grows out of bed-wetting. When treating ADHD, the medicine may be needed for a longer time. Some people may need to take the medicine even as adults.

What Else Should I Know About This Medicine?

In youth who have bipolar disorder or who are at risk for bipolar disorder, any antidepressant medicine may increase the risk of hypomania or mania (excitement, agitation, increased activity, decreased sleep).

An overdose by accident or on purpose with this medicine is very dangerous! You must closely supervise the medicine. You may have to lock up the medicine if your child or teenager is suicidal or if young children live in or visit your home.

Tricyclic antidepressants may cause dry mouth, which could increase the chance of tooth decay. Regular brushing of teeth and checkups with the dentist are especially important.

This medicine causes increased risk of sunburn. Be sure that your child wears sunscreen or protective clothing or stays out of the sun.

People who take tricyclic antidepressants must not drink alcohol or use tranquilizers. Severe sleepiness, loss of consciousness, or even death may result.

Black Box Antidepressant Warning

In 2004, an advisory committee to the FDA decided that there might be an increased risk of suicidal behavior for some youth taking medicines called *antidepressants*. In the research studies that the committee reviewed, about 3%–4% of youth with depression who took an antidepressant medicine—and 1%–2% of youth with depression who took a placebo (pill without active medicine)—talked about suicidal thoughts (thinking about killing themselves or wishing they were dead) or did something to harm themselves. This means that almost twice as many youth who were taking an antidepressant to treat their depression talked about suicide or had suicidal behavior compared with youth with depression who were taking inactive medicine. There were *no* completed suicides in any of these research studies, which included more than 4,000 children and adolescents. For youth being treated for anxiety, there was no difference in suicidal talking or behavior between those taking antidepressant medication and those taking placebo.

The FDA told drug companies to add a *black box warning* label to all antidepressant medicines. Because of this label, a doctor (or advanced practice nurse) prescribing one of these medicines has to warn youth and their families that there might be more suicidal thoughts and actions in youth taking these medicines.

On the other hand, in places where more youth are taking the newer antidepressant medicines, the number of adolescents who commit suicide has gotten smaller. Also, thinking about or attempting suicide is more common in surveys of teenagers in the community than it is in depressed youth treated in research studies with antidepressant medicine.

If a youth is being treated with this medicine and is doing well, then no changes are needed as a result of this warning. Increased suicidal talk or action is most likely to happen in the first few months of treatment with a medicine. If your child has recently started this medicine or is about to start, then you and your doctor (or advanced practice nurse) should watch for any changes in behavior. People who are depressed often have suicidal thoughts or actions. It is hard to know whether suicidal thoughts or actions in depressed people are caused by the depression itself or by the medicine. Also, as their depression is getting better, some people talk more about the suicidal thoughts that they had before but did not talk about. As young people get better from depression, they might be at higher risk of doing something about suicidal thoughts that they have had for some time, because they have more energy.

What Should a Parent Do?

1. Be honest with your child about possible risks and benefits of medicine.
2. Talk to your child about whether he or she is having any suicidal thoughts, and tell your child to come to you if he or she is having such thoughts.
3. You, your child, and your child's doctor or nurse should develop a safety plan. Pick adults whom your child can tell if he or she is thinking about suicide.
4. Be sure to tell your child's doctor, nurse, or therapist if you suspect that your child is using alcohol or drugs or if something has happened that might make your child feel worse, such as a family separation, breaking up with a boyfriend or girlfriend, someone close dying or attempting suicide, physical or sexual abuse, or failure in school.
5. Be sure that there are no guns in the home and that all medicines (including over-the-counter medicines like Tylenol) are closely supervised by an adult and kept in a safe place.
6. Watch for new or worse thoughts of suicide, self-harm, depression, anxiety (nerves), feeling very agitated or restless, being angry or aggressive, having more trouble sleeping, or anything else that you see for the first time, seems worse, or worries your child or you. If these appear, contact a mental health professional **right away.** Do not just stop or change the dose of the medicine on your own. If the problems are serious, and you cannot reach one of your clinicians, call a 24-hour psychiatry emergency telephone number or take your child to an emergency room.

Youth taking antidepressant medicine should be watched carefully by their parent(s), clinician(s) (doctor, advanced practice nurse, nurse, therapist), and other concerned adults for the first weeks of treatment. It is a good idea to have regular contact with the doctor, APN, nurse, or therapist for the first months to check for feelings of depression or sadness, thoughts of killing or harming himself or herself, and any problems with the medication. If you have questions, be sure to ask the doctor, APN, nurse, or therapist.

For more information, see http://www.parentsmedguide.org/.

Notes

Use this space to take notes or to write down questions you want to ask the doctor.

_____

_____

_____

_____

_____

_____

_____

_____

_____

_____

_____

_____

_____

From Dulcan MK, Ballard R (editors): _Helping Parents and Teachers Understand Medications for Behavioral and Emotional Problems: A Resource Book of Medication Information Handouts_, Fourth Edition. Washington, DC, American Psychiatric Publishing, 2015

Medication Information for Parents and Teachers

Lamotrigine—Lamictal, Lamictal XR

General Information About Medication

Each child and adolescent is different. No one has exactly the same combination of medical and psychological problems. It is a good idea to talk with the doctor or nurse about the reasons a medicine is being used. It is very important to keep all appointments and to be in touch by telephone if you have concerns. It is important to communicate with the doctor, nurse, or therapist. An *advanced practice nurse* (APN) has additional education and training after becoming a registered nurse (RN). Your child's medication may be prescribed by a medical doctor (MD or DO) or an APN. In addition, a *physician assistant* (PA) working with a physician may prescribe certain medications. In this information sheet, "doctor" includes medical doctors as well as APNs and PAs who prescribe medication. Often a nurse (RN) will be part of the team and answer questions and give information.

It is very important that the medicine be taken exactly as the doctor instructs. However, once in a while, everyone forgets to give a medicine on time. It is a good idea to ask the doctor or nurse what to do if this happens. Do not stop or change a medicine without asking the doctor or nurse first.

If the medicine seems to stop working, it may be because it is not being taken regularly. The youth may be "cheeking" or hiding the medicine or forgetting to take it (especially at school). The doses may be too far apart or a different dose or medicine may be needed. Something at school, at home, or in the neighborhood may be upsetting the youth, or he or she may need special help for learning disabilities or tutoring. Please discuss your concerns with the doctor. **Do not just increase the dose.** It is also very important not to decrease the dose or stop the medicine without talking to the doctor first. The problem being treated may come back, or there could be uncomfortable or even dangerous results.

All medicines should be kept in a safe place, out of the reach of children, and should be supervised by an adult. If someone takes too much of a medicine, call the doctor, the poison control center, or a hospital emergency room.

Each medicine has a "generic" or chemical name. Just like laundry detergents or paper towels, some medicines are sold by more than one company under different brand names. The same medicine may be available under a generic name and several brand names. The generic medications are usually less expensive than the brand name ones. The generic medications have the same chemical formula, but they may or may not be exactly the same strength as the brand-name medications. Also, some brands of pills contain dye or other things that can cause allergic reactions. It is a good idea to talk to the doctor and the pharmacist about whether it is important to use a specific brand of medicine.

Any medicine can cause an allergic reaction. Examples are hives, itching, rashes, swelling, and trouble breathing. Even a tiny amount of a medicine can cause a reaction in patients who are allergic to that medicine. Be *sure* to talk to the doctor before restarting a medicine that has caused an allergic reaction and tell the doctor about any reactions to medicine that your child has had before.

Taking more than one medicine at the same time may cause more side effects or cause one of the medicines to not work as well. Always ask the doctor, nurse, or pharmacist before adding another medicine, either prescription or bought without a prescription in a store or on the Internet. Be sure

that each doctor knows about *all* of the medicines your child is taking. **Also tell the doctor about any vitamins, herbal medicines, or supplements your child may be taking.** Some of these may have side effects alone or when taken with this medication. It is a very good idea to keep a list with you of the names and doses of all medicines that your child is taking.

Everyone taking medicine should have a physical examination at least once a year.

If you think that your child may be using drugs or alcohol, please tell the doctor right away.

Pregnancy requires special care in the use of medicine. Some medicines can cause birth defects if taken by a pregnant mother. **Please tell the doctor immediately if you suspect the teenager is at risk of becoming pregnant.** The doctor may wish to discuss sexual behavior and/or birth control with your daughter.

Printed information like this applies to children and adolescents in general. If you have questions about the medicine, or if you notice changes or anything unusual, please ask the doctor or nurse. As scientific research advances, knowledge increases and advice changes. Even experts do not always agree. Many medicines have not been "approved" by the U.S. Food and Drug Administration (FDA) for use in children or use for particular problems. For this reason, use of the medicine for a problem or age group often is not listed in the *Physicians' Desk Reference*. This does not necessarily mean that the medicine is dangerous or does not work, only that the company that makes the medicine has not received permission to advertise the medicine for use in children. Companies often do not apply for this permission because it is expensive to do the tests needed to apply for approval for use in children. Once a medication is approved by the FDA for any purpose, a doctor is allowed to prescribe it according to research and clinical experience.

Note to Teachers

It is a good idea to talk with the parent(s) about the reason(s) that a medication is being used. If the parent(s) sign consent to release information, it is often helpful for you to talk with the doctor. If the parent(s) give permission, the doctor may ask you to fill out rating forms about your experience with the student's behavior, feelings, academic performance, and medication side effects. This information is very useful in selecting and monitoring medication treatment. If you have observations that you think are important, do not hesitate to share these with the student's parent(s) and treating clinicians (with parental consent).

It is very important that the medicine be taken exactly as the doctor instructs. However, everyone forgets to give a medicine on time once in a while. It is a good idea to ask the parent(s) in advance what to do if this happens. Do not stop or change the time you are giving a medicine at school without parental permission. If a medication is to be taken with food, but lunchtime or snack time changes, be sure to notify the parent(s) so appropriate adjustments can be made.

All medicines should be kept in a secure place and should be supervised by an adult. If someone takes too much of a medicine, follow your school procedure for an urgent medical problem.

Taking medicine is a private matter and is best managed discreetly and confidentially. It is important to be sensitive to the student's feelings about taking medicine.

If you suspect that the student is using drugs or alcohol, please tell the parent(s) or a school counselor right away.

Please tell the parent(s) or school nurse if you suspect medication side effects.

Modifications of the classroom environment or assignments may be useful in addition to medication. The student may need to be evaluated for additional help or a 504 plan or an Individualized Education Plan for learning problems or emotional or behavioral issues.

Any expression of suicidal thoughts or feelings or self-harm by a child or adolescent is a signal of distress and should be taken seriously. These behaviors should not be dismissed as "attention seeking." School procedures for safety issues should be followed.

What Is Lamotrigine (Lamictal)?

Lamotrigine was first used to treat seizures (fits, convulsions), so it is sometimes called an *anticonvulsant* or an *antiepileptic drug* (AED). Now it is also used for behavioral problems, depression, or bipolar disorder, whether or not the patient has seizures. It also may be used when the patient has a history of severe mood changes, sometimes called *mood swings*. When used in psychiatry, this medicine is more commonly called a *mood stabilizer*.

Lamotrigine comes in brand name Lamictal and generic tablets and chewable tablets and Lamictal XR and generic extended-release tablets, as well as Lamictal tablets that dissolve under the tongue.

How Can This Medicine Help?

Lamotrigine can reduce aggression, anger, and severe mood swings. It can treat mania or prevent bipolar depression.

How Does This Medicine Work?

Lamotrigine is thought to work by stabilizing a part of the brain cell (the cell membrane or envelope) and by changing the concentration of a *neurotransmitter* (brain chemical) called *glutamate*.

How Long Does This Medicine Last?

Lamotrigine needs to be taken once or twice a day.

How Will the Doctor Monitor This Medicine?

The doctor will review your child's medical history and physical examination before starting lamotrigine. The doctor may order some blood tests to be sure your child does not have a hidden medical condition that would make it unsafe to use this medicine. The doctor or nurse may measure your child's pulse and blood pressure before starting lamotrigine.

After the medicine is started, the doctor will want to have regular appointments with you and your child to see how the medicine is working, to see if a dose change is needed, to watch for side effects, to see if lamotrigine is still needed, and to see if any other treatment is needed. The doctor or nurse may check your child's height, weight, pulse, and blood pressure. Blood tests are not usually needed during treatment with lamotrigine.

What Side Effects Can This Medicine Have?

Any medicine can have side effects, including an allergy to the medicine. Because each patient is different, the doctor will monitor the youth closely, especially when the medicine is started. The doctor will work with you to increase the positive effects and decrease the negative effects of the medicine. Please tell the doctor if any

271

of the listed side effects appear or if you think that the medicine is causing any other problems. Not all of the rare or unusual side effects are listed.

Side effects are most common after starting the medicine or after a dose increase. Many side effects can be avoided or lessened by starting with a very low dose and increasing it slowly—ask the doctor.

Allergic Reaction

Tell the doctor in a day or two (if possible, before the next dose of medicine):

- Hives
- Itching

Stop the medicine and get *immediate* medical care:

- Rash
- Trouble breathing or chest tightness
- Swelling of lips, tongue, or throat

General Side Effects

These side effects are more common when first starting the medicine. Tell the doctor within a week or two:

- Daytime sleepiness—Do not allow your child to drive, ride a bicycle or motorcycle, or operate machinery if this happens.
- Dizziness
- Headache
- Blurred vision
- Double vision
- Unsteadiness
- Nausea, vomiting
- Stomach cramps

Behavioral and Emotional Side Effects

Call the doctor within a day or two:

- Anxiety or nervousness
- Agitation or mania
- Tics (motor movements or sounds), thinking unwanted words or phrases over and over

Tell the doctor right away:

- Increased suicidal thoughts or behaviors or new or worse depression or anxiety

Possibly Dangerous Side Effects

Stop lamotrigine and go to an emergency room *immediately:*

- Vomiting
- Rash, especially when the rash is in the nose or mouth or there is also sore throat, fever, and/or generally feeling sick
- Severe headache together with pain in the neck, fever, nausea, vomiting, muscle pain

Some Interactions With Other Medicines or Food

Please note that the following are only the most likely interactions with other medicines or food.

Caffeine may increase side effects.

Lamotrigine interacts with many other medicines. Taking it with another medicine may make one or both not work as well or may cause more side effects. Be sure that each doctor knows about *all* of the medicines your child is taking.

Valproate (Depakote, Depakene) increases the level of lamotrigine, which increases the risk of very serious skin reaction.

When lamotrigine and birth control pills are taken together, neither one works very well. This could increase the risk of accidental pregnancy. An alternative form of birth control may be needed.

What Could Happen if This Medicine Is Stopped Suddenly?

Stopping lamotrigine suddenly may cause seizures or convulsions if your child is being treated for epilepsy (seizures).

How Long Will This Medicine Be Needed?

The length of time a person needs to take lamotrigine depends on what problem is being treated. For example, someone with an impulse control disorder usually takes the medicine only until behavioral therapy begins to work. Someone with bipolar disorder may need to take the medicine for many years. Please ask the doctor about the length of treatment needed.

What Else Should I Know About This Medicine?

Taking lamotrigine with food may decrease stomach upset.

There are four different formulations of lamotrigine (Lamictal). Be sure to check when you get a prescription or a new bottle of pills that you have the correct one.

The FDA has required a *black box warning* on lamotrigine because of the risk of an extreme skin reaction called *Stevens-Johnson syndrome*, a serious and potentially life-threatening condition. The risk is higher in children than in adults. This very serious blistering of skin and mucous membranes is more likely when lamotri-

273

gine is combined with valproate (Depakene or Depakote). Most rashes go away if the lamotrigine is stopped, but all rashes should be seen by a doctor. Some ways that the risk of serious reaction might be decreased include

- Increasing the dose of lamotrigine very slowly
- Avoiding other new medicines in the first 2 months of treatment with lamotrigine
- Avoiding new foods, cosmetics, deodorants, or clothes detergents or fabric softeners in the first 2 months of taking lamotrigine
- Not starting lamotrigine within 2 weeks of a rash, viral illness, or vaccination
- Avoiding sunburn
- Avoiding exposure to poison ivy or poison oak

Keep the medicine in a safe place under close supervision. Keep the pill container tightly closed and in a dry place, away from bathrooms, showers, and humidifiers.

People with kidney or liver problems may have more severe side effects from taking lamotrigine.

If your daughter becomes pregnant while taking lamotrigine, call the doctor right away.

Notes

Use this space to take notes or to write down questions you want to ask the doctor.

From Dulcan MK, Ballard R (editors): *Helping Parents and Teachers Understand Medications for Behavioral and Emotional Problems: A Resource Book of Medication Information Handouts*, Fourth Edition. Washington, DC, American Psychiatric Publishing, 2015

Medication Information for Parents and Teachers

Levomilnacipran—Fetzima

General Information About Medication

Each child and adolescent is different. No one has exactly the same combination of medical and psychological problems. It is a good idea to talk with the doctor or nurse about the reasons a medicine is being used. It is very important to keep all appointments and to be in touch by telephone if you have concerns. It is important to communicate with the doctor, nurse, or therapist. An *advanced practice nurse* (APN) has additional education and training after becoming a registered nurse (RN). Your child's medication may be prescribed by a medical doctor (MD or DO) or an APN. In addition, a *physician assistant* (PA) working with a physician may prescribe certain medications. In this information sheet, "doctor" includes medical doctors as well as APNs and PAs who prescribe medication. Often a nurse (RN) will be part of the team and answer questions and give information.

It is very important that the medicine be taken exactly as the doctor instructs. However, once in a while, everyone forgets to give a medicine on time. It is a good idea to ask the doctor or nurse what to do if this happens. Do not stop or change a medicine without asking the doctor or nurse first.

If the medicine seems to stop working, it may be because it is not being taken regularly. The youth may be "cheeking" or hiding the medicine or forgetting to take it (especially at school). The doses may be too far apart or a different dose or medicine may be needed. Something at school, at home, or in the neighborhood may be upsetting the youth, or he or she may need special help for learning disabilities or tutoring. Please discuss your concerns with the doctor. **Do not just increase the dose.** It is also very important not to decrease the dose or stop the medicine without talking to the doctor first. The problem being treated may come back, or there could be uncomfortable or even dangerous results.

All medicines should be kept in a safe place, out of the reach of children, and should be supervised by an adult. If someone takes too much of a medicine, call the doctor, the poison control center, or a hospital emergency room.

Each medicine has a "generic" or chemical name. Just like laundry detergents or paper towels, some medicines are sold by more than one company under different brand names. The same medicine may be available under a generic name and several brand names. The generic medications are usually less expensive than the brand name ones. The generic medications have the same chemical formula, but they may or may not be exactly the same strength as the brand-name medications. Also, some brands of pills contain dye or other things that can cause allergic reactions. It is a good idea to talk to the doctor and the pharmacist about whether it is important to use a specific brand of medicine.

Any medicine can cause an allergic reaction. Examples are hives, itching, rashes, swelling, and trouble breathing. Even a tiny amount of a medicine can cause a reaction in patients who are allergic to that medicine. Be *sure* to talk to the doctor before restarting a medicine that has caused an allergic reaction and tell the doctor about any reactions to medicine that your child has had before.

Taking more than one medicine at the same time may cause more side effects or cause one of the medicines to not work as well. Always ask the doctor, nurse, or pharmacist before adding another

medicine, either prescription or bought without a prescription in a store or on the Internet. **Be sure that each doctor knows about *all* of the medicines your child is taking. Also tell the doctor about any vitamins, herbal medicines, or supplements your child may be taking.** Some of these may have side effects alone or when taken with this medication. It is a very good idea to keep a list with you of the names and doses of all medicines that your child is taking.

Everyone taking medicine should have a physical examination at least once a year.

If you think that your child may be using drugs or alcohol, please tell the doctor right away.

Pregnancy requires special care in the use of medicine. Some medicines can cause birth defects if taken by a pregnant mother. **Please tell the doctor immediately if you suspect the teenager is at risk of becoming pregnant.** The doctor may wish to discuss sexual behavior and/or birth control with your daughter.

Printed information like this applies to children and adolescents in general. If you have questions about the medicine, or if you notice changes or anything unusual, please ask the doctor or nurse. As scientific research advances, knowledge increases and advice changes. Even experts do not always agree. Many medicines have not been "approved" by the U.S. Food and Drug Administration (FDA) for use in children or use for particular problems. For this reason, use of the medicine for a problem or age group often is not listed in the *Physicians' Desk Reference*. This does not necessarily mean that the medicine is dangerous or does not work, only that the company that makes the medicine has not received permission to advertise the medicine for use in children. Companies often do not apply for this permission because it is expensive to do the tests needed to apply for approval for use in children. Once a medication is approved by the FDA for any purpose, a doctor is allowed to prescribe it according to research and clinical experience.

Note to Teachers

It is a good idea to talk with the parent(s) about the reason(s) that a medication is being used. If the parent(s) sign consent to release information, it is often helpful for you to talk with the doctor. If the parent(s) give permission, the doctor may ask you to fill out rating forms about your experience with the student's behavior, feelings, academic performance, and medication side effects. This information is very useful in selecting and monitoring medication treatment. If you have observations that you think are important, do not hesitate to share these with the student's parent(s) and treating clinicians (with parental consent).

It is very important that the medicine be taken exactly as the doctor instructs. However, everyone forgets to give a medicine on time once in a while. It is a good idea to ask the parent(s) in advance what to do if this happens. Do not stop or change the time you are giving a medicine at school without parental permission. If a medication is to be taken with food, but lunchtime or snack time changes, be sure to notify the parent(s) so appropriate adjustments can be made.

All medicines should be kept in a secure place and should be supervised by an adult. If someone takes too much of a medicine, follow your school procedure for an urgent medical problem.

Taking medicine is a private matter and is best managed discreetly and confidentially. It is important to be sensitive to the student's feelings about taking medicine.

If you suspect that the student is using drugs or alcohol, please tell the parent(s) or a school counselor right away.

Please tell the parent(s) or school nurse if you suspect medication side effects.

Modifications of the classroom environment or assignments may be useful in addition to medication. The student may need to be evaluated for additional help or a 504 plan or an Individualized Education Plan for learning problems or emotional or behavioral issues.

Any expression of suicidal thoughts or feelings or self-harm by a child or adolescent is a signal of distress and should be taken seriously. These behaviors should not be dismissed as "attention seeking." School procedures for safety issues should be followed.

What Is Levomilnacipran (Fetzima)?

Levomilnacipran is an *antidepressant*. It is known as a *serotonin-norepinephrine reuptake inhibitor* (SNRI). It comes in brand name Fetzima extended-release capsules.

How Can This Medicine Help?

Levomilnacipran has been used successfully to treat depression in adults. There is currently little information on its use in children or adolescents. Levomilnacipran may take as long as 4–8 weeks to reach its full effect.

How Does This Medicine Work?

Levomilnacipran works by increasing the brain chemicals *serotonin* and *norepinephrine* (*neurotransmitters*) to more normal activity levels in certain parts of the brain and is referred to as a *serotonin-norepinephrine reuptake inhibitor* (SNRI). It has a somewhat different way of working than the antidepressants that are called *selective serotonin reuptake inhibitors* (SSRIs).

How Long Does This Medicine Last?

Levomilnacipran is taken once daily.

How Will the Doctor Monitor This Medicine?

The doctor will review your child's medical history and physical examination before starting levomilnacipran. The doctor may order some blood or urine tests to be sure your child does not have a hidden medical condition that would make it unsafe to use this medicine. This medication is eliminated from the body by the kidneys and should not be used in persons with severe kidney disease. It should not be used in children with known heart disease or an irregular heart rate. The doctor or nurse may measure your child's height and weight, and will check your child's pulse and blood pressure before starting levomilnacipran.

Be sure to tell the doctor if your child or anyone in the family has bipolar illness (manic-depressive illness) or has tried to kill himself or herself.

After the medicine is started, the doctor will want to have regular appointments with you and your child to see how the medicine is working, to see if a dose change is needed, to watch for side effects, to see if levomilnacipran is still needed, and to see if any other treatment is needed. The doctor or nurse may check your child's height, weight, pulse, and blood pressure. No blood tests are routinely required while taking levomilnacipran.

Before using medicine and at times afterward, the doctor may ask your child to fill out a rating scale about depression and anxiety, to help see how your child is doing.

What Side Effects Can This Medicine Have?

Any medicine can have side effects, including an allergy to the medicine. Because each patient is different, the doctor will monitor the youth closely, especially when the medicine is started. The doctor will work with you to increase the positive effects and decrease the negative effects of the medicine. Please tell the doctor if any of the listed side effects appear or if you think that the medicine is causing any other problems. Not all of the rare or unusual side effects are listed.

Side effects are most common after starting the medicine or after a dose increase. Many side effects can be avoided or lessened by starting with a very low dose and increasing it slowly—ask the doctor.

Allergic Reaction

Tell the doctor in a day or two (if possible, before the next dose of medicine):

- Hives
- Itching
- Rash

Stop the medicine and get *immediate* medical care:

- Trouble breathing or chest tightness
- Swelling of lips, tongue, or throat
- Severe skin rash or skin blisters

Common Side Effects

Tell the doctor within a week or two:

- Nausea
- Constipation—Encourage your child to drink more fluids and eat high-fiber foods; if necessary, the doctor may recommend a fiber medicine such as Benefiber or a stool softener such as Colace or mineral oil.
- Excessive sweating

Occasional Side Effects

Tell the doctor within a week or two:

- Increased blood pressure
- Rapid heart rate
- Abnormal bleeding—more common if the child is also taking aspirin or a nonsteroidal anti-inflammatory medication, such as ibuprofen or naproxen
- Difficulty passing urine
- Trouble with sexual functioning

Less Common, but More Serious, Side Effects

Call the doctor *immediately:*

• Seizure (fit, convulsion)

Serotonin Syndrome

A very serious side effect called *serotonin syndrome* can happen when certain kinds of medicines (including SSRI antidepressants, clomipramine, and other medicines, such as triptans for migraine headaches, buspirone, linezolid, tramadol, or St. John's wort) are taken by the same person. Very rarely, serotonin syndrome can happen at high doses of just one medicine. The early signs are restlessness, confusion, shaking, skin turning red, sweating, muscle stiffness, sweating, and jerking of muscles. If you see these symptoms, stop the medicine and send or take the youth to an emergency room right away.

Some Interactions With Other Medicines or Food

Please note that the following are only the most likely interactions with other medicines or food.

Levomilnacipran can be taken with or without food.

When the same person takes levomilnacipran and some medicines used to fight infection, the blood level of levomilnacipran and the risk of side effects may be increased. Talk with the doctor.

It can be *very dangerous* to take duloxetine at the same time as or even within a month of taking another type of medicine called a *monoamine oxidase inhibitor* (MAOI), such as selegiline (Eldepryl), phenelzine (Nardil), tranylcypromine (Parnate), or isocarboxazid (Marplan).

What Could Happen if This Medicine Is Stopped Suddenly?

No known serious medical withdrawal effects occur if levomilnacipran is stopped suddenly, but there may be uncomfortable feelings such as dizziness, insomnia, nausea, or nervousness, or the problem being treated may come back. Ask the doctor before stopping the medicine.

How Long Will This Medicine Be Needed?

Your child may need to keep taking the medicine for at least 6–12 months so that the emotional or behavioral problem does not come back. Please discuss this with the doctor.

What Else Should I Know About This Medicine?

Levomilnacipran must be swallowed whole and not be cut, chewed, or crushed.

In youth who have bipolar disorder or who may be at risk for bipolar disorder, any antidepressant medicine may increase the risk of hypomania or mania (excitement, agitation, increased activity, decreased sleep).

Black Box Antidepressant Warning

In 2004, an advisory committee to the FDA decided that there might be an increased risk of suicidal behavior for some youth taking medicines called *antidepressants*. In the research studies that the committee reviewed, about 3%–4% of youth with depression who took an antidepressant medicine—and 1%–2% of youth with depression who took a placebo (pill without active medicine)—talked about suicidal thoughts (thinking about killing themselves or wishing they were dead) or did something to harm themselves. This means that almost twice as many youth who were taking an antidepressant to treat their depression talked about suicide or had suicidal behavior compared with youth with depression who were taking inactive medicine. There were *no* completed suicides in any of these research studies, which included more than 4,000 children and adolescents. For youth being treated for anxiety, there was no difference in suicidal talking or behavior between those taking antidepressant medication and those taking placebo.

The FDA told drug companies to add a *black box warning* label to all antidepressant medicines. Because of this label, a doctor (or advanced practice nurse) prescribing one of these medicines has to warn youth and their families that there might be more suicidal thoughts and actions in youth taking these medicines.

On the other hand, in places where more youth are taking the newer antidepressant medicines, the number of adolescents who commit suicide has gotten smaller. Also, thinking about or attempting suicide is more common in surveys of teenagers in the community than it is in depressed youth treated in research studies with antidepressant medicine.

If a youth is being treated with this medicine and is doing well, then no changes are needed as a result of this warning. Increased suicidal talk or action is most likely to happen in the first few months of treatment with a medicine. If your child has recently started this medicine or is about to start, then you and your doctor (or advanced practice nurse) should watch for any changes in behavior. People who are depressed often have suicidal thoughts or actions. It is hard to know whether suicidal thoughts or actions in depressed people are caused by the depression itself or by the medicine. Also, as their depression is getting better, some people talk more about the suicidal thoughts that they had before but did not talk about. As young people get better from depression, they might be at higher risk of doing something about suicidal thoughts that they have had for some time, because they have more energy.

What Should A Parent Do?

1. Be honest with your child about possible risks and benefits of medicine.
2. Talk to your child about whether he or she is having any suicidal thoughts, and tell your child to come to you if he or she is having such thoughts.
3. You, your child, and your child's doctor or nurse should develop a safety plan. Pick adults whom your child can tell if he or she is thinking about suicide.
4. Be sure to tell your child's doctor, nurse, or therapist if you suspect that your child is using alcohol or drugs or if something has happened that might make your child feel worse, such as a family separation, breaking up with a boyfriend or girlfriend, someone close dying or attempting suicide, physical or sexual abuse, or failure in school.
5. Be sure that there are no guns in the home and that all medicines (including over-the-counter medicines like Tylenol) are closely supervised by an adult and kept in a safe place.
6. Watch for new or worse thoughts of suicide, self-harm, depression, anxiety (nerves), feeling very agitated or restless, being angry or aggressive, having more trouble sleeping, or anything else that you see for the first time, seems worse, or worries your child or you. If these appear, contact a mental health professional **right away.** Do not just stop or change the dose of the medicine on your own. If the problems are serious, and you cannot reach one of your clinicians, call a 24-hour psychiatry emergency telephone number or take your child to an emergency room.

Youth taking antidepressant medicine should be watched carefully by their parent(s), clinician(s) (doctor, advanced practice nurse, nurse, therapist), and other concerned adults for the first weeks of treatment. It is a good idea to have regular contact with the doctor, APN, nurse, or therapist for the first months to check for feelings of depression or sadness, thoughts of killing or harming himself or herself, and any problems with the medication. If you have questions, be sure to ask the doctor, APN, nurse, or therapist.

For more information, see http://www.parentsmedguide.org/.

Notes

Use this space to take notes or to write down questions you want to ask the doctor.

_____

_____

_____

_____

_____

_____

_____

_____

_____

_____

_____

chanical errors sometimes occur, we recommend that readers follow the advice of a physician who is directly involved in their care or the care of a member of their family.

From Dulcan MK, Ballard R (editors): *Helping Parents and Teachers Understand Medications for Behavioral and Emotional Problems: A Resource Book of Medication Information Handouts*, Fourth Edition. Washington, DC, American Psychiatric Publishing, 2015

Medication Information for Parents and Teachers

Lithium—Lithobid

General Information About Medication

Each child and adolescent is different. No one has exactly the same combination of medical and psychological problems. It is a good idea to talk with the doctor or nurse about the reasons a medicine is being used. It is very important to keep all appointments and to be in touch by telephone if you have concerns. It is important to communicate with the doctor, nurse, or therapist. An *advanced practice nurse* (APN) has additional education and training after becoming a registered nurse (RN). Your child's medication may be prescribed by a medical doctor (MD or DO) or an APN. In addition, a *physician assistant* (PA) working with a physician may prescribe certain medications. In this information sheet, "doctor" includes medical doctors as well as APNs and PAs who prescribe medication. Often a nurse (RN) will be part of the team and answer questions and give information.

It is very important that the medicine be taken exactly as the doctor instructs. However, once in a while, everyone forgets to give a medicine on time. It is a good idea to ask the doctor or nurse what to do if this happens. Do not stop or change a medicine without asking the doctor or nurse first.

If the medicine seems to stop working, it may be because it is not being taken regularly. The youth may be "cheeking" or hiding the medicine or forgetting to take it (especially at school). The doses may be too far apart or a different dose or medicine may be needed. Something at school, at home, or in the neighborhood may be upsetting the youth, or he or she may need special help for learning disabilities or tutoring. Please discuss your concerns with the doctor. **Do not just increase the dose.** It is also very important not to decrease the dose or stop the medicine without talking to the doctor first. The problem being treated may come back, or there could be uncomfortable or even dangerous results.

All medicines should be kept in a safe place, out of the reach of children, and should be supervised by an adult. If someone takes too much of a medicine, call the doctor, the poison control center, or a hospital emergency room.

Each medicine has a "generic" or chemical name. Just like laundry detergents or paper towels, some medicines are sold by more than one company under different brand names. The same medicine may be available under a generic name and several brand names. The generic medications are usually less expensive than the brand name ones. The generic medications have the same chemical formula, but they may or may not be exactly the same strength as the brand-name medications. Also, some brands of pills contain dye or other things that can cause allergic reactions. It is a good idea to talk to the doctor and the pharmacist about whether it is important to use a specific brand of medicine.

Any medicine can cause an allergic reaction. Examples are hives, itching, rashes, swelling, and trouble breathing. Even a tiny amount of a medicine can cause a reaction in patients who are allergic to that medicine. Be *sure* to talk to the doctor before restarting a medicine that has caused an allergic reaction and tell the doctor about any reactions to medicine that your child has had before.

Taking more than one medicine at the same time may cause more side effects or cause one of the medicines to not work as well. Always ask the doctor, nurse, or pharmacist before adding another medicine, either prescription or bought without a prescription in a store or on the Internet. Be sure

that each doctor knows about *all* of the medicines your child is taking. Also tell the doctor about any vitamins, herbal medicines, or supplements your child may be taking. Some of these may have side effects alone or when taken with this medication. It is a very good idea to keep a list with you of the names and doses of all medicines that your child is taking.

Everyone taking medicine should have a physical examination at least once a year.

If you think that your child may be using drugs or alcohol, please tell the doctor right away.

Pregnancy requires special care in the use of medicine. Some medicines can cause birth defects if taken by a pregnant mother. **Please tell the doctor immediately if you suspect the teenager is at risk of becoming pregnant.** The doctor may wish to discuss sexual behavior and/or birth control with your daughter.

Printed information like this applies to children and adolescents in general. If you have questions about the medicine, or if you notice changes or anything unusual, please ask the doctor or nurse. As scientific research advances, knowledge increases and advice changes. Even experts do not always agree. Many medicines have not been "approved" by the U.S. Food and Drug Administration (FDA) for use in children or use for particular problems. For this reason, use of the medicine for a problem or age group often is not listed in the *Physicians' Desk Reference*. This does not necessarily mean that the medicine is dangerous or does not work, only that the company that makes the medicine has not received permission to advertise the medicine for use in children. Companies often do not apply for this permission because it is expensive to do the tests needed to apply for approval for use in children. Once a medication is approved by the FDA for any purpose, a doctor is allowed to prescribe it according to research and clinical experience.

Note to Teachers

It is a good idea to talk with the parent(s) about the reason(s) that a medication is being used. If the parent(s) sign consent to release information, it is often helpful for you to talk with the doctor. If the parent(s) give permission, the doctor may ask you to fill out rating forms about your experience with the student's behavior, feelings, academic performance, and medication side effects. This information is very useful in selecting and monitoring medication treatment. If you have observations that you think are important, do not hesitate to share these with the student's parent(s) and treating clinicians (with parental consent).

It is very important that the medicine be taken exactly as the doctor instructs. However, everyone forgets to give a medicine on time once in a while. It is a good idea to ask the parent(s) in advance what to do if this happens. Do not stop or change the time you are giving a medicine at school without parental permission. If a medication is to be taken with food, but lunchtime or snack time changes, be sure to notify the parent(s) so appropriate adjustments can be made.

You may notice the following side effects at school:

Common Side Effects

The following side effects often go away after 2 weeks or so:

- Weight gain
- Stomachache
- Diarrhea
- Nausea, vomiting—The student may need to take the medicine after a meal or snack to decrease nausea.
- Increased thirst—Allow the student to make extra trips to the water fountain or carry a water bottle.
- Increased frequency of urination—The student may need to go to the bathroom more often.
- Shakiness of hands (tremor)—You may notice the student's handwriting getting worse.

- Tiredness, weakness
- Headache
- Dizziness (when standing up quickly)—This may happen in the classroom or during physical education. Suggest that the student stand up more slowly.

Occasional Side Effects

- Low thyroid function or goiter (enlarged thyroid)—You may notice that the student is tired, feels cold, gains weight, has coarsening of hair, or does less well academically.
- Acne
- Skin rash
- Hair loss
- Irritability

Signs That the Lithium Level May Be Too High–Early Symptoms of Lithium Toxicity

If the student has any of these signs, tell the parent(s) or school nurse immediately:

- Vomiting or diarrhea
- Trembling that is worse than usual or very severe
- Weakness
- Lack of coordination
- Unsteadiness when standing or walking
- Extreme sleepiness or tiredness
- Severe dizziness
- Trouble speaking or slurred speech
- Confusion

Serious (Toxic) Effects of Too Much Lithium–Dangerous Lithium Toxicity

Use your school procedure for a medical emergency if the student experiences any of the following side effects:

- Irregular heartbeat
- Fainting
- Staggering
- Blurred vision
- Ringing or buzzing sound in the ears
- Inability to urinate
- Muscle twitches
- High fever
- Seizure (fit, convulsion)
- Unconsciousness

Overdosing with lithium may cause death. Be sure the lithium bottle is in a secure place and medication is taken under supervision.

All medicines should be kept in a secure place and should be supervised by an adult. If someone takes too much of a medicine, follow your school procedure for an urgent medical problem.

Taking medicine is a private matter and is best managed discreetly and confidentially. It is important to be sensitive to the student's feelings about taking medicine.

If you suspect that the student is using drugs or alcohol, please tell the parent(s) or a school counselor right away.

Please tell the parent(s) or school nurse if you suspect medication side effects.

Modifications of the classroom environment or assignments may be useful in addition to medication. The student may need to be evaluated for additional help or a 504 plan or an Individualized Education Plan for learning problems or emotional or behavioral issues.

Any expression of suicidal thoughts or feelings or self-harm by a child or adolescent is a signal of distress and should be taken seriously. These behaviors should not be dismissed as "attention seeking." School procedures for safety issues should be followed.

What Is Lithium (Lithobid)?

Lithium is a naturally occurring salt similar to sodium. Lithium is available in the following forms:

Name	Form
Generic	Lithium carbonate tablets and capsules
Generic*	Slow-release lithium carbonate tablets
Lithobid*	Slow-release lithium carbonate tablets
Generic liquid	Lithium citrate syrup

*Do not cut or crush; must be swallowed whole.

How Can This Medicine Help?

Lithium can decrease mood swings. Lithium may be prescribed for bipolar disorder, certain types of depression, severe mood swings, or very serious aggression.

How Does This Medicine Work?

Lithium acts by stabilizing nerve cells in the brain. This action works in different ways depending on the problem that is being treated. For children with bipolar disorder, it works by reducing mood swings or treating mania or depression. In adults with bipolar disorder it has been shown to help prevent mania relapse and to reduce depression.

For children and adolescents with depression whose symptoms have not responded to treatment with an antidepressant used alone or if there is concern about developing mania, lithium can help the antidepressant work better.

For children with explosive aggression, lithium works by "turning down" the anger and decreasing impulsivity. Therapy is needed to help the youth develop more constructive ways to deal with severe anger.

How Long Does This Medicine Last?

Lithium is generally taken three or four times a day. The slow-release forms may be taken once or twice a day.

How Will the Doctor Monitor This Medicine?

The doctor will review your child's medical history and physical examination before starting lithium. The doctor may order some blood or urine tests to be sure your child does not have a hidden medical condition that would make it unsafe to use this medicine. Be sure to tell the doctor if your child or anyone in the family has a history of kidney or thyroid problems or diabetes. The doctor or nurse may measure your child's height, weight, pulse, and blood pressure before starting the medicine. The doctor may order other tests, such as an ECG (electrocardiogram or heart rhythm test) and an EEG (electroencephalogram or brain wave test).

After lithium is started, the doctor will want to have regular appointments with you and your child to see how the medicine is working, to see if a dose change is needed, to watch for side effects, to see if lithium is still needed, and to see if any other treatment is needed. The doctor will need to do blood tests (to check lithium levels) regularly to make sure that the medicine is at the right dose. These tests may be done once or twice a week at first and then once every month or two after the dose is set. Blood should be drawn first thing in the morning, 10–12 hours after the evening dose and before the morning dose. The doctor also will perform blood and urine tests regularly to check for kidney or thyroid side effects. The doctor or nurse may check your child's height, weight, pulse, and blood pressure.

What Side Effects Can This Medicine Have?

Any medicine can have side effects, including an allergy to the medicine. Because each patient is different, the doctor will monitor the youth closely, especially when the medicine is started. The doctor will work with you to increase the positive effects and decrease the negative effects of the medicine. Please tell the doctor if any of the listed side effects appear or if you think that the medicine is causing any other problems. Not all of the rare or unusual side effects are listed.

Side effects are most common after starting the medicine or after a dose increase. Many side effects can be avoided or lessened by starting with a very low dose and increasing it slowly—ask the doctor.

Allergic Reaction

Tell the doctor in a day or two (if possible, before the next dose of medicine):

- Hives
- Itching
- Rash

Stop the medicine and get *immediate* medical care:

- Trouble breathing or chest tightness
- Swelling of lips, tongue, or throat

Lithium should be taken with food to decrease side effects. Make sure that your child drinks plenty of water when taking lithium to prevent dehydration and lithium toxicity. If side effects appear, give your child one or two glasses of water.

Common Side Effects

The following side effects often go away after 2 weeks or so. If they are troublesome, ask the doctor about lowering the dose.

- Weight gain
- Stomachache
- Mild diarrhea
- Nausea
- Increased thirst
- Increased frequency of passing urine
- Shakiness of hands (tremor)—Another medication, such as propranolol (Inderal), may be added.
- Tiredness, weakness
- Headache
- Dizziness

Occasional Side Effects

Tell the doctor within a week or two:

- Tiredness, feeling cold, weight gain, dry skin, coarser hair, or decreased school performance—These could be signs of low thyroid function.
- A lump on the front of the neck—This could be a sign of enlarged thyroid gland (goiter).
- New or worse acne or psoriasis
- Hair loss
- Bed-wetting
- Metallic taste in the mouth
- Irritability

Signs That the Lithium Level May Be Too High—Early Symptoms of Lithium Toxicity

Call the doctor *immediately* and do not give lithium for at least 24 hours:

- Vomiting or diarrhea
- Trembling that is worse than usual or very severe
- Weakness
- Lack of coordination
- Unsteadiness when standing or walking
- Extreme sleepiness or tiredness
- Severe dizziness

- Trouble speaking or slurred speech
- Confusion

Serious (Toxic) Effects of Too Much Lithium—Dangerous Lithium Toxicity

If your child has any of the following, go to the doctor's office or to an emergency room *immediately!*

- Irregular heartbeat
- Fainting
- Staggering
- Blurred vision
- Ringing or buzzing sound in the ears
- Inability to pass urine
- Muscle twitches
- High fever
- Seizure (fit, convulsion)
- Unconsciousness

A lithium overdose may cause death. You must closely supervise the medicine. You should lock up the medicine if your child or teenager is suicidal or if a young child lives in or visits your home.

Some Interactions With Other Medicines or Food

Please note that the following are only the most likely interactions with other medicines or food.

Soft drinks with caffeine may make side effects worse.

Some anti-inflammatory medicines can increase lithium levels and make side effects worse. Examples are listed in the table below.

Brand name	Generic name
Advil, Motrin	Ibuprofen
Indocin	Indomethacin
Aleve, Anaprox, Naprosyn	Naproxen

Taking lithium with theophylline may decrease lithium levels so that it does not work as well. Certain diuretics such as hydrochlorothiazide can increase lithium levels.

Some medicines that work on the kidneys to lower blood pressure may increase lithium levels. Ask the doctor.

What Could Happen if This Medicine Is Stopped Suddenly?

There are no medical withdrawal effects if lithium is stopped suddenly. However, the problem being treated is likely to come back. If lithium is stopped suddenly, some patients with bipolar disorder may become manic more often and may be more difficult to treat. If your child has been taking lithium for 6–8 weeks or longer, the dose should be decreased gradually (tapered) over 8–16 weeks before stopping it to prevent this effect. Always check with your child's doctor before stopping or changing a medicine.

How Long Will This Medicine Be Needed?

How long your child will need to take lithium depends on the reason that it was prescribed. For children and adolescents with bipolar disorder, lithium is often prescribed for 2 years or longer. Depending on how many times your child has had depression or mania, he or she may need to take the medicine for many years. Some patients require lithium for their entire lives to function normally.

For children and adolescents with severe depression who need lithium plus an antidepressant, lithium is usually needed for at least 5–6 months after the child's mood returns to normal. This is necessary to prevent the depression from coming back.

For severe anger outbursts, lithium must be continued for several months to years until the patient, his or her family, and the doctor can find different ways to control aggressive behavior. The anger usually becomes more controllable as the child develops more effective problem-solving and coping skills. There are some other medicines that also may help.

What Else Should I Know About This Medicine?

Store the medicine at room temperature, away from moisture.

Make sure your child drinks plenty of water, especially in hot weather and when exercising. Avoid extremes of salt intake; large amounts of salty foods or a salt-free diet can make the lithium level too low or too high.

Tell the doctor if the pharmacy changes the brand of lithium—extra blood tests of the lithium level may be needed.

When lithium causes increased thirst, young people may drink large amounts of soft drinks. Drinking soft drinks is not a good idea because it can lead to weight gain (from sugar) or nervousness (from caffeine). Drinking water, fruit juice mixed with water, or salt-free seltzer is fine. Your child may need a note to allow frequent trips to the water fountain and bathroom at school.

Stop the lithium and call the doctor if your child develops an illness with vomiting, diarrhea, fever, or loss of appetite. Talk with the doctor if your child wants to diet to lose weight.

Lithium levels may change with the menstrual cycle. If you suspect that this is happening, keep a log or diary and discuss it with the doctor.

Lithium should not be taken during pregnancy because it can cause birth defects. Your doctor may consider doing a pregnancy test before your daughter starts this medication. If your daughter is sexually active, or decides to start sexual activity while taking this medication, she should talk with her doctor about birth control and other health issues related to sex.

Notes

Use this space to take notes or to write down questions you want to ask the doctor.

_____

_____

_____

_____

_____

_____

_____

_____

_____

_____

_____

_____

_____

From Dulcan MK, Ballard R (editors): _Helping Parents and Teachers Understand Medications for Behavioral and Emotional Problems: A Resource Book of Medication Information Handouts_, Fourth Edition. Washington, DC, American Psychiatric Publishing, 2015

Medication Information for Parents and Teachers

L-methylfolate—Deplin

General Information About Medication

Each child and adolescent is different. No one has exactly the same combination of medical and psychological problems. It is a good idea to talk with the doctor or nurse about the reasons a medicine is being used. It is very important to keep all appointments and to be in touch by telephone if you have concerns. It is important to communicate with the doctor, nurse, or therapist. An *advanced practice nurse* (APN) has additional education and training after becoming a registered nurse (RN). Your child's medication may be prescribed by a medical doctor (MD or DO) or an APN. In addition, a *physician assistant* (PA) working with a physician may prescribe certain medications. In this information sheet, "doctor" includes medical doctors as well as APNs and PAs who prescribe medication. Often a nurse (RN) will be part of the team and answer questions and give information.

It is very important that the medicine be taken exactly as the doctor instructs. However, once in a while, everyone forgets to give a medicine on time. It is a good idea to ask the doctor or nurse what to do if this happens. Do not stop or change a medicine without asking the doctor or nurse first.

If the medicine seems to stop working, it may be because it is not being taken regularly. The youth may be "cheeking" or hiding the medicine or forgetting to take it (especially at school). The doses may be too far apart or a different dose or medicine may be needed. Something at school, at home, or in the neighborhood may be upsetting the youth, or he or she may need special help for learning disabilities or tutoring. Please discuss your concerns with the doctor. **Do not just increase the dose.** It is also very important not to decrease the dose or stop the medicine without talking to the doctor first. The problem being treated may come back, or there could be uncomfortable or even dangerous results.

All medicines should be kept in a safe place, out of the reach of children, and should be supervised by an adult. If someone takes too much of a medicine, call the doctor, the poison control center, or a hospital emergency room.

Each medicine has a "generic" or chemical name. Just like laundry detergents or paper towels, some medicines are sold by more than one company under different brand names. The same medicine may be available under a generic name and several brand names. The generic medications are usually less expensive than the brand name ones. The generic medications have the same chemical formula, but they may or may not be exactly the same strength as the brand-name medications. Also, some brands of pills contain dye or other things that can cause allergic reactions. It is a good idea to talk to the doctor and the pharmacist about whether it is important to use a specific brand of medicine.

Any medicine can cause an allergic reaction. Examples are hives, itching, rashes, swelling, and trouble breathing. Even a tiny amount of a medicine can cause a reaction in patients who are allergic to that medicine. Be *sure* to talk to the doctor before restarting a medicine that has caused an allergic reaction and tell the doctor about any reactions to medicine that your child has had before.

Taking more than one medicine at the same time may cause more side effects or cause one of the medicines to not work as well. Always ask the doctor, nurse, or pharmacist before adding another medicine, either prescription or bought without a prescription in a store or on the Internet. Be sure

that each doctor knows about *all* of the medicines your child is taking. Also tell the doctor about any vitamins, herbal medicines, or supplements your child may be taking. Some of these may have side effects alone or when taken with this medication. It is a very good idea to keep a list with you of the names and doses of all medicines that your child is taking.

Everyone taking medicine should have a physical examination at least once a year.

If you think that your child may be using drugs or alcohol, please tell the doctor right away.

Pregnancy requires special care in the use of medicine. Some medicines can cause birth defects if taken by a pregnant mother. **Please tell the doctor immediately if you suspect the teenager is at risk of becoming pregnant.** The doctor may wish to discuss sexual behavior and/or birth control with your daughter.

Printed information like this applies to children and adolescents in general. If you have questions about the medicine, or if you notice changes or anything unusual, please ask the doctor or nurse. As scientific research advances, knowledge increases and advice changes. Even experts do not always agree. Many medicines have not been "approved" by the U.S. Food and Drug Administration (FDA) for use in children or use for particular problems. For this reason, use of the medicine for a problem or age group often is not listed in the *Physicians' Desk Reference*. This does not necessarily mean that the medicine is dangerous or does not work, only that the company that makes the medicine has not received permission to advertise the medicine for use in children. Companies often do not apply for this permission because it is expensive to do the tests needed to apply for approval for use in children. Once a medication is approved by the FDA for any purpose, a doctor is allowed to prescribe it according to research and clinical experience.

Note to Teachers

It is a good idea to talk with the parent(s) about the reason(s) that a medication is being used. If the parent(s) sign consent to release information, it is often helpful for you to talk with the doctor. If the parent(s) give permission, the doctor may ask you to fill out rating forms about your experience with the student's behavior, feelings, academic performance, and medication side effects. This information is very useful in selecting and monitoring medication treatment. If you have observations that you think are important, do not hesitate to share these with the student's parent(s) and treating clinicians (with parental consent).

It is very important that the medicine be taken exactly as the doctor instructs. However, everyone forgets to give a medicine on time once in a while. It is a good idea to ask the parent(s) in advance what to do if this happens. Do not stop or change the time you are giving a medicine at school without parental permission. If a medication is to be taken with food, but lunchtime or snack time changes, be sure to notify the parent(s) so appropriate adjustments can be made.

All medicines should be kept in a secure place and should be supervised by an adult. If someone takes too much of a medicine, follow your school procedure for an urgent medical problem.

Taking medicine is a private matter and is best managed discreetly and confidentially. It is important to be sensitive to the student's feelings about taking medicine.

If you suspect that the student is using drugs or alcohol, please tell the parent(s) or a school counselor right away.

Please tell the parent(s) or school nurse if you suspect medication side effects.

Modifications of the classroom environment or assignments may be useful in addition to medication. The student may need to be evaluated for additional help or a 504 plan or an Individualized Education Plan for learning problems or emotional or behavioral issues.

Any expression of suicidal thoughts or feelings or self-harm by a child or adolescent is a signal of distress and should be taken seriously. These behaviors should not be dismissed as "attention seeking." School procedures for safety issues should be followed.

What Is L-methylfolate?

L-methylfolate is a *medical food* or *supplement* that is used to treat conditions related to folate deficiency. It is a form of folate (vitamin B_9) that is active in the brain. Most L-methylfolate comes as a prescription medicine (such as Deplin). It is not the same as over-the-counter folate.

How Can This Medicine Help?

L-methylfolate can improve depressed mood in people who have folate deficiency and depression or in people who have not had a good response to treatment with an antidepressant medication. Studies in adults have shown that when L-methylfolate is added to an antidepressant medication, many people who were not improving on the antidepressant alone did better with the combination.

How Does This Medicine Work?

L-methylfolate is the form of folate that works in the brain to regulate the production of the *neurotransmitters* serotonin, dopamine, and norepinephrine. Folate or folic acid can be taken as a supplement, but it has to be converted to L-methylfolate to get into the brain. In many people, this does not work well. Examples are people who take certain medications including lamotrigine, valproate, metformin, warfarin, or birth control pills and people who are obese.

How Long Does This Medicine Last?

L-methylfolate is generally taken once a day.

How Will the Doctor Monitor This Medicine?

The doctor will review your child's medical history and physical examination before starting L-methylfolate. The doctor may order some blood or urine tests to be sure your child does not have a hidden medical condition. The doctor or nurse may measure your child's pulse and blood pressure before starting L-methylfolate. The doctor may order other tests, such as a folate level or B_{12} level.

After the medicine is started, the doctor will want to have regular appointments with you and your child to see how the medicine is working, to see if a dose change is needed, to watch for side effects, to see if L-methylfolate is still needed, and to see if any other treatment is needed. The doctor or nurse may check your child's height, weight, pulse, and blood pressure or order tests, such as a follow-up folate level.

What Side Effects Can This Medicine Have?

In most studies, L-methylfolate has no more side effects than a placebo (sugar pill).

Any medicine can have side effects, including an allergy to the medicine. Because each patient is different, the doctor will monitor the youth closely, especially when the medicine is started. The doctor will work with you to increase the positive effects and decrease the negative effects of the medicine. Please tell the doctor if any of the listed side effects appear or if you think that the medicine is causing any other problem. Not all of the rare or unusual side effects are listed.

Allergic Reaction

Tell the doctor in a day or two (if possible, before the next dose of medicine):

- Hives
- Itching
- Rash

Get *immediate* medical care:

- Trouble breathing or chest tightness
- Swelling of lips, tongue, or throat

Some Interactions With Other Medicines or Food

Please note that the following is only the most likely interaction with food or other medicines.
L-methylfolate may decrease blood levels of the seizure medication phenytoin (Dilantin).

What Could Happen if This Medicine Is Stopped Suddenly?

There are no known problems resulting from stopping L-methylfolate suddenly.

How Long Will This Medicine Be Needed?

There have not been a lot of studies that tell us how long L-methylfolate should be taken. If it is added to an antidepressant medication, then it should be taken as long as the antidepressant is taken. Your doctor could do follow-up folate levels after the L-methylfolate is stopped to see if your child's level decreases.

What Else Should I Know About This Medicine?

Your doctor can prescribe L-methylfolate, but it can also be bought over the counter or online without a prescription. Buying L-methylfolate can be confusing because there are several similar products. Folate or folic acid is the form of the vitamin that the body changes into L-methylfolate. For many people, taking folate supplements does not work as well as taking L-methylfolate because their body does not convert the vitamin effectively. Ask your doctor to write down the name and dose of the product that you should look for if you are buying over the counter.

Notes

Use this space to take notes or to write down questions you want to ask the doctor.

_____

_____

_____

_____

_____

_____

_____

_____

_____

_____

_____

Medication Information for Parents and Teachers

Lorazepam—Ativan

General Information About Medication

Each child and adolescent is different. No one has exactly the same combination of medical and psychological problems. It is a good idea to talk with the doctor or nurse about the reasons a medicine is being used. It is very important to keep all appointments and to be in touch by telephone if you have concerns. It is important to communicate with the doctor, nurse, or therapist. An *advanced practice nurse* (APN) has additional education and training after becoming a registered nurse (RN). Your child's medication may be prescribed by a medical doctor (MD or DO) or an APN. In addition, a *physician assistant* (PA) working with a physician may prescribe certain medications. In this information sheet, "doctor" includes medical doctors as well as APNs and PAs who prescribe medication. Often a nurse (RN) will be part of the team and answer questions and give information.

It is very important that the medicine be taken exactly as the doctor instructs. However, once in a while, everyone forgets to give a medicine on time. It is a good idea to ask the doctor or nurse what to do if this happens. Do not stop or change a medicine without asking the doctor or nurse first.

If the medicine seems to stop working, it may be because it is not being taken regularly. The youth may be "cheeking" or hiding the medicine or forgetting to take it (especially at school). The doses may be too far apart or a different dose or medicine may be needed. Something at school, at home, or in the neighborhood may be upsetting the youth, or he or she may need special help for learning disabilities or tutoring. Please discuss your concerns with the doctor. **Do not just increase the dose.** It is also very important not to decrease the dose or stop the medicine without talking to the doctor first. The problem being treated may come back, or there could be uncomfortable or even dangerous results.

All medicines should be kept in a safe place, out of the reach of children, and should be supervised by an adult. If someone takes too much of a medicine, call the doctor, the poison control center, or a hospital emergency room.

Each medicine has a "generic" or chemical name. Just like laundry detergents or paper towels, some medicines are sold by more than one company under different brand names. The same medicine may be available under a generic name and several brand names. The generic medications are usually less expensive than the brand name ones. The generic medications have the same chemical formula, but they may or may not be exactly the same strength as the brand-name medications. Also, some brands of pills contain dye or other things that can cause allergic reactions. It is a good idea to talk to the doctor and the pharmacist about whether it is important to use a specific brand of medicine.

Any medicine can cause an allergic reaction. Examples are hives, itching, rashes, swelling, and trouble breathing. Even a tiny amount of a medicine can cause a reaction in patients who are allergic to that medicine. Be *sure* to talk to the doctor before restarting a medicine that has caused an allergic reaction and tell the doctor about any reactions to medicine that your child has had before.

Taking more than one medicine at the same time may cause more side effects or cause one of the medicines to not work as well. Always ask the doctor, nurse, or pharmacist before adding another

medicine, either prescription or bought without a prescription in a store or on the Internet. Be sure that each doctor knows about *all* of the medicines your child is taking. Also tell the doctor about any vitamins, herbal medicines, or supplements your child may be taking. Some of these may have side effects alone or when taken with this medication. It is a very good idea to keep a list with you of the names and doses of all medicines that your child is taking.

Everyone taking medicine should have a physical examination at least once a year.

If you think that your child may be using drugs or alcohol, please tell the doctor right away.

Pregnancy requires special care in the use of medicine. Some medicines can cause birth defects if taken by a pregnant mother. **Please tell the doctor immediately if you suspect the teenager is at risk of becoming pregnant.** The doctor may wish to discuss sexual behavior and/or birth control with your daughter.

Printed information like this applies to children and adolescents in general. If you have questions about the medicine, or if you notice changes or anything unusual, please ask the doctor or nurse. As scientific research advances, knowledge increases and advice changes. Even experts do not always agree. Many medicines have not been "approved" by the U.S. Food and Drug Administration (FDA) for use in children or use for particular problems. For this reason, use of the medicine for a problem or age group often is not listed in the *Physicians' Desk Reference*. This does not necessarily mean that the medicine is dangerous or does not work, only that the company that makes the medicine has not received permission to advertise the medicine for use in children. Companies often do not apply for this permission because it is expensive to do the tests needed to apply for approval for use in children. Once a medication is approved by the FDA for any purpose, a doctor is allowed to prescribe it according to research and clinical experience.

Note to Teachers

It is a good idea to talk with the parent(s) about the reason(s) that a medication is being used. If the parent(s) sign consent to release information, it is often helpful for you to talk with the doctor. If the parent(s) give permission, the doctor may ask you to fill out rating forms about your experience with the student's behavior, feelings, academic performance, and medication side effects. This information is very useful in selecting and monitoring medication treatment. If you have observations that you think are important, do not hesitate to share these with the student's parent(s) and treating clinicians (with parental consent).

It is very important that the medicine be taken exactly as the doctor instructs. However, everyone forgets to give a medicine on time once in a while. It is a good idea to ask the parent(s) in advance what to do if this happens. Do not stop or change the time you are giving a medicine at school without parental permission. If a medication is to be taken with food, but lunchtime or snack time changes, be sure to notify the parent(s) so appropriate adjustments can be made.

All medicines should be kept in a secure place and should be supervised by an adult. If someone takes too much of a medicine, follow your school procedure for an urgent medical problem.

Taking medicine is a private matter and is best managed discreetly and confidentially. It is important to be sensitive to the student's feelings about taking medicine.

If you suspect that the student is using drugs or alcohol, please tell the parent(s) or a school counselor right away.

Please tell the parent(s) or school nurse if you suspect medication side effects.

Modifications of the classroom environment or assignments may be useful in addition to medication. The student may need to be evaluated for additional help or a 504 plan or an Individualized Education Plan for learning problems or emotional or behavioral issues.

Any expression of suicidal thoughts or feelings or self-harm by a child or adolescent is a signal of distress and should be taken seriously. These behaviors should not be dismissed as "attention seeking." School procedures for safety issues should be followed.

What Is Lorazepam (Ativan)?

Lorazepam is a *benzodiazepine* or *antianxiety* medicine. It used to be called a *minor tranquilizer*. It is sometimes called an *anxiolytic* or *sedative*. It comes in brand name Ativan and generic tablets and liquid. There are other forms used for medical problems.

How Can This Medicine Help?

Lorazepam can decrease anxiety, nervousness, fears, and excessive worrying. It can help anxious people to be calm enough to learn—with therapy and practice (exposure to feared things or situations)—to understand and tolerate their worries or fears and even to overcome them. People with generalized anxiety disorder, social phobia, posttraumatic stress disorder (PTSD), or panic disorder can be helped by lorazepam. Most often, it is used for a short time when symptoms are very uncomfortable or frightening or when they make it hard to do important things such as going to school. Lorazepam can decrease the severe physical symptoms (rapid heartbeat, trouble breathing, dizziness, sweating) of panic attacks and phobias.

Lorazepam also can be used for sleep problems, such as night terrors (sudden waking up from sleep with great fear) or sleepwalking, when these problems put the youth at risk of an accident or make it impossible for other family members to get enough sleep. Lorazepam can help with insomnia (difficulty falling asleep) when used for a short time along with a behavioral program, such as regular soothing routines at bedtime and increased exercise in the daytime.

Sometimes lorazepam is used for a few days to treat agitation in mania or psychosis until other medicines start to work.

Lorazepam can be used to treat seizures (epilepsy).

Occasionally the benzodiazepines are used to reduce the side effects of other medicines.

How Does This Medicine Work?

Lorazepam works by calming the parts of the brain that are too excitable in anxious people. The medicine does this by working on *receptors* (special places on brain cells) in certain parts of the brain to change the action of *GABA*, a *neurotransmitter*—a chemical that the brain makes for brain cells to communicate with each other.

How Long Does This Medicine Last?

Lorazepam usually needs to be taken three times a day. For acute symptoms of anxiety or agitation, it can be taken occasionally, as needed. When used for sleep, it is taken at bedtime. There may still be some effects in the morning.

How Will the Doctor Monitor This Medicine?

The doctor will review your child's medical history and physical examination before starting lorazepam. The doctor may order some blood or urine tests or an ECG (electrocardiogram or heart rhythm test) to be sure your child does not have a hidden medical condition. The doctor or nurse may measure your child's height, weight, pulse, and blood pressure before starting lorazepam.

After the medicine is started, the doctor will want to have regular appointments with you and your child to see how the medicine is working, to see if a dose change is needed, to watch for side effects, to see if lorazepam is still needed, and to see if any other treatment is needed. The doctor or nurse may check your child's height, weight, pulse, and blood pressure.

What Side Effects Can This Medicine Have?

Any medicine can have side effects, including an allergy to the medicine. Because each patient is different, the doctor will monitor the youth closely, especially when the medicine is started. The doctor will work with you to increase the positive effects and decrease the negative effects of the medicine. Please tell the doctor if any of the listed side effects appear or if you think that the medicine is causing any other problems. Not all of the rare or unusual side effects are listed.

Side effects are most common after starting the medicine or after a dose increase. Many side effects can be avoided or lessened by starting with a very low dose and increasing it slowly—ask the doctor.

Allergic Reaction

Tell the doctor in a day or two (if possible, before the next dose of medicine):

- Hives
- Itching
- Rash

Stop the medicine and get *immediate* medical care:

- Trouble breathing or chest tightness
- Swelling of lips, tongue, or throat

Lorazepam is usually very safe when used for short periods as the doctor prescribes.

The most common side effect is daytime sleepiness. Lorazepam can also cause dizziness, feeling "spacey," or decreased coordination. If the medicine is causing any of these problems it is very important not to drive a car, ride a bicycle or motorcycle, or operate machinery.

Lorazepam can cause decreased concentration and memory. These problems, along with daytime sleepiness, may decrease learning and performance in school.

People who take lorazepam must not drink alcohol. Severe sleepiness or even loss of consciousness may result.

It is possible to become psychologically and physically dependent on lorazepam, but that is not a common problem for patients who see their doctors regularly. Because some people abuse benzodiazepines, it is illegal to give or sell these medicines to someone other than the patient for whom they were prescribed.

Very rarely, lorazepam causes excitement, irritability, anger, aggression, trouble sleeping, nightmares, uncontrollable behavior, or memory loss. This is called *disinhibition* or a *paradoxical effect*. Stop the medicine and call the doctor if this happens.

Some Interactions With Other Medicines or Food

Please note that the following are only the most likely interactions with other medicines or food.

Lorazepam may be taken with or without food.

It is important not to use other sedatives, tranquilizers, or sleeping pills or antihistamines (such as Benadryl) when taking lorazepam because of greatly increased side effects.

It is better to limit drinks with caffeine (coffee, tea, soft drinks) because caffeine works in the opposite way from this medicine, and the positive effects might be decreased.

What Could Happen if This Medicine Is Stopped Suddenly?

Many medicines cause problems if stopped suddenly. Lorazepam must be decreased slowly (tapered) rather than stopped suddenly. When lorazepam is stopped suddenly, there are withdrawal symptoms that are uncomfortable and may even be dangerous. Problems are more likely in patients taking high doses of lorazepam for 2 months or longer, but even after taking lorazepam for just a few weeks, it is important to stop it slowly. Withdrawal symptoms may include anxiety, irritability, shaking, sweating, aches and pains, muscle cramps, vomiting, confusion, and trouble sleeping. If large doses taken for a long time are stopped suddenly, seizures (fits, convulsions), hallucinations (hearing voices or seeing things that are not there), or out-of-control behavior may result.

How Long Will This Medicine Be Needed?

Lorazepam is usually prescribed for only a few weeks to allow the patient to be calm enough to learn new ways to cope with anxiety and to allow the nervous system to become less excitable. Sometimes antianxiety medicines are used for longer periods to treat panic attacks or anxiety that remain after therapy is completed. Each person is unique, and some people may need these medicines for months or years.

What Else Should I Know About This Medicine?

Because benzodiazepines can be abused (especially by people who abuse alcohol or drugs) and can cause psychological dependence or physical dependence (addiction), they are regulated by special state and federal laws as *controlled substances*. These laws place limitations on telephone prescriptions and refills, and prescriptions expire if they are not filled promptly.

Sometimes alprazolam (Xanax) and lorazepam (Ativan) get mixed up; be sure to check the medicine when you get it from the pharmacy.

People with sleep apnea (breathing stops while they are asleep) should not take lorazepam. Tell the doctor if your child snores very loudly.

Lorazepam should be avoided during pregnancy, especially in the first 3 months, because it may cause birth defects in the baby. If taken regularly at the end of pregnancy, lorazepam may cause withdrawal symptoms in the baby. If you think that your daughter might be pregnant, tell the doctor right away.

Notes

Use this space to take notes or to write down questions you want to ask the doctor.

_____

_____

_____

_____

_____

_____

_____

_____

_____

_____

_____

_____

_____

_____

From Dulcan MK, Ballard R (editors): _Helping Parents and Teachers Understand Medications for Behavioral and Emotional Problems: A Resource Book of Medication Information Handouts_, Fourth Edition. Washington, DC, American Psychiatric Publishing, 2015

Medication Information for Parents and Teachers

Loxapine—Loxitane, Adasuve

General Information About Medication

Each child and adolescent is different. No one has exactly the same combination of medical and psychological problems. It is a good idea to talk with the doctor or nurse about the reasons a medicine is being used. It is very important to keep all appointments and to be in touch by telephone if you have concerns. It is important to communicate with the doctor, nurse, or therapist. An *advanced practice nurse* (APN) has additional education and training after becoming a registered nurse (RN). Your child's medication may be prescribed by a medical doctor (MD or DO) or an APN. In addition, a *physician assistant* (PA) working with a physician may prescribe certain medications. In this information sheet, "doctor" includes medical doctors as well as APNs and PAs who prescribe medication. Often a nurse (RN) will be part of the team and answer questions and give information.

It is very important that the medicine be taken exactly as the doctor instructs. However, once in a while, everyone forgets to give a medicine on time. It is a good idea to ask the doctor or nurse what to do if this happens. Do not stop or change a medicine without asking the doctor or nurse first.

If the medicine seems to stop working, it may be because it is not being taken regularly. The youth may be "cheeking" or hiding the medicine or forgetting to take it (especially at school). The doses may be too far apart or a different dose or medicine may be needed. Something at school, at home, or in the neighborhood may be upsetting the youth, or he or she may need special help for learning disabilities or tutoring. Please discuss your concerns with the doctor. **Do not just increase the dose.** It is also very important not to decrease the dose or stop the medicine without talking to the doctor first. The problem being treated may come back, or there could be uncomfortable or even dangerous results.

All medicines should be kept in a safe place, out of the reach of children, and should be supervised by an adult. If someone takes too much of a medicine, call the doctor, the poison control center, or a hospital emergency room.

Each medicine has a "generic" or chemical name. Just like laundry detergents or paper towels, some medicines are sold by more than one company under different brand names. The same medicine may be available under a generic name and several brand names. The generic medications are usually less expensive than the brand name ones. The generic medications have the same chemical formula, but they may or may not be exactly the same strength as the brand-name medications. Also, some brands of pills contain dye or other things that can cause allergic reactions. It is a good idea to talk to the doctor and the pharmacist about whether it is important to use a specific brand of medicine.

Any medicine can cause an allergic reaction. Examples are hives, itching, rashes, swelling, and trouble breathing. Even a tiny amount of a medicine can cause a reaction in patients who are allergic to that medicine. Be *sure* to talk to the doctor before restarting a medicine that has caused an allergic reaction and tell the doctor about any reactions to medicine that your child has had before.

Taking more than one medicine at the same time may cause more side effects or cause one of the medicines to not work as well. Always ask the doctor, nurse, or pharmacist before adding another

medicine, either prescription or bought without a prescription in a store or on the Internet. Be sure that each doctor knows about *all* of the medicines your child is taking. Also tell the doctor about any vitamins, herbal medicines, or supplements your child may be taking. Some of these may have side effects alone or when taken with this medication. It is a very good idea to keep a list with you of the names and doses of all medicines that your child is taking.

Everyone taking medicine should have a physical examination at least once a year.

If you think that your child may be using drugs or alcohol, please tell the doctor right away.

Pregnancy requires special care in the use of medicine. Some medicines can cause birth defects if taken by a pregnant mother. **Please tell the doctor immediately if you suspect the teenager is at risk of becoming pregnant.** The doctor may wish to discuss sexual behavior and/or birth control with your daughter.

Printed information like this applies to children and adolescents in general. If you have questions about the medicine, or if you notice changes or anything unusual, please ask the doctor or nurse. As scientific research advances, knowledge increases and advice changes. Even experts do not always agree. Many medicines have not been "approved" by the U.S. Food and Drug Administration (FDA) for use in children or use for particular problems. For this reason, use of the medicine for a problem or age group often is not listed in the *Physicians' Desk Reference*. This does not necessarily mean that the medicine is dangerous or does not work, only that the company that makes the medicine has not received permission to advertise the medicine for use in children. Companies often do not apply for this permission because it is expensive to do the tests needed to apply for approval for use in children. Once a medication is approved by the FDA for any purpose, a doctor is allowed to prescribe it according to research and clinical experience.

Note to Teachers

It is a good idea to talk with the parent(s) about the reason(s) that a medication is being used. If the parent(s) sign consent to release information, it is often helpful for you to talk with the doctor. If the parent(s) give permission, the doctor may ask you to fill out rating forms about your experience with the student's behavior, feelings, academic performance, and medication side effects. This information is very useful in selecting and monitoring medication treatment. If you have observations that you think are important, do not hesitate to share these with the student's parent(s) and treating clinicians (with parental consent).

It is very important that the medicine be taken exactly as the doctor instructs. However, everyone forgets to give a medicine on time once in a while. It is a good idea to ask the parent(s) in advance what to do if this happens. Do not stop or change the time you are giving a medicine at school without parental permission. If a medication is to be taken with food, but lunchtime or snack time changes, be sure to notify the parent(s) so appropriate adjustments can be made.

All medicines should be kept in a secure place and should be supervised by an adult. If someone takes too much of a medicine, follow your school procedure for an urgent medical problem.

Taking medicine is a private matter and is best managed discreetly and confidentially. It is important to be sensitive to the student's feelings about taking medicine.

If you suspect that the student is using drugs or alcohol, please tell the parent(s) or a school counselor right away.

Please tell the parent(s) or school nurse if you suspect medication side effects.

Modifications of the classroom environment or assignments may be useful in addition to medication. The student may need to be evaluated for additional help or a 504 plan or an Individualized Education Plan for learning problems or emotional or behavioral issues.

Any expression of suicidal thoughts or feelings or self-harm by a child or adolescent is a signal of distress and should be taken seriously. These behaviors should not be dismissed as "attention seeking." School procedures for safety issues should be followed.

What Is Loxapine (Loxitane, Adasuve)?

Loxapine is sometimes called a *typical, conventional,* or *first-generation antipsychotic* medicine. It is also called a *neuroleptic.* It used to be called a *major tranquilizer.* It comes in brand name Loxitane and generic capsules and as Adasuve brand name inhaled powder. Adasuve must be administered by a health care professional.

How Can This Medicine Help?

Loxapine is used to treat psychosis, such as in schizophrenia, mania, or very severe depression. It can reduce hallucinations (hearing voices or seeing things that are not there) and delusions (troubling beliefs that other people do not share). It can help the patient be less upset and agitated. It can improve the patient's ability to think clearly.

Sometimes loxapine is used to decrease severe aggression or very serious behavioral problems in young people with conduct disorder, intellectual disability, or autism spectrum disorder.

Adasuve is sometimes used to treat acute agitation. It is given by a doctor or nurse using an inhaler and works very fast.

This medicine is very powerful and should be used to treat very serious problems or symptoms that other medicines do not help. Be patient; the positive effects of this medicine may not appear for 2–3 weeks.

How Does This Medicine Work?

Cells in the brain (neurons) communicate using chemicals called *neurotransmitters.* Too much or too little of these substances in certain parts of the brain can cause problems. Loxapine reduces the activity of one of these neurotransmitters, *dopamine.* Blocking the effect of dopamine in certain parts of the brain reduces what have been called *positive symptoms* of psychosis: delusions; hallucinations; disorganized and unusual thinking, speaking, and behavior; excessive activity (agitation); and lack of activity (catatonia). Reducing dopamine action in other parts of the brain may lead to the side effects of this medicine.

How Long Does This Medicine Last?

Loxapine is usually taken several times a day. The inhaled form, Adasuve, is taken only once a day.

How Will the Doctor Monitor This Medicine?

The doctor will review your child's medical history and physical examination before starting loxapine. The doctor may order some blood or urine tests to be sure your child does not have a hidden medical condition. The doctor or nurse may measure your child's pulse and blood pressure before starting loxapine.

Before your child starts taking loxapine and every so often afterward, the doctor may perform a test such as the AIMS (Abnormal Involuntary Movement Scale) to check your child's tongue, legs, and arms for unusual movements that could be caused by the medicine.

After the medicine is started, the doctor will want to have regular appointments with you and your child to see how the medicine is working, to see if a dose change is needed, to watch for side effects, to see if loxapine is still needed, and to see if any other treatment is needed. The doctor or nurse may check your child's height, weight, pulse, and blood pressure, and watch for abnormal movements.

What Side Effects Can This Medicine Have?

Any medicine can have side effects, including an allergy to the medicine. Because each patient is different, the doctor will monitor the youth closely, especially when the medicine is started. The doctor will work with you to increase the positive effects and decrease the negative effects of the medicine. Please tell the doctor if any of the listed side effects appear or if you think that the medicine is causing any other problems. Not all of the rare or unusual side effects are listed.

Side effects are most common after starting the medicine or after a dose increase. Many side effects can be avoided or lessened by starting with a very low dose and increasing it slowly—ask the doctor.

Allergic Reaction

Tell the doctor in a day or two (if possible, before the next dose of medicine):

- Hives
- Itching
- Rash

Stop the medicine and get *immediate* medical care:

- Trouble breathing or chest tightness
- Swelling of lips, tongue, or throat

Common, but Not Usually Serious, Side Effects

Discuss the following side effects with your child's doctor within a week or two. They often can be helped by lowering the dose of medicine, changing the times medicine is taken, or adding another medicine.

- Dry mouth—Have your child try using sugar-free gum or candy.
- Constipation—Encourage your child to drink more fluids and eat high-fiber foods; if necessary, the doctor may recommend a fiber medicine such as Benefiber or a stool softener such as Colace or mineral oil.
- Increased risk of sunburn—Have your child wear sunscreen or protective clothing or stay out of the sun.
- Mild trouble urinating
- Blurred vision
- Weight gain—Seek nutritional counseling; provide your child with low-calorie snacks and encourage regular exercise.
- Sadness, irritability, nervousness, clinginess, not wanting to go to school
- Restlessness or inability to sit still
- Shaking of hands and fingers

Less Common, but Not Usually Serious, Side Effects

Discuss the following side effects with your child's doctor within a week or two. They often can be helped by lowering the dose of medicine, changing the times medicine is taken, or adding another medicine.

- Daytime sleepiness or tiredness—Do not allow your child to drive, ride a bicycle or motorcycle, or operate machinery if this happens. This problem may be lessened by taking the medicine at bedtime.
- Dizziness—This side effect is worse when the child stands up quickly, especially when getting out of bed in the morning; try having the child stand up slowly.
- Decreased or slowed movement and decreased facial expressions
- Drooling
- Decreased sexual interest or ability
- Changes in menstrual cycle
- Increase in breast size or discharge from the breasts (in both boys and girls)—This may go away with time.

Less Common, but Potentially Serious, Side Effects

Call the doctor or go to an emergency room *right away*:

- Stiffness of the tongue, jaw, neck, back, or legs
- Overheating or heatstroke—Prevent by decreasing activity in hot weather, staying out of the sun, and drinking water.
- Seizure (fit, convulsion)—This is more likely in people with a history of seizures or head injury.
- Severe confusion

Rare, but Serious, Side Effects

- Extreme stiffness or lack of movement, very high fever, mental confusion, irregular pulse rate, or eye pain—**This is a medical emergency. Go to an emergency room *right away*.**
- Sudden stiffness and inability to breathe or swallow—**Go to an emergency room or call 911.** Tell the paramedics, nurses, and doctors that the patient is taking loxapine. Other medicines can be used to treat this problem fast.
- Very rare: increased thirst, frequent urination, lethargy, tiredness, dizziness—These could be signs of diabetes (especially if your child is overweight or there is a family history of diabetes). **Talk to a doctor within a day.**

What Else Should I Know About Side Effects?

Most side effects lessen over time. If they are troublesome, talk with your child's doctor. Some side effects can be decreased by taking a smaller dose of medicine, by stopping the medicine, by changing to another medicine, or by adding another medicine (see the table).

Adasuve should not be used if a person has asthma or other breathing disease.

One side effect that may not go away is *tardive dyskinesia* (or TD). Patients with tardive dyskinesia have involuntary movements of the body, especially the mouth and tongue. The patient may look as though he or she is making faces over and over again. Jerky movements of the arms, legs, or body may occur. There may be fine, wormlike, or sudden repeated movements of the tongue, or the person may appear to be chewing

311

something or smacking or puckering his or her lips. The fingers may look as though they are rolling something. If you notice any unusual movements, be sure to tell the doctor. The doctor may use the AIMS test to look for these movements.

The medicine may increase the level of *prolactin*, a natural hormone made in the part of the brain called the *pituitary*. This may cause side effects such as breast tenderness or swelling or production of milk, in both boys and girls. It also may interfere with sexual functioning in teenage boys and with regular menstrual cycles (periods) in teenage girls. A blood test can measure the level of prolactin. If these side effects do not go away and are troublesome, talk with your child's doctor about substituting another medicine for loxapine.

Heart problems are more common if other medicines are being taken also. Be sure to tell all your child's doctors and your pharmacist about all medications your child is taking.

Neuroleptic malignant syndrome is a very rare side effect that can lead to death. The symptoms are severe muscle stiffness, high fever, increased heart rate and blood pressure, irregular heartbeat (pulse), and sweating. It may lead to unconsciousness. If you suspect this, **call 911 or go to an emergency room right away.**

Some Interactions With Other Medicines or Food

Please note that the following are only the most likely interactions with other medicines or food.

Loxapine may be taken with or without food. If the medicine causes stomach upset, taking it with food may help.

It is better to limit drinks with caffeine (coffee, tea, soft drinks) because caffeine works in the opposite way from this medicine, and the positive effects might be decreased.

What Could Happen if This Medicine Is Stopped Suddenly?

Involuntary movements, or *withdrawal dyskinesias*, may appear within 1–4 weeks of lowering the dose or stopping the medicine. Usually these go away, but they can last for days to months. If loxapine is stopped suddenly, emotional problems such as irritability, nervousness, moodiness; behavior problems; or physical problems such as stomachache, loss of appetite, nausea, vomiting, diarrhea, sweating, indigestion, trouble sleeping, trembling, or shaking may appear. These problems usually last only a few days to a few weeks. If they happen, tell your child's doctor. The medicine dose may need to be lowered more slowly (tapered). Always check with the doctor before stopping a medicine.

How Long Will This Medicine Be Needed?

How long your child will need to be on loxapine depends partly on the reason that it was prescribed. Some problems last for only a few months, whereas others last much longer. Sometimes loxapine is used for only a short time until other medicines or behavioral treatments start to work. Some people need to take loxapine for years. It is especially important with medicines as powerful as this one to ask the doctor whether it is still needed. Every few months, you should discuss with your child's doctor the reasons for using loxapine and whether it is time for a trial of lowering the dose.

What Else Should I Know About This Medicine?

There are many older and newer medicines that are used for the same kinds of problems. If your child is having bad side effects or the medicine does not seem to be working, ask the doctor if another medicine in this group might work as well or better and have fewer side effects for your child.

Be sure to tell the doctor if there is anyone in your family who died suddenly or had a heart problem.

Sometimes this medicine can cause a *dystonic reaction*. This is a sudden stiffening of the muscles, most often in the jaw, neck, tongue, face, or shoulders. If this happens, and your child is not having trouble breathing, you may give a dose of diphenhydramine (Benadryl). Follow the dose instructions on the package for your child's age. This should relax the muscles in a few minutes. Then call your doctor to tell him or her what happened. If the muscles do not relax, take your child to the emergency department.

Notes

Use this space to take notes or to write down questions you want to ask the doctor.

_____

_____

_____

_____

_____

_____

_____

_____

_____

_____

all the possible uses, precautions, side effects, or interactions of this drug. For a complete listing of side effects, see the manufacturer's package insert, which can be obtained from your physician or pharmacist. As medical research and practice advance, therapeutic standards may change. For this reason and because human and mechanical errors sometimes occur, we recommend that readers follow the advice of a physician who is directly involved in their care or the care of a member of their family.

From Dulcan MK, Ballard R (editors): *Helping Parents and Teachers Understand Medications for Behavioral and Emotional Problems: A Resource Book of Medication Information Handouts*, Fourth Edition. Washington, DC, American Psychiatric Publishing, 2015

Lurasidone—Latuda

General Information About Medication

Each child and adolescent is different. No one has exactly the same combination of medical and psychological problems. It is a good idea to talk with the doctor or nurse about the reasons a medicine is being used. It is very important to keep all appointments and to be in touch by telephone if you have concerns. It is important to communicate with the doctor, nurse, or therapist. An *advanced practice nurse* (APN) has additional education and training after becoming a registered nurse (RN). Your child's medication may be prescribed by a medical doctor (MD or DO) or an APN. In addition, a *physician assistant* (PA) working with a physician may prescribe certain medications. In this information sheet, "doctor" includes medical doctors as well as APNs and PAs who prescribe medication. Often a nurse (RN) will be part of the team and answer questions and give information.

It is very important that the medicine be taken exactly as the doctor instructs. However, once in a while, everyone forgets to give a medicine on time. It is a good idea to ask the doctor or nurse what to do if this happens. Do not stop or change a medicine without asking the doctor or nurse first.

If the medicine seems to stop working, it may be because it is not being taken regularly. The youth may be "cheeking" or hiding the medicine or forgetting to take it (especially at school). The doses may be too far apart or a different dose or medicine may be needed. Something at school, at home, or in the neighborhood may be upsetting the youth, or he or she may need special help for learning disabilities or tutoring. Please discuss your concerns with the doctor. **Do not just increase the dose.** It is also very important not to decrease the dose or stop the medicine without talking to the doctor first. The problem being treated may come back, or there could be uncomfortable or even dangerous results.

All medicines should be kept in a safe place, out of the reach of children, and should be supervised by an adult. If someone takes too much of a medicine, call the doctor, the poison control center, or a hospital emergency room.

Each medicine has a "generic" or chemical name. Just like laundry detergents or paper towels, some medicines are sold by more than one company under different brand names. The same medicine may be available under a generic name and several brand names. The generic medications are usually less expensive than the brand name ones. The generic medications have the same chemical formula, but they may or may not be exactly the same strength as the brand-name medications. Also, some brands of pills contain dye or other things that can cause allergic reactions. It is a good idea to talk to the doctor and the pharmacist about whether it is important to use a specific brand of medicine.

Any medicine can cause an allergic reaction. Examples are hives, itching, rashes, swelling, and trouble breathing. Even a tiny amount of a medicine can cause a reaction in patients who are allergic to that medicine. Be *sure* to talk to the doctor before restarting a medicine that has caused an allergic reaction and tell the doctor about any reactions to medicine that your child has had before.

Taking more than one medicine at the same time may cause more side effects or cause one of the medicines to not work as well. Always ask the doctor, nurse, or pharmacist before adding another medicine, either prescription or bought without a prescription in a store or on the Internet. Be sure

that each doctor knows about *all* of the medicines your child is taking. Also tell the doctor about any vitamins, herbal medicines, or supplements your child may be taking. Some of these may have side effects alone or when taken with this medication. It is a very good idea to keep a list with you of the names and doses of all medicines that your child is taking.

Everyone taking medicine should have a physical examination at least once a year.

If you think that your child may be using drugs or alcohol, please tell the doctor right away.

Pregnancy requires special care in the use of medicine. Some medicines can cause birth defects if taken by a pregnant mother. **Please tell the doctor immediately if you suspect the teenager is at risk of becoming pregnant.** The doctor may wish to discuss sexual behavior and/or birth control with your daughter.

Printed information like this applies to children and adolescents in general. If you have questions about the medicine, or if you notice changes or anything unusual, please ask the doctor or nurse. As scientific research advances, knowledge increases and advice changes. Even experts do not always agree. Many medicines have not been "approved" by the U.S. Food and Drug Administration (FDA) for use in children or use for particular problems. For this reason, use of the medicine for a problem or age group often is not listed in the *Physicians' Desk Reference*. This does not necessarily mean that the medicine is dangerous or does not work, only that the company that makes the medicine has not received permission to advertise the medicine for use in children. Companies often do not apply for this permission because it is expensive to do the tests needed to apply for approval for use in children. Once a medication is approved by the FDA for any purpose, a doctor is allowed to prescribe it according to research and clinical experience.

Note to Teachers

It is a good idea to talk with the parent(s) about the reason(s) that a medication is being used. If the parent(s) sign consent to release information, it is often helpful for you to talk with the doctor. If the parent(s) give permission, the doctor may ask you to fill out rating forms about your experience with the student's behavior, feelings, academic performance, and medication side effects. This information is very useful in selecting and monitoring medication treatment. If you have observations that you think are important, do not hesitate to share these with the student's parent(s) and treating clinicians (with parental consent).

It is very important that the medicine be taken exactly as the doctor instructs. However, everyone forgets to give a medicine on time once in a while. It is a good idea to ask the parent(s) in advance what to do if this happens. Do not stop or change the time you are giving a medicine at school without parental permission. If a medication is to be taken with food, but lunchtime or snack time changes, be sure to notify the parent(s) so appropriate adjustments can be made.

All medicines should be kept in a secure place and should be supervised by an adult. If someone takes too much of a medicine, follow your school procedure for an urgent medical problem.

Taking medicine is a private matter and is best managed discreetly and confidentially. It is important to be sensitive to the student's feelings about taking medicine.

If you suspect that the student is using drugs or alcohol, please tell the parent(s) or a school counselor right away.

Please tell the parent(s) or school nurse if you suspect medication side effects.

Modifications of the classroom environment or assignments may be useful in addition to medication. The student may need to be evaluated for additional help or a 504 plan or an Individualized Education Plan for learning problems or emotional or behavioral issues.

Any expression of suicidal thoughts or feelings or self-harm by a child or adolescent is a signal of distress and should be taken seriously. These behaviors should not be dismissed as "attention seeking." School procedures for safety issues should be followed.

What Is Lurasidone (Latuda)?

This medicine is called an *atypical* or *second-generation antipsychotic*. It is sometimes called an *atypical psychotropic agent*, or simply an *atypical*. It comes in brand name Latuda tablets.

How Can This Medicine Help?

Lurasidone is used to treat psychosis, such as in schizophrenia, mania, or very severe depression. It can reduce *positive symptoms* such as hallucinations (hearing voices or seeing things that are not there); delusions (troubling beliefs that other people do not share); agitation; and very unusual thinking, speech, and behavior. It is also used to lessen the *negative symptoms* of schizophrenia, such as lack of interest in doing things (apathy), lack of motivation, social withdrawal, and lack of energy.

Lurasidone may be used as a *mood stabilizer* in patients with bipolar disorder or severe mood swings. It can reduce mania and may be able to help maintain a stable mood.

In adults, lurasidone has been used alone or together with another medicine (such as lithium or valproate) to help depression in people with bipolar disorder.

Sometimes lurasidone is used to reduce severe aggression or very serious behavioral problems in young people with conduct disorder, intellectual disability, or autism spectrum disorder.

This medicine is very powerful and is used to treat very serious problems or symptoms that other medicines do not help. Be patient; the positive effects of this medicine may not appear for 2–3 weeks.

How Does This Medicine Work?

Cells in the brain communicate using chemicals called *neurotransmitters*. Too much or too little of these substances in parts of the brain can cause problems. Lurasidone works by blocking the action of one of these neurotransmitters—*dopamine*—in certain areas of the brain.

How Long Does This Medicine Last?

Lurasidone is usually taken once a day.

How Will the Doctor Monitor This Medicine?

The doctor will review your child's medical history and physical examination before starting lurasidone. The doctor may order some blood or urine tests to be sure your child does not have a hidden medical condition that would make it unsafe to use this medicine. The doctor or nurse may measure your child's pulse and blood pressure before starting lurasidone. The doctor may order other tests, such as baseline tests for blood sugar and cholesterol. An ECG (electrocardiogram or heart rhythm test) may be done before and after starting the medicine. A blood test for potassium may also be done.

Be sure to tell the doctor if anyone in the family has diabetes, high blood pressure, high cholesterol, or heart disease or if a family member died suddenly.

Before your child starts taking lurasidone and every so often afterward, a test such as the Abnormal Involuntary Movement Scale (AIMS) may be used to check your child's tongue, legs, and arms for unusual movements that could be caused by the medicine.

After the medicine is started, the doctor will want to have regular appointments with you and your child to see how the medicine is working, to see if a dose change is needed, to watch for side effects, to see if lurasidone is still needed, and to see if any other treatment is needed. The doctor or nurse will check your child's height, weight, pulse, and blood pressure and watch for abnormal movements. Sometimes blood tests are needed to watch for diabetes or increased cholesterol.

What Side Effects Can This Medicine Have?

Any medicine can have side effects, including an allergy to the medicine. Because each patient is different, the doctor will monitor the youth closely, especially when the medicine is started. The doctor will work with you to increase the positive effects and decrease the negative effects of the medicine. Please tell the doctor if any of the listed side effects appear or if you think that the medicine is causing any other problems. Not all of the rare or unusual side effects are listed.

Side effects are most common after starting the medicine or after a dose increase. Many side effects can be avoided or lessened by starting with a very low dose and increasing it slowly—ask the doctor.

Allergic Reaction

Tell the doctor in a day or two (if possible, before the next dose of medicine):

- Hives
- Itching
- Rash

Stop the medicine and get *immediate* medical care:

- Trouble breathing or chest tightness
- Swelling of lips, tongue, or throat

Common, but Not Usually Serious, Side Effects

Discuss the following side effects with your child's doctor when convenient. These side effects often can be helped by lowering the dose of medicine, changing the times medicine is taken, or adding another medicine.

- Daytime sleepiness or tiredness—Do not allow your child to drive, ride a bicycle or motorcycle, or operate machinery if this happens. This problem may be lessened by taking the medicine at bedtime.
- Dry mouth—Have your child try using sugar-free gum or candy.
- Constipation—Encourage your child to drink more fluids and eat high-fiber foods; if necessary, the doctor may recommend a fiber medicine such as Benefiber or a stool softener such as Colace or mineral oil.
- Upset stomach, nausea
- Headache

- Increased appetite
- Weight gain—Seek nutritional counseling; provide your child with low-calorie snacks and encourage regular exercise.

Rare, but Not Usually Serious, Side Effects

Discuss the following side effects with your child's doctor when convenient. These side effects often can be helped by lowering the dose of medicine, changing the times medicine is taken, or adding another medicine.

- Dizziness—This side effect is worse when the child stands up quickly, especially when getting out of bed in the morning; try having the child stand up slowly.
- Increased restlessness or inability to sit still
- Shaking of hands and fingers
- Decreased or slowed movement and decreased facial expressions

Less Common, but Potentially Serious, Side Effects

Call the doctor *immediately*:

- Stiffness of the tongue, jaw, neck, back, or legs
- Seizure (fit, convulsion)—This is more common in people with a history of seizures or head injury.
- Increased thirst, frequent urination (having to go to the bathroom often), lethargy, tiredness, dizziness, and blurred vision—These could be signs of diabetes, especially if your child is overweight or there is a family history of diabetes. **Talk to a doctor within a day.**

Very Rare, but Serious, Side Effects

- Extreme stiffness or lack of movement, very high fever, mental confusion, irregular pulse rate, or eye pain—**This is a medical emergency. Go to an emergency room right away.**
- Sudden stiffness and inability to breathe or swallow—**Go to an emergency room or call 911.** Tell the paramedics, nurses, and doctors that the patient is taking lurasidone. Other medicines can be used to treat this problem quickly.

What Else Should I Know About Side Effects?

Most side effects lessen over time. If they are troublesome, talk with your child's doctor. Some side effects can be decreased by taking a smaller dose of medicine, by stopping the medicine, by changing to another medicine, or by adding another medicine.

Many young people who take lurasidone gain weight. The weight gain may be from increased appetite and also from ways that the medicine changes how the body processes food. Lurasidone may also change the way that the body handles glucose (sugar) and cause high levels of blood sugar (*hyperglycemia*). People who take lurasidone, especially those who gain a lot of weight, might be at increased risk of developing *diabetes* and of having increased fats (*lipids—cholesterol and triglycerides*) in their blood. Over time, both diabetes and increased fats in the blood may lead to heart disease, stroke, and other complications. The FDA has put warnings on all atypical agents about the increased risks of hyperglycemia, diabetes, and increased blood cholesterol and triglycerides when taking one of these medicines. It is much easier to prevent weight gain than to lose weight later. When your child first starts taking lurasidone, it is a good idea to be sure that he or she eats a well-balanced diet without "junk food" and with healthy snacks like fruits and vegetables, not sweets or fried foods. He or she should drink water or skim milk, not pop, sodas, soft drinks, or sugary juices. Regular exercise is important for maintaining a healthy weight (and may also help with sleep).

One very rare side effect that may not go away is *tardive dyskinesia* (or TD). Patients with tardive dyskinesia have involuntary movements (movements that they cannot help making) of the body, especially the mouth and tongue. The patient may look as though he or she is making faces over and over again. Jerky movements of the arms, legs, or body may occur. There may be fine, wormlike or sudden repeated movements of the tongue, or the person may appear to be chewing something or smacking or puckering his or her lips. The fingers may look as though they are rolling something. If you notice any unusual movements, be sure to tell the doctor. The doctor may use the AIMS test to look for these movements.

Neuroleptic malignant syndrome is a very rare side effect that can lead to death. The symptoms are severe muscle stiffness, high fever, increased heart rate and blood pressure, irregular heartbeat (pulse), and sweating. It may lead to unconsciousness. If you suspect this, **call 911 or go to an emergency room right away.**

The medicine may increase the level of *prolactin*, a natural hormone made in the part of the brain called the *pituitary*. This may cause side effects such as breast tenderness or swelling or production of milk in both boys and girls. It also may interfere with sexual functioning in teenage boys and with regular menstrual cycles (periods) in teenage girls. A blood test can measure the level of prolactin. If these side effects do not go away and are troublesome, talk with your child's doctor about substituting another medicine for lurasidone.

Sometimes this medicine can cause a *dystonic reaction*. This is a sudden stiffening of the muscles, most often in the jaw, neck, tongue, face, or shoulders. If this happens, and your child is not having trouble breathing, you may give a dose of diphenhydramine (Benadryl). Follow the dose instructions on the package for your child's age. This should relax the muscles in a few minutes. Then call your doctor to tell him or her what happened. If the muscles do not relax, take your child to the emergency department.

Some Interactions With Other Medicines or Food

Please note that the following are only the most likely interactions with other medicines or food.

Heart problems are more common if other medicines that affect the heart or antibiotics such as erythromycin are being taken as well. Be sure to tell all your child's doctors and your pharmacist about all medications your child is taking.

Lurasidone should be taken with food (at least 350 calories). Grapefruit juice may increase lurasidone blood levels and possibly side effects. It is better to limit drinks with caffeine (coffee, tea, soft drinks) because caffeine works in the opposite way from this medicine, and the positive effects might be decreased.

Many medicines used to fight infections may increase levels of lurasidone and increase side effects. Ask the doctor.

What Could Happen if This Medicine Is Stopped Suddenly?

Involuntary movements, or *withdrawal dyskinesias*, may appear within 1–4 weeks of lowering the dose or stopping the medicine. Usually these go away, but they can last for days to months. If lurasidone is stopped suddenly, emotional disturbance (such as irritability, nervousness, moodiness, or oppositional behavior) or physical problems (such as stomachache, loss of appetite, nausea, vomiting, diarrhea, sweating, indigestion, trouble sleeping, trembling, or shaking) may appear. These problems usually last only a few days to a few weeks. If they happen, you should tell your child's doctor. The medicine dose may need to be lowered more slowly (tapered). Always check with the doctor before stopping a medicine.

How Long Will This Medicine Be Needed?

How long your child will need to take this medicine depends partly on the reason that it was prescribed. Some problems last for only a few months, whereas others last much longer. It is important to ask the doctor whether medicine is still needed, especially with medicines as powerful as this one. Every few months, you should discuss with your child's doctor the reasons for using lurasidone and whether the medicine may be stopped or the dose lowered.

What Else Should I Know About This Medicine?

There are other medicines that are used for the same kinds of problems. If your child is having bad side effects or the medicine does not seem to be working, ask the doctor if another medicine might work as well or better and have fewer side effects for your child. Each person reacts differently to medicines.

Taking this medicine could make overheating or heatstroke more likely. Have your child decrease activity in hot weather, stay out of the sun, and drink water to prevent this.

Notes

Use this space to take notes or to write down questions you want to ask the doctor.

_____

_____

_____

_____

_____

_____

_____

_____

_____

_____

_____

From Dulcan MK, Ballard R (editors): *Helping Parents and Teachers Understand Medications for Behavioral and Emotional Problems: A Resource Book of Medication Information Handouts*, Fourth Edition. Washington, DC, American Psychiatric Publishing, 2015

Melatonin

General Information About Medication

Each child and adolescent is different. No one has exactly the same combination of medical and psychological problems. It is a good idea to talk with the doctor or nurse about the reasons a medicine is being used. It is very important to keep all appointments and to be in touch by telephone if you have concerns. It is important to communicate with the doctor, nurse, or therapist. An *advanced practice nurse* (APN) has additional education and training after becoming a registered nurse (RN). Your child's medication may be prescribed by a medical doctor (MD or DO) or an APN. In addition, a *physician assistant* (PA) working with a physician may prescribe certain medications. In this information sheet, "doctor" includes medical doctors as well as APNs and PAs who prescribe medication. Often a nurse (RN) will be part of the team and answer questions and give information.

It is very important that the medicine be taken exactly as the doctor instructs. However, once in a while, everyone forgets to give a medicine on time. It is a good idea to ask the doctor or nurse what to do if this happens. Do not stop or change a medicine without asking the doctor or nurse first.

If the medicine seems to stop working, it may be because it is not being taken regularly. The youth may be "cheeking" or hiding the medicine or forgetting to take it (especially at school). The doses may be too far apart or a different dose or medicine may be needed. Something at school, at home, or in the neighborhood may be upsetting the youth, or he or she may need special help for learning disabilities or tutoring. Please discuss your concerns with the doctor. **Do not just increase the dose.** It is also very important not to decrease the dose or stop the medicine without talking to the doctor first. The problem being treated may come back, or there could be uncomfortable or even dangerous results.

All medicines should be kept in a safe place, out of the reach of children, and should be supervised by an adult. If someone takes too much of a medicine, call the doctor, the poison control center, or a hospital emergency room.

Each medicine has a "generic" or chemical name. Just like laundry detergents or paper towels, some medicines are sold by more than one company under different brand names. The same medicine may be available under a generic name and several brand names. The generic medications are usually less expensive than the brand name ones. The generic medications have the same chemical formula, but they may or may not be exactly the same strength as the brand-name medications. Also, some brands of pills contain dye or other things that can cause allergic reactions. It is a good idea to talk to the doctor and the pharmacist about whether it is important to use a specific brand of medicine.

Any medicine can cause an allergic reaction. Examples are hives, itching, rashes, swelling, and trouble breathing. Even a tiny amount of a medicine can cause a reaction in patients who are allergic to that medicine. Be *sure* to talk to the doctor before restarting a medicine that has caused an allergic reaction and tell the doctor about any reactions to medicine that your child has had before.

Taking more than one medicine at the same time may cause more side effects or cause one of the medicines to not work as well. Always ask the doctor, nurse, or pharmacist before adding another

medicine, either prescription or bought without a prescription in a store or on the Internet. Be sure that each doctor knows about *all* of the medicines your child is taking. Also tell the doctor about any vitamins, herbal medicines, or supplements your child may be taking. Some of these may have side effects alone or when taken with this medication. It is a very good idea to keep a list with you of the names and doses of all medicines that your child is taking.

Everyone taking medicine should have a physical examination at least once a year.

If you think that your child may be using drugs or alcohol, please tell the doctor right away.

Pregnancy requires special care in the use of medicine. Some medicines can cause birth defects if taken by a pregnant mother. **Please tell the doctor immediately if you suspect the teenager is at risk of becoming pregnant.** The doctor may wish to discuss sexual behavior and/or birth control with your daughter.

Printed information like this applies to children and adolescents in general. If you have questions about the medicine, or if you notice changes or anything unusual, please ask the doctor or nurse. As scientific research advances, knowledge increases and advice changes. Even experts do not always agree. Many medicines have not been "approved" by the U.S. Food and Drug Administration (FDA) for use in children or use for particular problems. For this reason, use of the medicine for a problem or age group often is not listed in the *Physicians' Desk Reference*. This does not necessarily mean that the medicine is dangerous or does not work, only that the company that makes the medicine has not received permission to advertise the medicine for use in children. Companies often do not apply for this permission because it is expensive to do the tests needed to apply for approval for use in children. Once a medication is approved by the FDA for any purpose, a doctor is allowed to prescribe it according to research and clinical experience.

Note to Teachers

It is a good idea to talk with the parent(s) about the reason(s) that a medication is being used. If the parent(s) sign consent to release information, it is often helpful for you to talk with the doctor. If the parent(s) give permission, the doctor may ask you to fill out rating forms about your experience with the student's behavior, feelings, academic performance, and medication side effects. This information is very useful in selecting and monitoring medication treatment. If you have observations that you think are important, do not hesitate to share these with the student's parent(s) and treating clinicians (with parental consent).

It is very important that the medicine be taken exactly as the doctor instructs. However, everyone forgets to give a medicine on time once in a while. It is a good idea to ask the parent(s) in advance what to do if this happens. Do not stop or change the time you are giving a medicine at school without parental permission. If a medication is to be taken with food, but lunchtime or snack time changes, be sure to notify the parent(s) so appropriate adjustments can be made.

All medicines should be kept in a secure place and should be supervised by an adult. If someone takes too much of a medicine, follow your school procedure for an urgent medical problem.

Taking medicine is a private matter and is best managed discreetly and confidentially. It is important to be sensitive to the student's feelings about taking medicine.

If you suspect that the student is using drugs or alcohol, please tell the parent(s) or a school counselor right away.

Please tell the parent(s) or school nurse if you suspect medication side effects.

Modifications of the classroom environment or assignments may be useful in addition to medication. The student may need to be evaluated for additional help or a 504 plan or an Individualized Education Plan for learning problems or emotional or behavioral issues.

Any expression of suicidal thoughts or feelings or self-harm by a child or adolescent is a signal of distress and should be taken seriously. These behaviors should not be dismissed as "attention seeking." School procedures for safety issues should be followed.

What Is Melatonin?

Melatonin is a natural hormone produced by the body. Melatonin is produced by the *pineal gland*, which is located just above the middle of the brain. During the day, the pineal gland is not active. It starts producing melatonin after sunset, usually around 9:00 P.M. As a result, melatonin levels in the brain rise sharply, and the person begins to feel less alert and more sleepy. Melatonin levels remain high through the night and fall to low daytime levels by the morning hours, usually around 9:00 A.M.

Melatonin is available in the United States without a prescription as a nutritional supplement. It comes in tablets, capsules, and liquid form.

Melatonin is not a sedative, hypnotic, or tranquilizer.

How Can This Medicine Help?

Melatonin can improve sleep by returning a person to a more natural sleep cycle. It can help with falling asleep and with staying asleep for long enough to be rested. It has been shown to work in children without psychiatric problems who have severe sleep problems as well as in children with attention-deficit/hyperactivity disorder (ADHD), developmental delays, or autism spectrum disorder who have severe sleep problems.

Melatonin can reset the body's clock and help to regulate the *circadian cycle*. Many adolescents have *delayed sleep phase syndrome*, a disorder of the biological clock in which the youth is not sleepy until very late at night and is unable to get up early in the morning. This causes problems with school attendance and performance. Melatonin is helpful in shifting sleep to a more regular time schedule.

How Does This Medicine Work?

Synthetic (man-made) melatonin can improve sleep in both children and adults. The exact way in which this happens is not known, but it is thought that the synthetic melatonin copies the effects of natural melatonin in the brain. It starts working 1–2 hours after taking it. It is usually given 30 minutes to 1 hour before bedtime.

A behavioral program, such as regular soothing routines at bedtime and increased exercise in the daytime, should be used in combination with the medicine to improve sleep. Finding developmentally appropriate bed- and wake-times and sticking to them is very important. These strategies should be continued after the medicine is stopped or when the medicine is used only occasionally.

How Will the Doctor Monitor This Medicine?

The doctor will review your child's medical history and physical examination before starting melatonin. The doctor may order some blood or urine tests to be sure your child does not have a hidden medical condition.

After the medicine is started, the doctor will want to have regular appointments with you and your child to see how the medicine is working, to see if a dose change is needed, to watch for side effects, to see if melatonin is still needed, and to see if any other treatment is needed.

What Side Effects Can This Medicine Have?

Any medicine can have side effects, including an allergy to the medicine. Because each patient is different, the doctor will monitor the youth closely, especially when the medicine is started. The doctor will work with you to increase the positive effects and decrease the negative effects of the medicine. Please tell the doctor if any of the listed side effects appear or if you think that the medicine is causing any other problems. Not all of the rare or unusual side effects are listed.

Side effects are most common after starting the medicine or after a dose increase. Many side effects can be avoided or lessened by starting with a very low dose and increasing it slowly—ask the doctor.

Allergic Reaction

Tell the doctor in a day or two (if possible, before the next dose of medicine):

- Hives
- Itching
- Rash

Stop the medicine and get *immediate* medical care:

- Trouble breathing or chest tightness
- Swelling of lips, tongue, or throat

Other Possible Side Effects

Melatonin appears to be well tolerated, with no significant side effects reported. There has not been a lot of research on the safety of melatonin in children. Some children may be sleepy in the morning when it is time to get up and go to school or may have a headache or upset stomach. Dreams or nightmares may be more intense.

Some Interactions With Other Medicines or Food

Please note that the following are only the most likely interactions with other medicines or food.

Most interactions of melatonin with other drugs are mild, but melatonin can interfere with anticoagulant medications like warfarin (Coumadin), making it more likely that a person would develop a blood clot. Melatonin can also decrease the levels of some antidepressants and some blood pressure medications.

Caffeine may interfere with sleep and make it more difficult for the melatonin to work.

What Could Happen if This Medicine Is Stopped Suddenly?

There are no known effects from stopping melatonin suddenly, although the original sleep problem might return.

How Long Will This Medicine Be Needed?

Some people may need melatonin for a long time (years), but others may need it only until the sleep rhythm improves.

What Else Should I Know About This Medicine?

Buy melatonin labeled USP to be sure that the amount of melatonin that is actually in the pill is the same as listed on the package.

Notes

Use this space to take notes or to write down questions you want to ask the doctor.

_____

_____

_____

_____

_____

_____

_____

_____

_____

_____

_____

_____

From Dulcan MK, Ballard R (editors): *Helping Parents and Teachers Understand Medications for Behavioral and Emotional Problems: A Resource Book of Medication Information Handouts*, Fourth Edition. Washington, DC, American Psychiatric Publishing, 2015

Medication Information for Parents and Teachers

Metformin—Glucophage, Glucophage XR, Fortamet, Glumetza, Riomet

General Information About Medication

Each child and adolescent is different. No one has exactly the same combination of medical and psychological problems. It is a good idea to talk with the doctor or nurse about the reasons a medicine is being used. It is very important to keep all appointments and to be in touch by telephone if you have concerns. It is important to communicate with the doctor, nurse, or therapist. An *advanced practice nurse* (APN) has additional education and training after becoming a registered nurse (RN). Your child's medication may be prescribed by a medical doctor (MD or DO) or an APN. In addition, a *physician assistant* (PA) working with a physician may prescribe certain medications. In this information sheet, "doctor" includes medical doctors as well as APNs and PAs who prescribe medication. Often a nurse (RN) will be part of the team and answer questions and give information.

It is very important that the medicine be taken exactly as the doctor instructs. However, once in a while, everyone forgets to give a medicine on time. It is a good idea to ask the doctor or nurse what to do if this happens. Do not stop or change a medicine without asking the doctor or nurse first.

If the medicine seems to stop working, it may be because it is not being taken regularly. The youth may be "cheeking" or hiding the medicine or forgetting to take it (especially at school). The doses may be too far apart or a different dose or medicine may be needed. Something at school, at home, or in the neighborhood may be upsetting the youth, or he or she may need special help for learning disabilities or tutoring. Please discuss your concerns with the doctor. **Do not just increase the dose.** It is also very important not to decrease the dose or stop the medicine without talking to the doctor first. The problem being treated may come back, or there could be uncomfortable or even dangerous results.

All medicines should be kept in a safe place, out of the reach of children, and should be supervised by an adult. If someone takes too much of a medicine, call the doctor, the poison control center, or a hospital emergency room.

Each medicine has a "generic" or chemical name. Just like laundry detergents or paper towels, some medicines are sold by more than one company under different brand names. The same medicine may be available under a generic name and several brand names. The generic medications are usually less expensive than the brand name ones. The generic medications have the same chemical formula, but they may or may not be exactly the same strength as the brand-name medications. Also, some brands of pills contain dye or other things that can cause allergic reactions. It is a good idea to talk to the doctor and the pharmacist about whether it is important to use a specific brand of medicine.

Any medicine can cause an allergic reaction. Examples are hives, itching, rashes, swelling, and trouble breathing. Even a tiny amount of a medicine can cause a reaction in patients who are allergic to that medicine. Be *sure* to talk to the doctor before restarting a medicine that has caused an allergic reaction and tell the doctor about any reactions to medicine that your child has had before.

Taking more than one medicine at the same time may cause more side effects or cause one of the medicines to not work as well. Always ask the doctor, nurse, or pharmacist before adding another medicine, either prescription or bought without a prescription in a store or on the Internet. Be sure that each doctor knows about *all* of the medicines your child is taking. Also tell the doctor about any vitamins, herbal medicines, or supplements your child may be taking. Some of these may have side effects alone or when taken with this medication. It is a very good idea to keep a list with you of the names and doses of all medicines that your child is taking.

Everyone taking medicine should have a physical examination at least once a year.

If you think that your child may be using drugs or alcohol, please tell the doctor right away.

Pregnancy requires special care in the use of medicine. Some medicines can cause birth defects if taken by a pregnant mother. **Please tell the doctor immediately if you suspect the teenager is at risk of becoming pregnant.** The doctor may wish to discuss sexual behavior and/or birth control with your daughter.

Printed information like this applies to children and adolescents in general. If you have questions about the medicine, or if you notice changes or anything unusual, please ask the doctor or nurse. As scientific research advances, knowledge increases and advice changes. Even experts do not always agree. Many medicines have not been "approved" by the U.S. Food and Drug Administration (FDA) for use in children or use for particular problems. For this reason, use of the medicine for a problem or age group often is not listed in the *Physicians' Desk Reference*. This does not necessarily mean that the medicine is dangerous or does not work, only that the company that makes the medicine has not received permission to advertise the medicine for use in children. Companies often do not apply for this permission because it is expensive to do the tests needed to apply for approval for use in children. Once a medication is approved by the FDA for any purpose, a doctor is allowed to prescribe it according to research and clinical experience.

Note to Teachers

It is a good idea to talk with the parent(s) about the reason(s) that a medication is being used. If the parent(s) sign consent to release information, it is often helpful for you to talk with the doctor. If the parent(s) give permission, the doctor may ask you to fill out rating forms about your experience with the student's behavior, feelings, academic performance, and medication side effects. This information is very useful in selecting and monitoring medication treatment. If you have observations that you think are important, do not hesitate to share these with the student's parent(s) and treating clinicians (with parental consent).

It is very important that the medicine be taken exactly as the doctor instructs. However, everyone forgets to give a medicine on time once in a while. It is a good idea to ask the parent(s) in advance what to do if this happens. Do not stop or change the time you are giving a medicine at school without parental permission. If a medication is to be taken with food, but lunchtime or snack time changes, be sure to notify the parent(s) so appropriate adjustments can be made.

All medicines should be kept in a secure place and should be supervised by an adult. If someone takes too much of a medicine, follow your school procedure for an urgent medical problem.

Taking medicine is a private matter and is best managed discreetly and confidentially. It is important to be sensitive to the student's feelings about taking medicine.

If you suspect that the student is using drugs or alcohol, please tell the parent(s) or a school counselor right away.

Please tell the parent(s) or school nurse if you suspect medication side effects.

Modifications of the classroom environment or assignments may be useful in addition to medication. The student may need to be evaluated for additional help or a 504 plan or an Individualized Education Plan for learning problems or emotional or behavioral issues.

Any expression of suicidal thoughts or feelings or self-harm by a child or adolescent is a signal of distress and should be taken seriously. These behaviors should not be dismissed as "attention seeking." School procedures for safety issues should be followed.

What Is Metformin (Glucophage, Glucophage XR, Fortamet, Glumetza, Riomet)?

Metformin is a medication used to treat diabetes and to prevent diabetes in people who are at high risk for it. Metformin comes in brand name Glucophage and generic tablets, brand name Glucophage XR, Fortamet, and Glumetza and generic extended-release form, and brand name Riomet cherry-flavored liquid.

How Can This Medicine Help?

Many people who take psychiatric medications called *atypical antipsychotics* gain weight and have increased blood sugar or increased lipids (fats) in their blood. (Some examples of atypical antipsychotic medications are risperidone and aripiprazole.) These changes can increase the risk of diabetes or heart disease or increase the risk of *metabolic syndrome*. Studies have shown that when metformin is taken along with the atypical antipsychotic, patients may have reduced weight gain and their blood sugar and lipids improve. Metformin can help the most if your child also eats a healthy diet and has regular physical exercise. Your doctor will review diet and exercise recommendations with you.

How Does This Medicine Work?

Metformin is in the class of medications called *biguanides*. It decreases absorption of glucose from the intestines and increases uptake and use of glucose by the body's cells. It also increases the body's sensitivity to insulin, the hormone that regulates blood glucose.

How Long Does This Medicine Last?

Metformin tablets and liquid are taken twice daily, with meals. The extended-release tablet is taken once a day.

How Will the Doctor Monitor This Medicine?

The doctor will review your child's medical history and physical examination before starting metformin. The doctor may order some blood or urine tests to be sure your child does not have a hidden medical condition that would make it unsafe to use this medicine. The doctor or nurse may measure your child's height, weight, pulse, and blood pressure before starting metformin. The doctor may order other tests, such as fasting blood sugar, electrolytes, lipids, and insulin.

After the medicine is started, the doctor will want to have regular appointments with you and your child to see how the medicine is working, to see if a dose change is needed, to watch for side effects, to see if metformin is still needed, and to see if any other treatment is needed. The doctor or nurse may check your child's height, weight, pulse, and blood pressure or order tests to keep track of your child's blood sugar, lipids, and electrolytes.

331

What Side Effects Can This Medicine Have?

Any medicine can have side effects, including an allergy to the medicine. Because each patient is different, the doctor will monitor the youth closely, especially when the medicine is started. The doctor will work with you to increase the positive effects and decrease the negative effects of the medicine. Please tell the doctor if any of the listed side effects appear or if you think that the medicine is causing any other problems. Not all of the rare or unusual side effects are listed.

Allergic Reaction

Tell the doctor in a day or two (if possible, before the next dose of medicine):

- Hives
- Itching
- Rash

Get *immediate* medical care:

- Trouble breathing or chest tightness
- Swelling of lips, tongue, or throat
- Body aches, nausea, deep or labored breathing, somnolence

Common Side Effects

- Heartburn
- Abdominal fullness
- Nausea, vomiting, or diarrhea—These are common in the first weeks of treatment but usually go away. If they happen later in treatment, tell your doctor.
- Metallic taste in the mouth

Rare, But Serious, Side Effects

Metformin can cause a condition caused *lactic acidosis*. This is rare in healthy young people. Symptoms are vague at first but can include weakness, nausea, body aches, deep or labored breathing, unusual sleepiness, or decreased consciousness. **If this occurs, take your child to the emergency room right away.** Drinking alcohol can be dangerous in a person taking metformin because of the risk of lactic acidosis. If your child develops an illness with vomiting and diarrhea, he or she may become dehydrated, which increases the risk of lactic acidosis. If your child has vomiting or diarrhea, stop the metformin and contact your doctor right away.

Some Interactions With Other Medicines or Food

Please note that the following are only the most likely interactions with other medicines or food.

If a person taking metformin is given intravenous (IV) contrast dye for an X-ray or computed tomography (CT) scan, there can be a serious reaction. If your child is going to have this kind of test, be sure to tell the doctor or nurse or technician that he or she is taking metformin.

Metformin does not usually lower the blood sugar so much that a person becomes hypoglycemic (blood sugar too low), but if taken with other diabetes medications that lower blood sugar it can make the blood sugar level fall more rapidly.

Metformin should not be taken with alcohol because it can increase the risk of lactic acidosis (see above).

What Could Happen if This Medicine Is Stopped Suddenly?

If metformin is being used to help control weight gain in a person without diabetes, there should be no problems from stopping it suddenly. In a person with diabetes, stopping metformin suddenly could result in changes in blood sugar control.

How Long Will This Medicine Be Needed?

Metformin may be given for as long as the atypical antipsychotic medication that is causing the weight gain is given or for as long as there is concern about weight gain or increased blood sugar or lipids. Following a healthy diet and exercise program can decrease the need for metformin.

What Else Should I Know About This Medicine?

Metformin is also prescribed for young women who have polycystic ovarian syndrome (PCOS) to help regulate their female hormones and their periods. It can improve fertility in these young women. Any young woman who is taking psychiatric medication and who is sexually active should discuss this with her doctor.

Notes

Use this space to take notes or to write down questions you want to ask the doctor.

_____

_____

_____

_____

_____

_____

_____

_____

_____

_____

Medication Information for Parents and Teachers

Methylphenidate—Methylin, Ritalin, Metadate, Concerta, Daytrana, Quillivant, Focalin

General Information About Medication

Each child and adolescent is different. No one has exactly the same combination of medical and psychological problems. It is a good idea to talk with the doctor or nurse about the reasons a medicine is being used. It is very important to keep all appointments and to be in touch by telephone if you have concerns. It is important to communicate with the doctor, nurse, or therapist. An *advanced practice nurse* (APN) has additional education and training after becoming a registered nurse (RN). Your child's medication may be prescribed by a medical doctor (MD or DO) or an APN. In addition, a *physician assistant* (PA) working with a physician may prescribe certain medications. In this information sheet, "doctor" includes medical doctors as well as APNs and PAs who prescribe medication. Often a nurse (RN) will be part of the team and answer questions and give information.

It is very important that the medicine be taken exactly as the doctor instructs. However, once in a while, everyone forgets to give a medicine on time. It is a good idea to ask the doctor or nurse what to do if this happens. Do not stop or change a medicine without asking the doctor or nurse first.

If the medicine seems to stop working, it may be because it is not being taken regularly. The youth may be "cheeking" or hiding the medicine or forgetting to take it (especially at school). The doses may be too far apart or a different dose or medicine may be needed. Something at school, at home, or in the neighborhood may be upsetting the youth, or he or she may need special help for learning disabilities or tutoring. Please discuss your concerns with the doctor. **Do not just increase the dose.** It is also very important not to decrease the dose or stop the medicine without talking to the doctor first. The problem being treated may come back, or there could be uncomfortable or even dangerous results.

All medicines should be kept in a safe place, out of the reach of children, and should be supervised by an adult. If someone takes too much of a medicine, call the doctor, the poison control center, or a hospital emergency room.

Each medicine has a "generic" or chemical name. Just like laundry detergents or paper towels, some medicines are sold by more than one company under different brand names. The same medicine may be available under a generic name and several brand names. The generic medications are usually less expensive than the brand name ones. The generic medications have the same chemical formula, but they may or may not be exactly the same strength as the brand-name medications. Also, some brands of pills contain dye or other things that can cause allergic reactions. It is a good idea to talk to the doctor and the pharmacist about whether it is important to use a specific brand of medicine.

Any medicine can cause an allergic reaction. Examples are hives, itching, rashes, swelling, and trouble breathing. Even a tiny amount of a medicine can cause a reaction in patients who are allergic to that medicine. Be *sure* to talk to the doctor before restarting a medicine that has caused an allergic reaction and tell the doctor about any reactions to medicine that your child has had before.

Taking more than one medicine at the same time may cause more side effects or cause one of the medicines to not work as well. Always ask the doctor, nurse, or pharmacist before adding another medicine, either prescription or bought without a prescription in a store or on the Internet. Be sure that each doctor knows about *all* **of the medicines your child is taking. Also tell the doctor about any vitamins, herbal medicines, or supplements your child may be taking.** Some of these may have side effects alone or when taken with this medication. It is a very good idea to keep a list with you of the names and doses of all medicines that your child is taking.

Everyone taking medicine should have a physical examination at least once a year.

If you think that your child may be using drugs or alcohol, please tell the doctor right away.

Pregnancy requires special care in the use of medicine. Some medicines can cause birth defects if taken by a pregnant mother. **Please tell the doctor immediately if you suspect the teenager is at risk of becoming pregnant.** The doctor may wish to discuss sexual behavior and/or birth control with your daughter.

Printed information like this applies to children and adolescents in general. If you have questions about the medicine, or if you notice changes or anything unusual, please ask the doctor or nurse. As scientific research advances, knowledge increases and advice changes. Even experts do not always agree. Many medicines have not been "approved" by the U.S. Food and Drug Administration (FDA) for use in children or use for particular problems. For this reason, use of the medicine for a problem or age group often is not listed in the *Physicians' Desk Reference*. This does not necessarily mean that the medicine is dangerous or does not work, only that the company that makes the medicine has not received permission to advertise the medicine for use in children. Companies often do not apply for this permission because it is expensive to do the tests needed to apply for approval for use in children. Once a medication is approved by the FDA for any purpose, a doctor is allowed to prescribe it according to research and clinical experience.

Note to Teachers

It is a good idea to talk with the parent(s) about the reason(s) that a medication is being used. If the parent(s) sign consent to release information, it is often helpful for you to talk with the doctor. If the parent(s) give permission, the doctor may ask you to fill out rating forms about your experience with the student's behavior, feelings, academic performance, and medication side effects. This information is very useful in selecting and monitoring medication treatment. If you have observations that you think are important, do not hesitate to share these with the student's parent(s) and treating clinicians (with parental consent).

It is very important that the medicine be taken exactly as the doctor instructs. However, everyone forgets to give a medicine on time once in a while. It is a good idea to ask the parent(s) in advance what to do if this happens. Do not stop or change the time you are giving a medicine at school without parental permission. If a medication is to be taken with food, but lunchtime or snack time changes, be sure to notify the parent(s) so appropriate adjustments can be made.

All medicines should be kept in a secure place and should be supervised by an adult. If someone takes too much of a medicine, follow your school procedure for an urgent medical problem.

Taking medicine is a private matter and is best managed discreetly and confidentially. It is important to be sensitive to the student's feelings about taking medicine.

If you suspect that the student is using drugs or alcohol, please tell the parent(s) or a school counselor right away.

Please tell the parent(s) or school nurse if you suspect medication side effects.

Modifications of the classroom environment or assignments may be useful in addition to medication. The student may need to be evaluated for additional help or a 504 plan or an Individualized Education Plan for learning problems or emotional or behavioral issues.

Any expression of suicidal thoughts or feelings or self-harm by a child or adolescent is a signal of distress and should be taken seriously. These behaviors should not be dismissed as "attention seeking." School procedures for safety issues should be followed.

What Is Methylphenidate (Methylin, Ritalin, Metadate, Concerta, Daytrana, Quillivant, Focalin)?

Methylphenidate is called a *stimulant*. It is used to treat attention-deficit/hyperactivity disorder (ADHD), whether the person has hyperactivity (increased moving around) or not. It comes in a generic form and several brand name formulations (see table below). Although all of these medicines have methylphenidate as the active ingredient, they are made differently, so that there are many different ways to take methylphenidate. This helps the doctor to find just the right form of the medicine for each person.

Generic and brand name formulations
Short-acting or immediate-release methylphenidate (3–4 hours)
Generic methylphenidate
Methylin tablets
Methylin CT chewable tablets
Methylin oral solution (grape flavored)
Ritalin
Long-acting methylphenidate
Ritalin SR (sustained-release; 6–8 hours) (wax matrix)
Metadate ER (extended-release; 6–8 hours) (wax matrix)
Metadate CD (controlled-delivery; 8 hours) (capsule Diffucap with beads; may be sprinkled on food)
Very long-acting methylphenidate
Ritalin LA (long-acting; 8–10 hours) (capsule with beads; may be sprinkled on food)
Concerta (osmotic controlled-release tablet [OROS]; 10–12 hours)
Daytrana Transdermal System (skin patch; worn for 9 hours; lasts 12 hours)
Quillivant XR (long-acting liquid; 12 hours)

Extended-release methylphenidate comes in brand name Concerta and several different generic forms. Only the generics from Actavis and Watson use the same OROS technology as Concerta. The others may not work as long.

Dexmethylphenidate is a form of methylphenidate that has only one of the two chemical shapes (called a *dextroisomer*) of methylphenidate. Dexmethylphenidate is given at half the dose of methylphenidate and may have fewer side effects. Dexmethylphenidate comes in brand name Focalin and generic (immediate-release, short-acting tablets; 3–4 hours) and Focalin XR and generic (extended-release, very long-acting capsules that contain beads of medicine; 8–10 hours; may be sprinkled on food).

How Can This Medicine Help?

Methylphenidate can increase attention and the ability to follow instructions. It can improve attention span, decrease distractibility, increase the ability to finish things, decrease hyperactivity, and improve the ability to think before acting (decrease impulsivity). Handwriting and completion of schoolwork and homework can improve. Methylphenidate can improve willingness to follow directions and decrease stubbornness in youngsters with both ADHD and oppositional defiant disorder.

Many people with Tourette's disorder (chronic motor and vocal tics) also have symptoms of ADHD. Methylphenidate may be used cautiously to reduce the symptoms of hyperactivity, impulsivity, and trouble paying attention and usually does not make the tics worse. If the tics get worse, talk with your child's doctor. Lowering the dose or stopping the methylphenidate will usually lead to the tics decreasing again. Tics also increase and decrease for a lot of reasons that are not related to medicine.

Medicine may not resolve all symptoms in children with ADHD. These youth may also need special help in school and behavior modification at home and at school. Some youngsters and families are helped by family therapy or group social skills therapy.

Stimulant medicines last for different amounts of time. ADHD symptoms may come back when the medicine wears off. This does not mean the medicine is not working but that longer coverage may be needed.

Methylphenidate is also used to help people with narcolepsy (sudden and uncontrollable episodes of deep sleep) to stay awake.

How Does This Medicine Work?

In people who have ADHD, parts of the brain are not working as well as they should. An example would be the part that controls impulsive actions ("the brakes"). Methylphenidate helps these parts of the brain work better by acting as a *stimulant*, increasing the activity of neurotransmitters—mostly *dopamine* but also *norepinephrine*. *Neurotransmitters* are the chemicals that the brain makes for the nerve cells to communicate with each other.

Methylphenidate is not a tranquilizer or sedative. It works in the same way in children and adults and in people with or without ADHD.

Methylphenidate and amphetamine are both stimulant medicines, but they work in different ways on the neurotransmitters. A person with ADHD might be helped by one stimulant but not the other, so if one is not working, the doctor may try the other one.

How Long Does This Medicine Last?

All pill types of methylphenidate start working within 30–60 minutes after taking them.

Different forms of methylphenidate last for different lengths of time. The immediate-release or short-acting forms last for 3–4 hours. The long-acting forms last for 6–8 hours. Ritalin LA and Focalin XR last for 8–10 hours, and Concerta lasts for 10–12 hours. Quillivant XR lasts for 12 hours. The length of time is different for different people, and the medicine may work longer for some symptoms than for others. An advantage of the longer-acting forms is that they do not have to be given during the school day.

Daytrana (the skin patch) may take longer to start working (1–2 hours after being put on the skin). It is designed to be worn for 9 hours. The effects of the medicine last as long as 3 hours after the skin patch is taken off. If there are too many side effects in the evening, the patch can be taken off earlier in the day.

How Will the Doctor Monitor This Medicine?

The doctor will review your child's medical history and physical examination before starting methylphenidate. The doctor may order some blood or urine tests to be sure your child does not have a hidden medical condition. Be sure to tell the doctor if your child or anyone in the family was born with or has had heart problems; seizures; very fast or irregular heartbeat; high blood pressure (hypertension); dizziness; fainting; shortness of breath; glaucoma; narrowing of the stomach, esophagus, or intestines; or severe tiredness. Tell the doctor if anyone in the family has died suddenly. Talk to your doctor if your child has a history of seizures. Also tell the doctor if your child or anyone in the family has had motor or vocal tics (hard-to-control repeated movements or sounds) or Tourette's disorder (also called Tourette's syndrome). The doctor or nurse will measure your child's height, weight, pulse, and blood pressure before starting the medicine. The doctor will usually ask parents and teachers to fill out behavior rating scales (checklists).

After the medicine is started, the doctor will want to have regular appointments with you and your child to see how the medicine is working, to see if a dose change is needed, to watch for side effects, to see if methylphenidate is still needed, and to see if any other treatment is needed. The doctor or nurse may check your child's height, weight, pulse, and blood pressure. With parental permission, the doctor will usually ask for reports (rating scale, checklist, testing results, comments) from the teacher(s) to keep track of progress in learning and behavior. Some young people take the medicine three or four times a day, every day. Others need to take it only once or twice a day, or only on school days. You and your child's doctor will work out the dose, timing, and type of methylphenidate that is best for your child and his or her symptoms and schedule.

What Side Effects Can This Medicine Have?

Any medicine can have side effects, including an allergy to the medicine. Because each patient is different, the doctor will monitor the youth closely, especially when the medicine is started. The doctor will work with you to increase the positive effects and decrease the negative effects of the medicine. Please tell the doctor if any of the listed side effects appear or if you think that the medicine is causing any other problems. Not all of the rare or unusual side effects are listed.

Side effects are most common after starting the medicine or after a dose increase. Many side effects can be avoided or lessened by starting with a very low dose and increasing it slowly—ask the doctor.

Allergic Reaction

Tell the doctor in a day or two (if possible, before the next dose of medicine):

- Hives
- Itching
- Rash

A rash under the patch may be a problem with the skin patch, and there may also be bumps, blisters, or swelling. After using the skin patch, a new allergy to methylphenidate pills may develop.

Stop the medicine and get *immediate* medical care:

- Trouble breathing or chest tightness
- Swelling of lips, tongue, or throat

Common Side Effects

If the following side effects do not go away after about 2 weeks, ask the doctor about lowering your child's dose.

- Lack of appetite and weight loss—Encourage your child to eat a good breakfast and afternoon and evening snacks; give medicine during or after meals.

- Insomnia (trouble falling asleep)—This may be the ADHD coming back and not a side effect. Talk with your child's doctor. Changing the time or dose of medicine, starting a bedtime routine, or adding another medicine may help.
- Headaches
- Stomachaches
- Irritability, crankiness, crying, emotional sensitivity
- Loss of interest in friends
- Staring into space
- Rapid pulse rate (heartbeat) or increased blood pressure

Preschool-age children are more likely than older children to have irritability, emotional sensitivity, lack of appetite, and/or insomnia.

Less Common Side Effects

Tell the doctor within a week or two:

- Rebound—As the medicine is wearing off, hyperactivity or bad mood may get worse than before the medicine was taken. The doctor can make adjustments to help this problem.
- Slowing of growth—This is why your child's height and weight are checked regularly; if this is a problem, growth usually catches up if the medicine is stopped or the dose is decreased.
- Nervous habits—Examples are picking at skin or biting nails (although these habits are also common in children with ADHD who do not take medicine).
- Stuttering

Rare, but Serious, Side Effects

If any of the following occur, call the doctor or go to an emergency room *right away:*

- Chest pain that doesn't go away after a few minutes
- Very fast or irregular heart beat not related to exercise or exertion
- Shortness of breath not related to exercise or exertion
- Fainting
- Seizures (fits, convulsions)
- In boys, a painful, prolonged erection that lasts longer than a few hours (called *priapism*)—This is very rare, but if untreated, this could lead to permanent damage to the penis. Boys may be embarrassed to talk about this, so both the patient and parents/caregivers should be aware of this possible problem and the importance of seeking immediate medical care if it happens.

Call the doctor within a day or two:

- Motor or vocal tics (fast, repeated movements or sounds) or muscle twitches (jerking movements) of parts of the body
- Sadness that lasts more than a few days
- Auditory, visual, or tactile hallucinations (hearing, seeing, or feeling things that are not there)
- Any behavior that is very unusual for your child

Some Interactions With Other Medicines or Food

Please note that the following are only the most likely interactions with other medicines or food.

Caffeine may increase side effects.

Methylphenidate may be taken with or without food. Appetite is better if methylphenidate is taken after the meal (breakfast, lunch). Avoid taking an antacid for 2 hours before or after taking methylphenidate.

The combination of methylphenidate with medicines such as imipramine (Tofranil), amitriptyline (Elavil), or nortriptyline (Pamelor) may cause irritability and confusion or severe emotional and behavioral problems (such as hallucinations and fighting).

It is not a good idea to combine stimulants with nasal decongestants or cough and cold medicines that contain ingredients such as pseudoephedrine or phenylephrine because rapid pulse rate (heartbeat) or high blood pressure may develop. If a stuffy nose is really troublesome, it is better to use a nasal spray. Check with the pharmacist before giving an over-the-counter medicine. Also, many children with ADHD become cranky or more hyperactive while taking antihistamines (such as Benadryl). If medicine for allergies is needed, ask your child's doctor.

Methylphenidate may increase the levels of selective serotonin reuptake inhibitor (SSRI) antidepressants such as fluoxetine (Prozac), escitalopram (Lexapro), paroxetine (Paxil), sertraline (Zoloft), and citalopram (Celexa).

Methylphenidate should not be taken at the same time as or even within a month of taking another type of medicine called a *monoamine oxidase inhibitor* (MAOI), such as selegiline (Eldepryl), phenelzine (Nardil), tranylcypromine (Parnate), or isocarboxazid (Marplan). The combination could cause severe high blood pressure.

What Could Happen if This Medicine Is Stopped Suddenly?

No medical withdrawal effects occur if methylphenidate is stopped suddenly. The ADHD will come back as soon as the medicine wears off. Some people may have irritability, trouble sleeping, or increased hyperactivity for a day or two if they have been taking the medicine every day for a long time, especially at high doses. It may be better to decrease the medicine slowly (taper) over a week or so.

How Long Will This Medicine Be Needed?

There is no way to know how long a person will need to take methylphenidate. The parent(s), the doctor, and the school will work together to determine what is right for each patient. Sometimes the medicine is needed for a few years, but many people need to take medicine for ADHD even as adults.

What Else Should I Know About This Medicine?

Many people have incorrect information about stimulants. If you hear anything that worries you, please check with your doctor.

Although the FDA has not approved methylphenidate for use in children younger than 6 years, this is not because it is dangerous or does not work. It is because there was not enough research on young children at the time that methylphenidate was approved by the FDA. Now there is research that shows that methylphenidate can be used safely and effectively in preschool children with ADHD. Amphetamines are FDA approved for children younger than 6 years, but this is a historical accident that happened as rules changed for approval of medicines. There is actually less research on amphetamines for ADHD in young children than there is for methylphenidate.

Stimulants do not *cause* drug use or addiction. However, because the patient or other people (especially if they have a history of drug abuse) may abuse these medicines, adult supervision is especially important. Some teenagers may try to sell or share their medicine, so it should be kept in a secure place and given by an adult. Methylphenidate will not help people who do not have ADHD to get better grades or do better on tests, but some people think that it will, so they try to take someone else's medicine. It is important to talk to your teen-ager about why he or she should never give away or sell medication. This is called *diversion* and can be considered a federal crime.

The government considers methylphenidate to be a *controlled substance*. There are special rules for how much of this medicine may be prescribed at one time and how soon prescriptions must be filled after they are written. Prescriptions may not have refills and may not be telephoned to the pharmacy. The doctor must write a new prescription for stimulants each time. Prescriptions may be mailed or picked up at the doctor's office.

It is important for the child *not* to chew or crush any of the long-acting tablets or capsules because doing so releases too much medicine all at once. Empty Concerta shells will pass through the digestive system and may be seen in bowel movements. This is harmless. If the patient has trouble swallowing, Concerta may be difficult to swallow or may even get stuck.

For children who cannot swallow pills, several options are available. The capsule long-acting forms may be opened and the tiny beads inside sprinkled onto a spoonful of applesauce. The mixture of applesauce and medicine should be swallowed right away, without chewing. The medicine should *not* be mixed into food and stored for later use. The beads should not be mixed in liquid. The skin patch may be useful for children who need a long-acting form but who cannot or will not swallow pills. Short-acting methylphenidate in chewable and liquid forms is also available.

A long-acting liquid form is also available (Quillivant XR). Quillivant comes in a powder that is mixed with water by the pharmacist, and it should be in liquid form when you receive it. Shake the bottle well for at least 10 seconds before each dose is given. Be sure that the bottle adapter (plug that fits the syringe dispenser) is in the bottle and stays there—do not remove it. Use the oral dosing dispenser (syringe without a needle). Fill the dispenser to the amount prescribed and slowly squirt the medicine into the child's mouth. After each use clean the dispenser in the dishwasher or by rinsing with tap water. In between uses, cap the bottle tightly and store it upright at room temperature (do not store it in freezing or very hot temperatures). If you have not used this type of dispenser before, be sure to ask the pharmacist for instructions.

When using Daytrana (the patch), a new patch is applied to the skin each day. Put the patch on 2 hours before the medicine needs to work. Remove half the liner and put the patch onto clean, dry skin on the hip area, below the waist. Peel off the rest of the liner and stick the whole patch onto the skin. Do not touch the sticky parts of the patch with the hands. Press the patch down with the palm of the hand for 30 seconds to be sure the patch is firmly attached. It is best to alternate sides daily and to put the patch onto a different part of the skin each day. Do not use a patch more than once. After taking the patch off, fold it in half, sticky side in, and throw it away. If a young child or a pet might take it out of the trash can, flush the patch down the toilet instead of throwing it into the trash.

Some of these medicines have similar names but have different strengths or last different amounts of time (for example, Metadate ER and Metadate CD, or Ritalin LA and Ritalin SR). Be sure to check your prescription to be sure you have the correct medicine from the pharmacy.

Notes

Use this space to take notes or to write down questions you want to ask the doctor.

_____

_____

_____

_____

_____

_____

_____

_____

_____

_____

From Dulcan MK, Ballard R (editors): _Helping Parents and Teachers Understand Medications for Behavioral and Emotional Problems: A Resource Book of Medication Information Handouts_, Fourth Edition. Washington, DC, American Psychiatric Publishing, 2015

Medication Information for Parents and Teachers

Mirtazapine—Remeron

General Information About Medication

Each child and adolescent is different. No one has exactly the same combination of medical and psychological problems. It is a good idea to talk with the doctor or nurse about the reasons a medicine is being used. It is very important to keep all appointments and to be in touch by telephone if you have concerns. It is important to communicate with the doctor, nurse, or therapist. An *advanced practice nurse* (APN) has additional education and training after becoming a registered nurse (RN). Your child's medication may be prescribed by a medical doctor (MD or DO) or an APN. In addition, a *physician assistant* (PA) working with a physician may prescribe certain medications. In this information sheet, "doctor" includes medical doctors as well as APNs and PAs who prescribe medication. Often a nurse (RN) will be part of the team and answer questions and give information.

It is very important that the medicine be taken exactly as the doctor instructs. However, once in a while, everyone forgets to give a medicine on time. It is a good idea to ask the doctor or nurse what to do if this happens. Do not stop or change a medicine without asking the doctor or nurse first.

If the medicine seems to stop working, it may be because it is not being taken regularly. The youth may be "cheeking" or hiding the medicine or forgetting to take it (especially at school). The doses may be too far apart or a different dose or medicine may be needed. Something at school, at home, or in the neighborhood may be upsetting the youth, or he or she may need special help for learning disabilities or tutoring. Please discuss your concerns with the doctor. **Do not just increase the dose.** It is also very important not to decrease the dose or stop the medicine without talking to the doctor first. The problem being treated may come back, or there could be uncomfortable or even dangerous results.

All medicines should be kept in a safe place, out of the reach of children, and should be supervised by an adult. If someone takes too much of a medicine, call the doctor, the poison control center, or a hospital emergency room.

Each medicine has a "generic" or chemical name. Just like laundry detergents or paper towels, some medicines are sold by more than one company under different brand names. The same medicine may be available under a generic name and several brand names. The generic medications are usually less expensive than the brand name ones. The generic medications have the same chemical formula, but they may or may not be exactly the same strength as the brand-name medications. Also, some brands of pills contain dye or other things that can cause allergic reactions. It is a good idea to talk to the doctor and the pharmacist about whether it is important to use a specific brand of medicine.

Any medicine can cause an allergic reaction. Examples are hives, itching, rashes, swelling, and trouble breathing. Even a tiny amount of a medicine can cause a reaction in patients who are allergic to that medicine. Be *sure* to talk to the doctor before restarting a medicine that has caused an allergic reaction and tell the doctor about any reactions to medicine that your child has had before.

Taking more than one medicine at the same time may cause more side effects or cause one of the medicines to not work as well. Always ask the doctor, nurse, or pharmacist before adding another

medicine, either prescription or bought without a prescription in a store or on the Internet. **Be sure that each doctor knows about** *all* **of the medicines your child is taking. Also tell the doctor about any vitamins, herbal medicines, or supplements your child may be taking.** Some of these may have side effects alone or when taken with this medication. It is a very good idea to keep a list with you of the names and doses of all medicines that your child is taking.

Everyone taking medicine should have a physical examination at least once a year.

If you think that your child may be using drugs or alcohol, please tell the doctor right away.

Pregnancy requires special care in the use of medicine. Some medicines can cause birth defects if taken by a pregnant mother. **Please tell the doctor immediately if you suspect the teenager is at risk of becoming pregnant.** The doctor may wish to discuss sexual behavior and/or birth control with your daughter.

Printed information like this applies to children and adolescents in general. If you have questions about the medicine, or if you notice changes or anything unusual, please ask the doctor or nurse. As scientific research advances, knowledge increases and advice changes. Even experts do not always agree. Many medicines have not been "approved" by the U.S. Food and Drug Administration (FDA) for use in children or use for particular problems. For this reason, use of the medicine for a problem or age group often is not listed in the *Physicians' Desk Reference*. This does not necessarily mean that the medicine is dangerous or does not work, only that the company that makes the medicine has not received permission to advertise the medicine for use in children. Companies often do not apply for this permission because it is expensive to do the tests needed to apply for approval for use in children. Once a medication is approved by the FDA for any purpose, a doctor is allowed to prescribe it according to research and clinical experience.

Note to Teachers

It is a good idea to talk with the parent(s) about the reason(s) that a medication is being used. If the parent(s) sign consent to release information, it is often helpful for you to talk with the doctor. If the parent(s) give permission, the doctor may ask you to fill out rating forms about your experience with the student's behavior, feelings, academic performance, and medication side effects. This information is very useful in selecting and monitoring medication treatment. If you have observations that you think are important, do not hesitate to share these with the student's parent(s) and treating clinicians (with parental consent).

It is very important that the medicine be taken exactly as the doctor instructs. However, everyone forgets to give a medicine on time once in a while. It is a good idea to ask the parent(s) in advance what to do if this happens. Do not stop or change the time you are giving a medicine at school without parental permission. If a medication is to be taken with food, but lunchtime or snack time changes, be sure to notify the parent(s) so appropriate adjustments can be made.

All medicines should be kept in a secure place and should be supervised by an adult. If someone takes too much of a medicine, follow your school procedure for an urgent medical problem.

Taking medicine is a private matter and is best managed discreetly and confidentially. It is important to be sensitive to the student's feelings about taking medicine.

If you suspect that the student is using drugs or alcohol, please tell the parent(s) or a school counselor right away.

Please tell the parent(s) or school nurse if you suspect medication side effects.

Modifications of the classroom environment or assignments may be useful in addition to medication. The student may need to be evaluated for additional help or a 504 plan or an Individualized Education Plan for learning problems or emotional or behavioral issues.

Any expression of suicidal thoughts or feelings or self-harm by a child or adolescent is a clear signal of distress and should be taken seriously. These behaviors should not be dismissed as "attention seeking." School safety procedures should be followed.

What Is Mirtazapine (Remeron)?

Mirtazapine is called an *antidepressant*. It is sometimes called a *norepinephrine-serotonin modulator*. It comes in brand name Remeron and generic tablets. The Remeron SolTab and generic orally disintegrating (quick-dissolving) tablets are dissolved in the mouth for people who cannot swallow pills.

How Can This Medicine Help?

Mirtazapine has been used successfully to treat depression and anxiety (nervousness) in adults. Now it is beginning to be used to treat emotional problems, including anxiety and depression, in children and adolescents. It may take as long as 4–8 weeks to work. Mirtazapine is sometimes used to treat problems with sleep in children with anxiety or depression. It may be helpful for youth with chronic or cyclic vomiting.

How Does This Medicine Work?

Mirtazapine works by increasing the brain chemicals *serotonin* and *norepinephrine (neurotransmitters)* to more normal functioning in certain parts of the brain. It has a somewhat different way of working than the antidepressants called selective serotonin reuptake inhibitors (SSRIs).

How Long Does This Medicine Last?

Mirtazapine generally can be taken only once a day.

How Will the Doctor Monitor This Medicine?

The doctor will review your child's medical history and physical examination before starting mirtazapine. The doctor may order some blood or urine tests to be sure your child does not have a hidden medical condition that would make it unsafe to use this medicine. The doctor or nurse may measure your child's height, weight, pulse, and blood pressure before starting mirtazapine. The doctor may order other tests, such as a blood cell count and levels of cholesterol and triglycerides (fats in the blood). If there is a family history of diabetes, the doctor may also want to measure sugar in the blood or urine before starting the medicine and at times afterward.

Be sure to tell the doctor if your child or anyone in the family has bipolar disorder or has tried to kill himself or herself. Also tell the doctor if there are concerns of heart, liver, or kidney problems or seizures.

After the medicine is started, the doctor will want to have regular appointments with you and your child to see how the medicine is working, to see if a dose change is needed, to watch for side effects, to see if mirtazapine is still needed, and to see if any other treatment is needed. The doctor or nurse may check your child's height, weight, pulse, and blood pressure or order tests, such as a blood cell count and levels of cholesterol and triglycerides.

Before using medicine and at times afterward, the doctor may ask your child to fill out a rating scale about depression, to help see how your child is doing.

What Side Effects Can This Medicine Have?

Any medicine can have side effects, including an allergy to the medicine. Because each patient is different, the doctor will monitor the youth closely, especially when the medicine is started. The doctor will work with you to increase the positive effects and decrease the negative effects of the medicine. Please tell the doctor if any of the listed side effects appear or if you think that the medicine is causing any other problems. Not all of the rare or unusual side effects are listed.

Side effects are most common after starting the medicine or after a dose increase. Many side effects can be avoided or lessened by starting with a very low dose and increasing it slowly—ask the doctor.

Allergic Reaction

Tell the doctor in a day or two (if possible, before the next dose of medicine):

- Hives
- Itching
- Rash

Stop the medicine and get *immediate* medical care:

- Trouble breathing or chest tightness
- Swelling of lips, tongue, or throat

Common Side Effects

Tell the doctor within a week or two (or sooner, if the problems are getting worse):

- Daytime sleepiness—Do not allow your child to drive, ride a bicycle or motorcycle, or operate machinery if this happens. This effect may be worse at the lowest dose and get better as the dose is increased.
- Nausea
- Increased appetite and weight gain
- Dry mouth—Have your child try using sugar-free gum or candy.
- Abnormal dreams

Occasional Side Effects

Tell the doctor within a week or two:

- Dizziness
- Constipation—Encourage your child to drink more fluids and eat high-fiber foods; if necessary, the doctor may recommend a fiber medicine such as Benefiber or a stool softener such as Colace or mineral oil.
- Lack of energy, tiredness
- Frequent urination

Less Common, but More Serious, Side Effects

Call the doctor *immediately* or go to an emergency room:

- Confusion
- Any infection, especially with sore throat and fever

Call the doctor within a day:

- Significant suicidal thoughts or self-injurious behavior
- Increased activity, rapid speech, feeling "speeded up," decreased need for sleep, being very excited or irritable (cranky), agitation, acting out of character

Serious Side Effects

Call the doctor *immediately* or go to an emergency room:

- Stiffness, high fever, confusion, tremors (shaking)
- Overheating or heatstroke—Prevent by decreasing activity in hot weather, staying out of the sun, and drinking water.

Serotonin Syndrome

A very serious side effect called *serotonin syndrome* can happen when certain kinds of medicines (including SSRI antidepressants, clomipramine, and other medicines, such as triptans for migraine headaches, buspirone, linezolid, tramadol, or St. John's wort) are taken by the same person. Very rarely, serotonin syndrome can happen at high doses of just one medicine. The early signs are restlessness, confusion, shaking, skin turning red, sweating, muscle stiffness, sweating, and jerking of muscles. If you see these symptoms, stop the medicine and send or take the youth to an emergency room right away.

Some Interactions With Other Medicines or Food

Please note that the following are only the most likely interactions with other medicines or food.

Mirtazapine may be taken with or without food.

Caffeine may increase side effects.

Cimetidine (Tagamet) should not be used with mirtazapine, because it increases the levels of mirtazapine and may increase side effects.

Carbamazepine (Tegretol) may decrease the levels of mirtazapine and make it not work as well.

It may be dangerous to take SSRI antidepressants, especially sertraline (Zoloft) or fluvoxamine (Luvox) together with mirtazapine. Mirtazapine should not be taken with pimozide (Orap).

It can be *very dangerous* to take mirtazapine at the same time as, or even within several weeks of, taking another type of medicine called a *monoamine oxidase inhibitor* (MAOI), such as selegiline (Eldepryl), phenelzine (Nardil), tranylcypromine (Parnate), or isocarboxazid (Marplan).

What Could Happen if This Medicine Is Stopped Suddenly?

No known serious medical withdrawal effects occur if mirtazapine is stopped suddenly, but there may be uncomfortable feelings, or the problem being treated may come back. Ask your child's doctor before stopping the medicine.

How Long Will This Medicine Be Needed?

Your child may need to keep taking the medicine for at least 6–12 months so that the emotional or behavioral problem does not come back. Be sure to discuss this with your child's doctor.

What Else Should I Know About This Medicine?

In youth who have bipolar disorder or who may be at risk for bipolar disorder, any antidepressant medicine may increase the risk of hypomania or mania (excitement, agitation, increased activity, decreased sleep).

Some people taking mirtazapine want to eat a lot more than usual and gain too much weight. It may be very important to be sure that your child has a healthy diet, without too many sweets or fast foods, and that your child has regular exercise.

Do not split the orally disintegrating tablets.

Black Box Antidepressant Warning

In 2004, an advisory committee to the FDA decided that there might be an increased risk of suicidal behavior for some youth taking medicines called *antidepressants*. In the research studies that the committee reviewed, about 3%–4% of youth with depression who took an antidepressant medicine—and 1%–2% of youth with depression who took a placebo (pill without active medicine)—talked about suicidal thoughts (thinking about killing themselves or wishing they were dead) or did something to harm themselves. This means that almost twice as many youth who were taking an antidepressant to treat their depression talked about suicide or had suicidal behavior compared with youth with depression who were taking inactive medicine. There were *no* completed suicides in any of these research studies, which included more than 4,000 children and adolescents. For youth being treated for anxiety, there was no difference in suicidal talking or behavior between those taking antidepressant medication and those taking placebo.

The FDA told drug companies to add a *black box warning* label to all antidepressant medicines. Because of this label, a doctor (or advanced practice nurse) prescribing one of these medicines has to warn youth and their families that there might be more suicidal thoughts and actions in youth taking these medicines.

On the other hand, in places where more youth are taking the newer antidepressant medicines, the number of adolescents who commit suicide has gotten smaller. Also, thinking about or attempting suicide is more common in surveys of teenagers in the community than it is in depressed youth treated in research studies with antidepressant medicine.

If a youth is being treated with this medicine and is doing well, then no changes are needed as a result of this warning. Increased suicidal talk or action is most likely to happen in the first few months of treatment with a medicine. If your child has recently started this medicine or is about to start, then you and your doctor (or advanced practice nurse) should watch for any changes in behavior. People who are depressed often have suicidal thoughts or actions. It is hard to know whether suicidal thoughts or actions in depressed people are caused by the depression itself or by the medicine. Also, as their depression is getting better, some people talk more about the suicidal thoughts that they had before but did not talk about. As young people get better from depression, they might be at higher risk of doing something about suicidal thoughts that they have had for some time, because they have more energy.

What Should a Parent Do?

1. Be honest with your child about possible risks and benefits of medicine.
2. Talk to your child about whether he or she is having any suicidal thoughts, and tell your child to come to you if he or she is having such thoughts.
3. You, your child, and your child's doctor or nurse should develop a safety plan. Pick adults whom your child can tell if he or she is thinking about suicide.
4. Be sure to tell your child's doctor, nurse, or therapist if you suspect that your child is using alcohol or drugs or if something has happened that might make your child feel worse, such as a family separation, breaking up with a boyfriend or girlfriend, someone close dying or attempting suicide, physical or sexual abuse, or failure in school.
5. Be sure that there are no guns in the home and that all medicines (including over-the-counter medicines like Tylenol) are closely supervised by an adult and kept in a safe place.
6. Watch for new or worse thoughts of suicide, self-harm, depression, anxiety (nerves), feeling very agitated or restless, being angry or aggressive, having more trouble sleeping, or anything else that you see for the first time, seems worse, or worries your child or you. If these appear, contact a mental health professional **right away.** Do not just stop or change the dose of the medicine on your own. If the problems are serious, and you cannot reach one of your clinicians, call a 24-hour psychiatry emergency telephone number or take your child to an emergency room.

Youth taking antidepressant medicine should be watched carefully by their parent(s), clinician(s) (doctor, advanced practice nurse, nurse, therapist), and other concerned adults for the first weeks of treatment. It is a good idea to have regular contact with the doctor, APN, nurse, or therapist for the first months to check for feelings of depression or sadness, thoughts of killing or harming himself or herself, and any problems with the medication. If you have questions, be sure to ask the doctor, APN, nurse, or therapist.

For more information, see http://www.parentsmedguide.org/.

Notes

Use this space to take notes or to write down questions you want to ask the doctor.

_____

_____

_____

_____

_____

_____

————————————————————————————

————————————————————————————

————————————————————————————

————————————————————————————

————————————————————————————

————————————————————————————

————————————————————————————

————————————————————————————

From Dulcan MK, Ballard R (editors): *Helping Parents and Teachers Understand Medications for Behavioral and Emotional Problems: A Resource Book of Medication Information Handouts*, Fourth Edition. Washington, DC, American Psychiatric Publishing, 2015

Medication Information for Parents and Teachers

Modafinil—Provigil
Armodafinil—Nuvigil

General Information About Medication

Each child and adolescent is different. No one has exactly the same combination of medical and psychological problems. It is a good idea to talk with the doctor or nurse about the reasons a medicine is being used. It is very important to keep all appointments and to be in touch by telephone if you have concerns. It is important to communicate with the doctor, nurse, or therapist. An *advanced practice nurse* (APN) has additional education and training after becoming a registered nurse (RN). Your child's medication may be prescribed by a medical doctor (MD or DO) or an APN. In addition, a *physician assistant* (PA) working with a physician may prescribe certain medications. In this information sheet, "doctor" includes medical doctors as well as APNs and PAs who prescribe medication. Often a nurse (RN) will be part of the team and answer questions and give information.

It is very important that the medicine be taken exactly as the doctor instructs. However, once in a while, everyone forgets to give a medicine on time. It is a good idea to ask the doctor or nurse what to do if this happens. Do not stop or change a medicine without asking the doctor or nurse first.

If the medicine seems to stop working, it may be because it is not being taken regularly. The youth may be "cheeking" or hiding the medicine or forgetting to take it (especially at school). The doses may be too far apart or a different dose or medicine may be needed. Something at school, at home, or in the neighborhood may be upsetting the youth, or he or she may need special help for learning disabilities or tutoring. Please discuss your concerns with the doctor. **Do not just increase the dose.** It is also very important not to decrease the dose or stop the medicine without talking to the doctor first. The problem being treated may come back, or there could be uncomfortable or even dangerous results.

All medicines should be kept in a safe place, out of the reach of children, and should be supervised by an adult. If someone takes too much of a medicine, call the doctor, the poison control center, or a hospital emergency room.

Each medicine has a "generic" or chemical name. Just like laundry detergents or paper towels, some medicines are sold by more than one company under different brand names. The same medicine may be available under a generic name and several brand names. The generic medications are usually less expensive than the brand name ones. The generic medications have the same chemical formula, but they may or may not be exactly the same strength as the brand-name medications. Also, some brands of pills contain dye or other things that can cause allergic reactions. It is a good idea to talk to the doctor and the pharmacist about whether it is important to use a specific brand of medicine.

Any medicine can cause an allergic reaction. Examples are hives, itching, rashes, swelling, and trouble breathing. Even a tiny amount of a medicine can cause a reaction in patients who are allergic to that medicine. Be *sure* to talk to the doctor before restarting a medicine that has caused an allergic reaction and tell the doctor about any reactions to medicine that your child has had before.

Taking more than one medicine at the same time may cause more side effects or cause one of the medicines to not work as well. Always ask the doctor, nurse, or pharmacist before adding another medicine, either prescription or bought without a prescription in a store or on the Internet. Be sure that each doctor knows about *all* of the medicines your child is taking. Also tell the doctor about any vitamins, herbal medicines, or supplements your child may be taking. Some of these may have side effects alone or when taken with this medication. It is a very good idea to keep a list with you of the names and doses of all medicines that your child is taking.

Everyone taking medicine should have a physical examination at least once a year.

If you think that your child may be using drugs or alcohol, please tell the doctor right away.

Pregnancy requires special care in the use of medicine. Some medicines can cause birth defects if taken by a pregnant mother. **Please tell the doctor immediately if you suspect the teenager is at risk of becoming pregnant.** The doctor may wish to discuss sexual behavior and/or birth control with your daughter.

Printed information like this applies to children and adolescents in general. If you have questions about the medicine, or if you notice changes or anything unusual, please ask the doctor or nurse. As scientific research advances, knowledge increases and advice changes. Even experts do not always agree. Many medicines have not been "approved" by the U.S. Food and Drug Administration (FDA) for use in children or use for particular problems. For this reason, use of the medicine for a problem or age group often is not listed in the *Physicians' Desk Reference*. This does not necessarily mean that the medicine is dangerous or does not work, only that the company that makes the medicine has not received permission to advertise the medicine for use in children. Companies often do not apply for this permission because it is expensive to do the tests needed to apply for approval for use in children. Once a medication is approved by the FDA for any purpose, a doctor is allowed to prescribe it according to research and clinical experience.

Note to Teachers

It is a good idea to talk with the parent(s) about the reason(s) that a medication is being used. If the parent(s) sign consent to release information, it is often helpful for you to talk with the doctor. If the parent(s) give permission, the doctor may ask you to fill out rating forms about your experience with the student's behavior, feelings, academic performance, and medication side effects. This information is very useful in selecting and monitoring medication treatment. If you have observations that you think are important, do not hesitate to share these with the student's parent(s) and treating clinicians (with parental consent).

It is very important that the medicine be taken exactly as the doctor instructs. However, everyone forgets to give a medicine on time once in a while. It is a good idea to ask the parent(s) in advance what to do if this happens. Do not stop or change the time you are giving a medicine at school without parental permission. If a medication is to be taken with food, but lunchtime or snack time changes, be sure to notify the parent(s) so appropriate adjustments can be made.

All medicines should be kept in a secure place and should be supervised by an adult. If someone takes too much of a medicine, follow your school procedure for an urgent medical problem.

Taking medicine is a private matter and is best managed discreetly and confidentially. It is important to be sensitive to the student's feelings about taking medicine.

If you suspect that the student is using drugs or alcohol, please tell the parent(s) or a school counselor right away.

Please tell the parent(s) or school nurse if you suspect medication side effects.

Modifications of the classroom environment or assignments may be useful in addition to medication. The student may need to be evaluated for additional help or a 504 plan or an Individualized Education Plan for learning problems or emotional or behavioral issues.

Any expression of suicidal thoughts or feelings or self-harm by a child or adolescent is a signal of distress and should be taken seriously. These behaviors should not be dismissed as "attention seeking." School procedures for safety issues should be followed.

What Are Modafinil (Provigil) and Armodafinil (Nuvigil)?

Modafinil and armodafinil are wake- and vigilance-promoting agents that increase alertness. They are not stimulant medicines, and they are chemically different from methylphenidate or amphetamine. Modafinil comes in brand name Provigil and generic tablets and armodafinil comes in brand name Nuvigil tablets. They are used for the treatment of excessive daytime sleepiness. Armodafinil has only one of the two chemical shapes (called *isomers*) of modafinil.

How Can These Medicines Help?

Modafinil and armodafinil are used to improve the ability to stay awake and alert in patients with excessive daytime sleepiness associated with narcolepsy or obstructive sleep apnea syndrome. Recently, research has shown that modafinil can improve the symptoms of attention-deficit/hyperactivity disorder (ADHD), such as trouble paying attention, thinking before acting (impulsivity), and hyperactivity.

How Do These Medicines Work?

Modafinil and armodafinil are thought to work by binding to the dopamine transporter, increasing alertness in certain parts of the brain. These medicines may decrease the action of some brain cells that promote sleep.

How Long Do These Medicines Last?

Modafinil is usually taken once or twice a day when treating excessive daytime sleepiness. The first dose is given in the morning, and if there is a second dose, it should be given before 2:00 P.M. because the medication stays in the body for a long time. If the medicine is given later, it can cause trouble sleeping at night. For ADHD, it can be given once a day in the morning.

Armodafinil is usually taken once daily in the morning and lasts the entire day.

How Will the Doctor Monitor These Medicines?

The doctor will review your child's medical history and physical examination before starting modafinil or armodafinil. The doctor may order some blood or urine tests to be sure your child does not have a hidden medical condition. The doctor or nurse may measure your child's height, weight, pulse, and blood pressure before starting modafinil or armodafinil. The doctor may order a sleep study if narcolepsy or sleep apnea is suspected.

After the medicine is started, the doctor will want to have regular appointments with you and your child to see how the medicine is working, to see if a dose change is needed, to watch for side effects, to see if the medicine is still needed, and to see if any other treatment is needed. The doctor or nurse may check your child's height, weight, pulse, and blood pressure.

What Side Effects Can These Medicines Have?

Any medicine can have side effects, including an allergy to the medicine. Because each patient is different, the doctor will monitor the youth closely, especially when the medicine is started. The doctor will work with you to increase the positive effects and decrease the negative effects of the medicine. Please tell the doctor if any of the listed side effects appear or if you think that the medicine is causing any other problems. Not all of the rare or unusual side effects are listed.

Side effects are most common after starting the medicine or after a dose increase. Many side effects can be avoided or lessened by starting with a very low dose and increasing it slowly—ask the doctor.

Allergic Reaction

Tell the doctor in a day or two (if possible, before the next dose of medicine):

- Hives
- Itching
- Rash

Stop the medicine and get *immediate* medical care:

- Trouble breathing or chest tightness
- Swelling of lips, tongue, or throat

Overall, modafinil and armodafinil have few side effects. Most of their side effects are not very bad, and they usually go away as soon as the medicine is stopped. Some people may have headaches, decreased appetite, nausea, diarrhea, stomachaches, nervousness (anxiety), or dizziness when taking modafinil or armodafinil.

When modafinil is used to treat ADHD, it may cause insomnia (trouble sleeping). Studies of modafinil to treat ADHD use a higher dose than when using modafinil to treat excessive daytime sleepiness.

Very rarely, youths being treated for ADHD with modafinil have developed a very bad skin reaction that could be dangerous. **If your child develops a skin rash with redness or blisters, stop the medicine and call the doctor right away.**

Potentially Severe Side Effects at Very High Doses

Seek medical care *right away*:

- Excitation or agitation
- High blood pressure
- Fast heart rate (pulse), palpitations
- Anxiety or nervousness
- Irritability

- Aggression
- Confusion
- Shaking
- Increased blood clotting

Some Interactions With Other Medicines or Food

Please note that the following are only the most likely interactions with other medicines or food.

Caution is needed if giving modafinil or armodafinil with medications such as carbamazepine (Tegretol) and antidepressants such as tricyclic antidepressants and selective serotonin reuptake inhibitors (SSRIs). With modafinil or armodafinil, the levels of these medicines may decrease, and they may be less effective.

Taking modafinil or armodafinil with diazepam, phenytoin, or propranolol may increase the levels of these medicines and increase the risk of side effects.

Taking modafinil or armodafinil together with birth control pills may result in reduced effectiveness of the birth control pills, leading to accidental pregnancy. An additional method of birth control is advised while using modafinil or armodafinil.

What Could Happen if These Medicines Are Stopped Suddenly?

There are no reported symptoms from stopping modafinil or armodafinil suddenly. The excessive daytime sleepiness or the ADHD symptoms are likely to return.

How Long Will These Medicines Be Needed?

Because the problems for which modafinil and armodafinil are used are chronic (long lasting), the medicine is likely to be needed for years.

What Else Should I Know About These Medicines?

Modafinil and armodafinil are not associated with drug abuse or dependency.

Notes

Use this space to take notes or to write down questions you want to ask the doctor.

_____

_____

_____

_____

_____

_____

_____

_____

_____

_____

_____

From Dulcan MK, Ballard R (editors): _Helping Parents and Teachers Understand Medications for Behavioral and Emotional Problems: A Resource Book of Medication Information Handouts_, Fourth Edition. Washington, DC, American Psychiatric Publishing, 2015

Medication Information for Parents and Teachers

N-acetylcysteine

General Information About Medication

Each child and adolescent is different. No one has exactly the same combination of medical and psychological problems. It is a good idea to talk with the doctor or nurse about the reasons a medicine is being used. It is very important to keep all appointments and to be in touch by telephone if you have concerns. It is important to communicate with the doctor, nurse, or therapist. An *advanced practice nurse* (APN) has additional education and training after becoming a registered nurse (RN). Your child's medication may be prescribed by a medical doctor (MD or DO) or an APN. In addition, a *physician assistant* (PA) working with a physician may prescribe certain medications. In this information sheet, "doctor" includes medical doctors as well as APNs and PAs who prescribe medication. Often a nurse (RN) will be part of the team and answer questions and give information.

It is very important that the medicine be taken exactly as the doctor instructs. However, once in a while, everyone forgets to give a medicine on time. It is a good idea to ask the doctor or nurse what to do if this happens. Do not stop or change a medicine without asking the doctor or nurse first.

If the medicine seems to stop working, it may be because it is not being taken regularly. The youth may be "cheeking" or hiding the medicine or forgetting to take it (especially at school). The doses may be too far apart or a different dose or medicine may be needed. Something at school, at home, or in the neighborhood may be upsetting the youth, or he or she may need special help for learning disabilities or tutoring. Please discuss your concerns with the doctor. **Do not just increase the dose.** It is also very important not to decrease the dose or stop the medicine without talking to the doctor first. The problem being treated may come back, or there could be uncomfortable or even dangerous results.

All medicines should be kept in a safe place, out of the reach of children, and should be supervised by an adult. If someone takes too much of a medicine, call the doctor, the poison control center, or a hospital emergency room.

Each medicine has a "generic" or chemical name. Just like laundry detergents or paper towels, some medicines are sold by more than one company under different brand names. The same medicine may be available under a generic name and several brand names. The generic medications are usually less expensive than the brand name ones. The generic medications have the same chemical formula, but they may or may not be exactly the same strength as the brand-name medications. Also, some brands of pills contain dye or other things that can cause allergic reactions. It is a good idea to talk to the doctor and the pharmacist about whether it is important to use a specific brand of medicine.

Any medicine can cause an allergic reaction. Examples are hives, itching, rashes, swelling, and trouble breathing. Even a tiny amount of a medicine can cause a reaction in patients who are allergic to that medicine. Be *sure* to talk to the doctor before restarting a medicine that has caused an allergic reaction and tell the doctor about any reactions to medicine that your child has had before.

Taking more than one medicine at the same time may cause more side effects or cause one of the medicines to not work as well. Always ask the doctor, nurse, or pharmacist before adding another medicine, either prescription or bought without a prescription in a store or on the Internet. Be sure

that each doctor knows about *all* of the medicines your child is taking. Also tell the doctor about any vitamins, herbal medicines, or supplements your child may be taking. Some of these may have side effects alone or when taken with this medication. It is a very good idea to keep a list with you of the names and doses of all medicines that your child is taking.

Everyone taking medicine should have a physical examination at least once a year.

If you think that your child may be using drugs or alcohol, please tell the doctor right away.

Pregnancy requires special care in the use of medicine. Some medicines can cause birth defects if taken by a pregnant mother. **Please tell the doctor immediately if you suspect the teenager is at risk of becoming pregnant.** The doctor may wish to discuss sexual behavior and/or birth control with your daughter.

Printed information like this applies to children and adolescents in general. If you have questions about the medicine, or if you notice changes or anything unusual, please ask the doctor or nurse. As scientific research advances, knowledge increases and advice changes. Even experts do not always agree. Many medicines have not been "approved" by the U.S. Food and Drug Administration (FDA) for use in children or use for particular problems. For this reason, use of the medicine for a problem or age group often is not listed in the *Physicians' Desk Reference*. This does not necessarily mean that the medicine is dangerous or does not work, only that the company that makes the medicine has not received permission to advertise the medicine for use in children. Companies often do not apply for this permission because it is expensive to do the tests needed to apply for approval for use in children. Once a medication is approved by the FDA for any purpose, a doctor is allowed to prescribe it according to research and clinical experience.

Note to Teachers

It is a good idea to talk with the parent(s) about the reason(s) that a medication is being used. If the parent(s) sign consent to release information, it is often helpful for you to talk with the doctor. If the parent(s) give permission, the doctor may ask you to fill out rating forms about your experience with the student's behavior, feelings, academic performance, and medication side effects. This information is very useful in selecting and monitoring medication treatment. If you have observations that you think are important, do not hesitate to share these with the student's parent(s) and treating clinicians (with parental consent).

It is very important that the medicine be taken exactly as the doctor instructs. However, everyone forgets to give a medicine on time once in a while. It is a good idea to ask the parent(s) in advance what to do if this happens. Do not stop or change the time you are giving a medicine at school without parental permission. If a medication is to be taken with food, but lunchtime or snack time changes, be sure to notify the parent(s) so appropriate adjustments can be made.

All medicines should be kept in a secure place and should be supervised by an adult. If someone takes too much of a medicine, follow your school procedure for an urgent medical problem.

Taking medicine is a private matter and is best managed discreetly and confidentially. It is important to be sensitive to the student's feelings about taking medicine.

If you suspect that the student is using drugs or alcohol, please tell the parent(s) or a school counselor right away.

Please tell the parent(s) or school nurse if you suspect medication side effects.

Modifications of the classroom environment or assignments may be useful in addition to medication. The student may need to be evaluated for additional help or a 504 plan or an Individualized Education Plan for learning problems or emotional or behavioral issues.

Any expression of suicidal thoughts or feelings or self-harm by a child or adolescent is a signal of distress and should be taken seriously. These behaviors should not be dismissed as "attention seeking." School procedures for safety issues should be followed.

What Is N-acetylcysteine?

N-acetylcysteine (sometimes called NAC) is a medicine made from the amino acid L-cysteine. *Amino acids* are building blocks of proteins in the body. N-acetylcysteine can be prescribed but is also available over the counter as a *supplement*. In children it is used mostly to treat overdoses of acetaminophen (Tylenol or combination medications), but it also helps with breathing problems in people with cystic fibrosis. In adults it is used to treat angina, kidney problems, reactions to certain drugs, and several other conditions. It has recently been found to be helpful for some mental health problems. For mental health problems N-acetylcysteine is given as a pill. It also comes in an IV form or a form to inhale.

How Can This Medicine Help?

N-acetylcysteine has been used in adults and children to treat several psychiatric conditions. It has been studied more in adults than in children and adolescents. It can decrease the urge to continue to use substances in people who abuse marijuana, cocaine, or nicotine. It can decrease the repetitive behaviors in obsessive-compulsive disorder (OCD). Adults with trichotillomania (hair pulling disorder) have improved when taking N-acetylcysteine, but it does not seem to work as well in children. In adults, it can reduce nail biting. It can decrease skin picking, including the skin picking that is seen in people with Prader-Willi syndrome. It may improve mood symptoms in people with bipolar disorder and can reduce irritability and self-injurious behavior in people with autism spectrum disorder.

How Does This Medicine Work?

N-acetylcysteine seems to work in two ways. It helps the brain make an important *antioxidant* that can reduce inflammation by clearing destructive oxygen molecules from cells. Research suggests that many psychiatric illnesses involve cellular inflammation in the brain. Another way that N-acetylcysteine works is by regulating the *neurotransmitters* glutamate and dopamine in the brain.

How Long Does This Medicine Last?

In most studies, N-acetylcysteine is taken 2 or 3 times daily.

How Will the Doctor Monitor This Medicine?

The doctor will review your child's medical history and physical examination before starting N-acetylcysteine. The doctor may order some blood or urine tests to be sure your child does not have a hidden medical condition that would make it unsafe to use this medicine. The doctor or nurse may measure your child's pulse and blood pressure before starting N-acetylcysteine.

After the medicine is started, the doctor will want to have regular appointments with you and your child to see how the medicine is working, to see if a dose change is needed, to watch for side effects, to see if N-acetylcysteine is still needed, and to see if any other treatment is needed. The doctor or nurse may check your child's height, weight, pulse, and blood pressure.

What Side Effects Can This Medicine Have?

Any medicine can have side effects, including an allergy to the medicine. Because each patient is different, the doctor will monitor the youth closely, especially when the medicine is started. The doctor will work with you to increase the positive effects and decrease the negative effects of the medicine. Please tell the doctor if any of the listed side effects appear or if you think that the medicine is causing any other problems. Not all of the rare or unusual side effects are listed.

Allergic Reaction

Tell the doctor in a day or two (if possible, before the next dose of medicine):

- Hives
- Itching
- Rash

Get *immediate* medical care:

- Trouble breathing or chest tightness
- Swelling of lips, tongue, or throat

Common Side Effects

- Stomachache
- Nausea

Some Interactions With Other Medicines or Food

Please note that the following are only the most likely interactions with other medicines or food.

There are few interactions of N-acetylcysteine with medications that children generally take. You should tell your doctor that your child is taking N-acetylcysteine if he or she needs to take a blood thinner like warfarin (Coumadin). It can also interact with nitroglycerin, which is given for chest pain.

What Could Happen if This Medicine Is Stopped Suddenly?

There should be no problems if N-acetylcysteine is stopped suddenly.

How Long Will This Medicine Be Needed?

It appears that N-acetylcysteine can be safely taken for as long as the symptoms it is treating are present. Symptoms may return when N-acetylcysteine is stopped.

What Else Should I Know About This Medicine?

When N-acetylcysteine is sold as a supplement, it is not regulated by the FDA. The amount of N-acetylcysteine in the pill may not be the same as that listed on the package. It is best to buy a brand that is labeled USP, because that shows that the contents meet uniform standards.

N-acetylcysteine has an unpleasant smell that can make it difficult to take.

Notes

Use this space to take notes or to write down questions you want to ask the doctor.

_____

_____

_____

_____

_____

_____

_____

_____

_____

_____

_____

concerning drug dosages, schedules, routes of administration, and side effects is accurate as of the time of publication and consistent with standards set by the U.S. Food and Drug Administration and the general medical community and accepted child psychiatric practice. The information on this medication sheet does not cover all the possible uses, precautions, side effects, or interactions of this drug. For a complete listing of side effects, see the manufacturer's package insert, which can be obtained from your physician or pharmacist. As medical research and practice advance, therapeutic standards may change. For this reason and because human and mechanical errors sometimes occur, we recommend that readers follow the advice of a physician who is directly involved in their care or the care of a member of their family.

From Dulcan MK, Ballard R (editors): *Helping Parents and Teachers Understand Medications for Behavioral and Emotional Problems: A Resource Book of Medication Information Handouts*, Fourth Edition. Washington, DC, American Psychiatric Publishing, 2015

Nortriptyline—Pamelor

General Information About Medication

Each child and adolescent is different. No one has exactly the same combination of medical and psychological problems. It is a good idea to talk with the doctor or nurse about the reasons a medicine is being used. It is very important to keep all appointments and to be in touch by telephone if you have concerns. It is important to communicate with the doctor, nurse, or therapist. An *advanced practice nurse* (APN) has additional education and training after becoming a registered nurse (RN). Your child's medication may be prescribed by a medical doctor (MD or DO) or an APN. In addition, a *physician assistant* (PA) working with a physician may prescribe certain medications. In this information sheet, "doctor" includes medical doctors as well as APNs and PAs who prescribe medication. Often a nurse (RN) will be part of the team and answer questions and give information.

It is very important that the medicine be taken exactly as the doctor instructs. However, once in a while, everyone forgets to give a medicine on time. It is a good idea to ask the doctor or nurse what to do if this happens. Do not stop or change a medicine without asking the doctor or nurse first.

If the medicine seems to stop working, it may be because it is not being taken regularly. The youth may be "cheeking" or hiding the medicine or forgetting to take it (especially at school). The doses may be too far apart or a different dose or medicine may be needed. Something at school, at home, or in the neighborhood may be upsetting the youth, or he or she may need special help for learning disabilities or tutoring. Please discuss your concerns with the doctor. **Do not just increase the dose.** It is also very important not to decrease the dose or stop the medicine without talking to the doctor first. The problem being treated may come back, or there could be uncomfortable or even dangerous results.

All medicines should be kept in a safe place, out of the reach of children, and should be supervised by an adult. If someone takes too much of a medicine, call the doctor, the poison control center, or a hospital emergency room.

Each medicine has a "generic" or chemical name. Just like laundry detergents or paper towels, some medicines are sold by more than one company under different brand names. The same medicine may be available under a generic name and several brand names. The generic medications are usually less expensive than the brand name ones. The generic medications have the same chemical formula, but they may or may not be exactly the same strength as the brand-name medications. Also, some brands of pills contain dye or other things that can cause allergic reactions. It is a good idea to talk to the doctor and the pharmacist about whether it is important to use a specific brand of medicine.

Any medicine can cause an allergic reaction. Examples are hives, itching, rashes, swelling, and trouble breathing. Even a tiny amount of a medicine can cause a reaction in patients who are allergic to that medicine. Be *sure* to talk to the doctor before restarting a medicine that has caused an allergic reaction and tell the doctor about any reactions to medicine that your child has had before.

Taking more than one medicine at the same time may cause more side effects or cause one of the medicines to not work as well. Always ask the doctor, nurse, or pharmacist before adding another

medicine, either prescription or bought without a prescription in a store or on the Internet. **Be sure that each doctor knows about** *all* **of the medicines your child is taking. Also tell the doctor about any vitamins, herbal medicines, or supplements your child may be taking.** Some of these may have side effects alone or when taken with this medication. It is a very good idea to keep a list with you of the names and doses of all medicines that your child is taking.

Everyone taking medicine should have a physical examination at least once a year.

If you think that your child may be using drugs or alcohol, please tell the doctor right away.

Pregnancy requires special care in the use of medicine. Some medicines can cause birth defects if taken by a pregnant mother. **Please tell the doctor immediately if you suspect the teenager is at risk of becoming pregnant.** The doctor may wish to discuss sexual behavior and/or birth control with your daughter.

Printed information like this applies to children and adolescents in general. If you have questions about the medicine, or if you notice changes or anything unusual, please ask the doctor or nurse. As scientific research advances, knowledge increases and advice changes. Even experts do not always agree. Many medicines have not been "approved" by the U.S. Food and Drug Administration (FDA) for use in children or use for particular problems. For this reason, use of the medicine for a problem or age group often is not listed in the *Physicians' Desk Reference*. This does not necessarily mean that the medicine is dangerous or does not work, only that the company that makes the medicine has not received permission to advertise the medicine for use in children. Companies often do not apply for this permission because it is expensive to do the tests needed to apply for approval for use in children. Once a medication is approved by the FDA for any purpose, a doctor is allowed to prescribe it according to research and clinical experience.

Note to Teachers

It is a good idea to talk with the parent(s) about the reason(s) that a medication is being used. If the parent(s) sign consent to release information, it is often helpful for you to talk with the doctor. If the parent(s) give permission, the doctor may ask you to fill out rating forms about your experience with the student's behavior, feelings, academic performance, and medication side effects. This information is very useful in selecting and monitoring medication treatment. If you have observations that you think are important, do not hesitate to share these with the student's parent(s) and treating clinicians (with parental consent).

It is very important that the medicine be taken exactly as the doctor instructs. However, everyone forgets to give a medicine on time once in a while. It is a good idea to ask the parent(s) in advance what to do if this happens. Do not stop or change the time you are giving a medicine at school without parental permission. If a medication is to be taken with food, but lunchtime or snack time changes, be sure to notify the parent(s) so appropriate adjustments can be made.

All medicines should be kept in a secure place and should be supervised by an adult. If someone takes too much of a medicine, follow your school procedure for an urgent medical problem.

Taking medicine is a private matter and is best managed discreetly and confidentially. It is important to be sensitive to the student's feelings about taking medicine.

If you suspect that the student is using drugs or alcohol, please tell the parent(s) or a school counselor right away.

Please tell the parent(s) or school nurse if you suspect medication side effects.

Modifications of the classroom environment or assignments may be useful in addition to medication. The student may need to be evaluated for additional help or a 504 plan or an Individualized Education Plan for learning problems or emotional or behavioral issues.

Any expression of suicidal thoughts or feelings or self-harm by a child or adolescent is a signal of distress and should be taken seriously. These behaviors should not be dismissed as "attention seeking." School procedures for safety issues should be followed.

You may notice the following side effects at school:

Common Side Effects

- Dry mouth—Allow the student to chew sugar-free gum, carry a water bottle, or make extra trips to the water fountain.
- Constipation—Allow the student to drink more fluids or to use the bathroom more often.
- Daytime sleepiness—The student should not drive, ride a bicycle or motorcycle, or operate machinery.
- Dizziness (especially when standing up quickly)—This may happen in the classroom or during physical education. Suggest that the student stand up more slowly.
- Irritability

Occasional Side Effects

- Stuttering
- Increased risk of sunburn (this may be a problem if recess or physical education is outdoors in warm weather)—The student should wear sunscreen or protective clothing or stay out of the sun.

Less Common Side Effects

- Nausea—The student may need to take the medicine after a meal or snack.
- Trouble urinating—The student may need more time in the bathroom.
- Blurred vision—The student may have trouble seeing the blackboard.
- Motor tics (fast, repeated movements) or muscle twitches (jerking movements) of parts of the body
- Increased activity, rapid speech, feeling "speeded up," being very excited or irritable (cranky)
- Skin rash

Rare, but Potentially Serious, Side Effects

Call the parent(s) or follow your school's emergency procedures *immediately*:

- Seizure (fit, convulsion) **(This is a medical emergency.)**
- Very fast or irregular heartbeat **(This is a medical emergency.)**
- Fainting
- Hallucinations (hearing voices or seeing things that are not there)
- Inability to urinate
- Confusion
- Severe change in behavior

What Is Nortriptyline (Pamelor)?

Nortriptyline is called a *tricyclic antidepressant*. It was first used to treat depression but is now used to treat attention-deficit/hyperactivity disorder (ADHD), school phobia, separation anxiety, panic disorder, and some sleep disorders (such as night terrors and sleepwalking). It is also sometimes used to treat fibromyalgia. It comes in brand name Pamelor and generic capsules and liquid.

How Can This Medicine Help?

Nortriptyline can decrease symptoms of ADHD, anxiety (nervousness), panic, and night terrors or sleepwalking. The medicine may take several weeks to work.

How Does This Medicine Work?

Tricyclic antidepressants affect *neurotransmitters*—the natural substances that are needed for certain parts of the brain to work more normally. They increase the activity of *serotonin* and *norepinephrine*.

How Long Does This Medicine Last?

In adults and older teenagers, one dose lasts for a whole day. In younger children, several doses a day may be needed.

How Will the Doctor Monitor This Medicine?

The doctor will review your child's medical history and physical examination, paying special attention to pulse rate, blood pressure, weight, and height, before starting nortriptyline. These measurements will be taken when the dose is increased and occasionally as long as the medicine is continued. The doctor may order some blood or urine tests to be sure your child does not have a hidden medical condition that would make it unsafe to use this medicine.

Tricyclic antidepressants can slow the speed at which signals move through the heart. This effect is not dangerous if the heart is normal, which is why an ECG (electrocardiogram or heart rhythm test) is done before starting the medicine. The ECG may be repeated as the dose is increased and occasionally while the medicine is being taken. Changes in the heart from the medicine usually can be seen on the ECG before they become a problem, so your child's doctor will order an ECG every so often. To find possible hidden heart risks, it is especially important to tell the doctor if your child or anyone in the family has a history of fainting, palpitations, or irregular heartbeat or if anyone in the family died suddenly.

Be sure to tell the doctor if your child or anyone in the family has bipolar disorder or has tried to kill himself or herself.

Because tricyclic antidepressants may increase the risk of seizures (fits, convulsions), the doctor will want to know whether your child has ever had a seizure or a head injury and if there is any family history of epilepsy. Your child's doctor may want to order an EEG (electroencephalogram or brain wave test) before starting the medicine.

Experts do not agree on whether blood tests are needed to measure the level of this medicine. Blood levels seem to be most useful when the doctor suspects that the dose of medicine is too high or too low. The most accurate level is obtained by drawing blood first thing in the morning after at least 5 days on the same dose, approximately 12 hours after the evening dose of medicine and before the morning dose.

After the medicine is started, the doctor will want to have regular appointments with you and your child to see how the medicine is working, to see if a dose change is needed, to watch for side effects, to see if nortriptyline is still needed, and to see if any other treatment is needed. The doctor or nurse may check your child's height, weight, pulse, and blood pressure or order tests, such as an ECG or blood level.

If nortriptyline is being used for ADHD, the doctor may ask for your child's teacher to fill out reports on your child's learning and behavior at school. Before using medicine and at times afterward, the doctor may ask your child to fill out a rating scale about anxiety and depression, to help see how your child is doing.

What Side Effects Can This Medicine Have?

Any medicine can have side effects, including an allergy to the medicine. Because each patient is different, the doctor will monitor the youth closely, especially when the medicine is started. The doctor will work with you to increase the positive effects and decrease the negative effects of the medicine. Please tell the doctor if any of the listed side effects appear or if you think that the medicine is causing any other problems. Not all of the rare or unusual side effects are listed.

Side effects are most common after starting the medicine or after a dose increase. Many side effects can be avoided or lessened by starting with a very low dose and increasing it slowly—ask the doctor.

Allergic Reaction

Tell the doctor in a day or two (if possible, before the next dose of medicine):

- Hives
- Itching
- Rash (may be caused by an allergy to the medicine or to a dye in the specific brand of pill)

  Stop medicine and get *immediate* medical care:

- Trouble breathing or chest tightness
- Swelling of lips, tongue, or throat

Common Side Effects

Tell the doctor within a week or two:

- Dry mouth—Have your child try using sugar-free gum or candy.
- Constipation—Encourage your child to drink more fluids and eat high-fiber foods; if necessary, the doctor may recommend a fiber medicine such as Benefiber or a stool softener such as Colace or mineral oil.
- Daytime sleepiness—Do not allow your child to drive, ride a bicycle or motorcycle, or operate machinery if this happens.
- Dizziness—This side effect is worse when the child stands up quickly, especially when getting out of bed in the morning; try having the child stand up slowly.
- Weight gain
- Loss of appetite and weight loss
- Irritability

Occasional Side Effects

Tell the doctor within a week or two:

- Nightmares
- Stuttering
- Blurred vision
- Increase in breast size, nipple discharge, or both (in girls)
- Increase in breast size (in boys)

Less Common, but More Serious, Side Effects

Call the doctor within a day or two:

- High or low blood pressure
- Nausea
- Trouble urinating
- Motor tics (fast, repeated movements) or muscle twitches (jerking movements)
- Increased activity, rapid speech, feeling "speeded up," decreased need for sleep, being very excited or irritable (cranky)

Rare, but Potentially Serious, Side Effects

Call the doctor *immediately*:

- Seizure (fit, convulsion)—**Go to an emergency room.**
- Very fast or irregular heartbeat—**Go to an emergency room.**
- Fainting
- Hallucinations (hearing voices or seeing things that are not there)
- Difficulty passing urine
- Confusion
- Severe change in behavior

Some Interactions With Other Medicines or Food

Please note that the following are only the most likely interactions with other medicines or food.

Check with your child's doctor before giving your child decongestants or over-the-counter cold medicine.

Taking another antidepressant or Depakote with nortriptyline may increase the level of nortriptyline and increase side effects.

Taking carbamazepine (Tegretol) with nortriptyline may decrease the positive effects of nortriptyline and increase the side effects of carbamazepine.

It can be *very dangerous* to take nortriptyline at the same time as or even within a month of taking another type of medicine called a *monoamine oxidase inhibitor* (MAOI), such as selegiline (Eldepryl), phenelzine (Nardil), tranylcypromine (Parnate), or isocarboxazid (Marplan).

Caffeine may worsen side effects on the heart or symptoms of anxiety. It is best not to drink coffee, tea, or soft drinks with caffeine while taking this medicine.

What Could Happen if This Medicine Is Stopped Suddenly?

Stopping the medicine suddenly or skipping a dose is not dangerous but can be very uncomfortable. Your child may feel like he or she has the flu—with a headache, muscle aches, stomachache, and upset stomach. Behavioral problems, sadness, nervousness, or trouble sleeping also may occur. If these feelings appear every day, the medicine may need to be given more often during each day.

How Long Will This Medicine Be Needed?

There is no way to know how long a person will need to take this medicine. Parents work together with the doctor to determine what is right for each child. The medicine may be needed for a long time. Some people may need to take the medicine even as adults.

What Else Should I Know About This Medicine?

In youth who have bipolar disorder or who are at risk for bipolar disorder, any antidepressant medicine may increase the risk of hypomania or mania (excitement, agitation, increased activity, decreased sleep).

An overdose by accident or on purpose with this medicine is *very dangerous*! You must closely supervise the medicine. You may have to lock up the medicine if your child or teenager is suicidal or if young children live in or visit your home.

Tricyclic antidepressants may cause dry mouth, which could increase the chance of tooth decay. Regular brushing of teeth and checkups with the dentist are especially important.

This medicine causes increased risk of sunburn. Be sure that your child wears sunscreen or protective clothing or stays out of the sun.

People who take tricyclic antidepressants must not drink alcohol or use tranquilizers. Severe sleepiness, loss of consciousness, or even death may result.

Black Box Antidepressant Warning

In 2004, an advisory committee to the FDA decided that there might be an increased risk of suicidal behavior for some youth taking medicines called *antidepressants*. In the research studies that the committee reviewed, about 3%–4% of youth with depression who took an antidepressant medicine—and 1%–2% of youth with depression who took a placebo (pill without active medicine)—talked about suicidal thoughts (thinking about killing themselves or wishing they were dead) or did something to harm themselves. This means that almost twice as many youth who were taking an antidepressant to treat their depression talked about suicide or had suicidal behavior compared with youth with depression who were taking inactive medicine. There were *no* completed suicides in any of these research studies, which included more than 4,000 children and adolescents. For youth being treated for anxiety, there was no difference in suicidal talking or behavior between those taking antidepressant medication and those taking placebo.

The FDA told drug companies to add a *black box warning* label to all antidepressant medicines. Because of this label, a doctor (or advanced practice nurse) prescribing one of these medicines has to warn youth and their families that there might be more suicidal thoughts and actions in youth taking these medicines.

On the other hand, in places where more youth are taking the newer antidepressant medicines, the number of adolescents who commit suicide has gotten smaller. Also, thinking about or attempting suicide is more common in surveys of teenagers in the community than it is in depressed youth treated in research studies with antidepressant medicine.

If a youth is being treated with this medicine and is doing well, then no changes are needed as a result of this warning. Increased suicidal talk or action is most likely to happen in the first few months of treatment with a medicine. If your child has recently started this medicine or is about to start, then you and your doctor (or advanced practice nurse) should watch for any changes in behavior. People who are depressed often have suicidal thoughts or actions. It is hard to know whether suicidal thoughts or actions in depressed people are caused by the depression itself or by the medicine. Also, as their depression is getting better, some people talk more about the suicidal thoughts that they had before but did not talk about. As young people get better from depression, they might be at higher risk of doing something about suicidal thoughts that they have had for some time, because they have more energy.

What Should a Parent Do?

1. Be honest with your child about possible risks and benefits of medicine.
2. Talk to your child about whether he or she is having any suicidal thoughts, and tell your child to come to you if he or she is having such thoughts.
3. You, your child, and your child's doctor or nurse should develop a safety plan. Pick adults whom your child can tell if he or she is thinking about suicide.
4. Be sure to tell your child's doctor, nurse, or therapist if you suspect that your child is using alcohol or drugs or if something has happened that might make your child feel worse, such as a family separation, breaking up with a boyfriend or girlfriend, someone close dying or attempting suicide, physical or sexual abuse, or failure in school.
5. Be sure that there are no guns in the home and that all medicines (including over-the-counter medicines like Tylenol) are closely supervised by an adult and kept in a safe place.
6. Watch for new or worse thoughts of suicide, self-harm, depression, anxiety (nerves), feeling very agitated or restless, being angry or aggressive, having more trouble sleeping, or anything else that you see for the first time, seems worse, or worries your child or you. If these appear, contact a mental health professional **right away.** Do not just stop or change the dose of the medicine on your own. If the problems are serious, and you cannot reach one of your clinicians, call a 24-hour psychiatry emergency telephone number or take your child to an emergency room.

Youth taking antidepressant medicine should be watched carefully by their parent(s), clinician(s) (doctor, advanced practice nurse, nurse, therapist), and other concerned adults for the first weeks of treatment. It is a good idea to have regular contact with the doctor, APN, nurse, or therapist for the first months to check for feelings of depression or sadness, thoughts of killing or harming himself or herself, and any problems with the medication. If you have questions, be sure to ask the doctor, APN, nurse, or therapist.

For more information, see http://www.parentsmedguide.org/.

Notes

Use this space to take notes or to write down questions you want to ask the doctor.

Medication Information for Parents and Teachers

Olanzapine—Zyprexa, Symbyax

General Information About Medication

Each child and adolescent is different. No one has exactly the same combination of medical and psychological problems. It is a good idea to talk with the doctor or nurse about the reasons a medicine is being used. It is very important to keep all appointments and to be in touch by telephone if you have concerns. It is important to communicate with the doctor, nurse, or therapist. An *advanced practice nurse* (APN) has additional education and training after becoming a registered nurse (RN). Your child's medication may be prescribed by a medical doctor (MD or DO) or an APN. In addition, a *physician assistant* (PA) working with a physician may prescribe certain medications. In this information sheet, "doctor" includes medical doctors as well as APNs and PAs who prescribe medication. Often a nurse (RN) will be part of the team and answer questions and give information.

It is very important that the medicine be taken exactly as the doctor instructs. However, once in a while, everyone forgets to give a medicine on time. It is a good idea to ask the doctor or nurse what to do if this happens. Do not stop or change a medicine without asking the doctor or nurse first.

If the medicine seems to stop working, it may be because it is not being taken regularly. The youth may be "cheeking" or hiding the medicine or forgetting to take it (especially at school). The doses may be too far apart or a different dose or medicine may be needed. Something at school, at home, or in the neighborhood may be upsetting the youth, or he or she may need special help for learning disabilities or tutoring. Please discuss your concerns with the doctor. **Do not just increase the dose.** It is also very important not to decrease the dose or stop the medicine without talking to the doctor first. The problem being treated may come back, or there could be uncomfortable or even dangerous results.

All medicines should be kept in a safe place, out of the reach of children, and should be supervised by an adult. If someone takes too much of a medicine, call the doctor, the poison control center, or a hospital emergency room.

Each medicine has a "generic" or chemical name. Just like laundry detergents or paper towels, some medicines are sold by more than one company under different brand names. The same medicine may be available under a generic name and several brand names. The generic medications are usually less expensive than the brand name ones. The generic medications have the same chemical formula, but they may or may not be exactly the same strength as the brand-name medications. Also, some brands of pills contain dye or other things that can cause allergic reactions. It is a good idea to talk to the doctor and the pharmacist about whether it is important to use a specific brand of medicine.

Any medicine can cause an allergic reaction. Examples are hives, itching, rashes, swelling, and trouble breathing. Even a tiny amount of a medicine can cause a reaction in patients who are allergic to that medicine. Be *sure* to talk to the doctor before restarting a medicine that has caused an allergic reaction and tell the doctor about any reactions to medicine that your child has had before.

Taking more than one medicine at the same time may cause more side effects or cause one of the medicines to not work as well. Always ask the doctor, nurse, or pharmacist before adding another

medicine, either prescription or bought without a prescription in a store or on the Internet. **Be sure that each doctor knows about** *all* **of the medicines your child is taking. Also tell the doctor about any vitamins, herbal medicines, or supplements your child may be taking.** Some of these may have side effects alone or when taken with this medication. It is a very good idea to keep a list with you of the names and doses of all medicines that your child is taking.

Everyone taking medicine should have a physical examination at least once a year.

If you think that your child may be using drugs or alcohol, please tell the doctor right away.

Pregnancy requires special care in the use of medicine. Some medicines can cause birth defects if taken by a pregnant mother. **Please tell the doctor immediately if you suspect the teenager is at risk of becoming pregnant.** The doctor may wish to discuss sexual behavior and/or birth control with your daughter.

Printed information like this applies to children and adolescents in general. If you have questions about the medicine, or if you notice changes or anything unusual, please ask the doctor or nurse. As scientific research advances, knowledge increases and advice changes. Even experts do not always agree. Many medicines have not been "approved" by the U.S. Food and Drug Administration (FDA) for use in children or use for particular problems. For this reason, use of the medicine for a problem or age group often is not listed in the *Physicians' Desk Reference*. This does not necessarily mean that the medicine is dangerous or does not work, only that the company that makes the medicine has not received permission to advertise the medicine for use in children. Companies often do not apply for this permission because it is expensive to do the tests needed to apply for approval for use in children. Once a medication is approved by the FDA for any purpose, a doctor is allowed to prescribe it according to research and clinical experience.

Note to Teachers

It is a good idea to talk with the parent(s) about the reason(s) that a medication is being used. If the parent(s) sign consent to release information, it is often helpful for you to talk with the doctor. If the parent(s) give permission, the doctor may ask you to fill out rating forms about your experience with the student's behavior, feelings, academic performance, and medication side effects. This information is very useful in selecting and monitoring medication treatment. If you have observations that you think are important, do not hesitate to share these with the student's parent(s) and treating clinicians (with parental consent).

It is very important that the medicine be taken exactly as the doctor instructs. However, everyone forgets to give a medicine on time once in a while. It is a good idea to ask the parent(s) in advance what to do if this happens. Do not stop or change the time you are giving a medicine at school without parental permission. If a medication is to be taken with food, but lunchtime or snack time changes, be sure to notify the parent(s) so appropriate adjustments can be made.

All medicines should be kept in a secure place and should be supervised by an adult. If someone takes too much of a medicine, follow your school procedure for an urgent medical problem.

Taking medicine is a private matter and is best managed discreetly and confidentially. It is important to be sensitive to the student's feelings about taking medicine.

If you suspect that the student is using drugs or alcohol, please tell the parent(s) or a school counselor right away.

Please tell the parent(s) or school nurse if you suspect medication side effects.

Modifications of the classroom environment or assignments may be useful in addition to medication. The student may need to be evaluated for additional help or a 504 plan or an Individualized Education Plan for learning problems or emotional or behavioral issues.

Any expression of suicidal thoughts or feelings or self-harm by a child or adolescent is a signal of distress and should be taken seriously. These behaviors should not be dismissed as "attention seeking." School procedures for safety issues should be followed.

What Is Olanzapine (Zyprexa, Symbyax)?

This medicine is called an *atypical* or *second-generation antipsychotic*. It is sometimes called an *atypical psychotropic agent* or simply an *atypical*. It comes in generic and brand name Zyprexa tablets, Zyprexa Zydis and generic rapid-dissolving tablets that melt quickly in the mouth, and a fast-acting injection (shot). Olanzapine also comes in a long-acting injectable (shot) form, Zyprexa Relprevv.

There is a combination capsule of fluoxetine and olanzapine that comes in brand name Symbyax and generic.

How Can This Medicine Help?

Olanzapine is used to treat psychosis, such as in schizophrenia, mania, or very severe depression. It can reduce *positive symptoms* such as hallucinations (hearing voices or seeing things that are not there); delusions (troubling beliefs that other people do not share); agitation; and very unusual thinking, speech, and behavior. It is also used to lessen the *negative symptoms* of schizophrenia, such as lack of interest in doing things (apathy), lack of motivation, social withdrawal, and lack of energy.

Olanzapine may be used as a *mood stabilizer* in patients with bipolar disorder or severe mood swings. It can reduce mania and may be able to help maintain a stable mood over the long term.

Sometimes olanzapine is used to reduce severe aggression or very serious behavioral problems in young people with conduct disorder, intellectual disability, or autism spectrum disorder.

Olanzapine may be used for behavior problems after a head injury.

It is also used to reduce motor and vocal tics (fast, repeated movements or sounds) and behavioral problems in people with Tourette's disorder.

This medicine is very powerful and is used to treat very serious problems or symptoms that other medicines do not help. Be patient; the positive effects of this medicine may not appear for 2–3 weeks.

Symbyax is used to treat depression in people with bipolar disorder.

How Does This Medicine Work?

Cells in the brain communicate using chemicals called *neurotransmitters*. Too much or too little of these substances in parts of the brain can cause problems. Olanzapine works by blocking the action of two of these neurotransmitters, *dopamine* and *serotonin*, in certain areas of the brain.

How Long Does This Medicine Last?

Olanzapine usually can be taken only once a day. The long-acting injection is generally used only in adults and is given every 2–4 weeks.

How Will the Doctor Monitor This Medicine?

The doctor will review your child's medical history and physical examination before starting olanzapine. The doctor may order some blood or urine tests to be sure your child does not have a hidden medical condition that would make it unsafe to use this medicine. The doctor or nurse will measure your child's height, weight, pulse, and blood pressure before starting olanzapine. The doctor may order other tests, such as baseline tests for blood sugar and cholesterol.

Be sure to tell the doctor if anyone in the family has diabetes, high blood pressure, high cholesterol, or heart disease.

Before starting olanzapine and every so often afterward, a test such as the AIMS (Abnormal Involuntary Movement Scale) may be used to check your child's tongue, legs, and arms for unusual movements that could be caused by the medicine.

After the medicine is started, the doctor will want to have regular appointments with you and your child to see how the medicine is working, to see if a dose change is needed, to watch for side effects, to see if olanzapine is still needed, and to see if any other treatment is needed. The doctor or nurse may check your child's height, weight, pulse, and blood pressure and watch for abnormal movements. Sometimes blood tests are needed to watch for diabetes or increased cholesterol.

What Side Effects Can This Medicine Have?

Any medicine can have side effects, including an allergy to the medicine. Because each patient is different, the doctor will monitor the youth closely, especially when the medicine is started. The doctor will work with you to increase the positive effects and decrease the negative effects of the medicine. Please tell the doctor if any of the listed side effects appear or if you think that the medicine is causing any other problems. Not all of the rare or unusual side effects are listed.

Side effects are most common after starting the medicine or after a dose increase. Many side effects can be avoided or lessened by starting with a very low dose and increasing it slowly—ask the doctor.

For the fluoxetine-olanzapine combination Symbyax, see also the information sheet for fluoxetine.

Allergic Reaction

Tell the doctor in a day or two (if possible, before the next dose of medicine):

- Hives
- Itching
- Rash

Stop the medicine and get *immediate* medical care:

- Trouble breathing or chest tightness
- Swelling of lips, tongue, or throat

Common, but Not Usually Serious, Side Effects

Discuss the following side effects with your child's doctor when convenient. Side effects often can be helped by lowering the dose of medicine, changing the times medicine is taken, or adding another medicine—ask the doctor.

- Daytime sleepiness or tiredness—Do not allow your child to drive, ride a bicycle or motorcycle, or operate machinery if this happens. This problem may be lessened by taking the medicine at bedtime.
- Dry mouth—Have your child try using sugar-free gum or candy.
- Constipation—Encourage your child to drink more fluids and eat high-fiber foods; if necessary, the doctor may recommend a fiber medicine such as Benefiber or a stool softener such as Colace or mineral oil.
- Dizziness—This side effect is worse when the child stands up quickly, especially when getting out of bed in the morning; try having the child stand up slowly.
- Increased appetite
- Weight gain—Seek nutritional counseling; provide your child with low-calorie snacks and encourage regular exercise.

Less Common, but Not Usually Serious, Side Effects

Discuss the following side effects with your child's doctor when convenient.

- Drooling
- Increased restlessness or inability to sit still
- Shaking of hands and fingers
- Decreased or slowed movement and decreased facial expressions
- Decreased sexual interest or ability
- Changes in menstrual cycle
- Increase in breast size or discharge from the breasts (in both boys and girls)—This may go away with time.

Less Common, but Potentially Serious, Side Effects

Call the doctor *immediately:*

- Stiffness of the tongue, jaw, neck, back, or legs
- Seizure (fit, convulsion)—This is more common in people with a history of seizures or head injury.
- Increased thirst, frequent urination (having to go to the bathroom often), lethargy, tiredness, dizziness, and blurred vision—These could be signs of diabetes (especially if your child is overweight or there is a family history of diabetes). **Talk to a doctor within a day.**

Very Rare, but Serious, Side Effects

- Extreme stiffness or lack of movement, very high fever, mental confusion, irregular pulse rate, or eye pain—**This is a medical emergency. Go to an emergency room right away.**
- Sudden stiffness and inability to breathe or swallow—**Go to an emergency room or call 911.** Tell the paramedics, nurses, and doctors that the patient is taking olanzapine. Other medicines can be used to treat this problem fast.

What Else Should I Know About Side Effects?

Most side effects lessen over time. If they are troublesome, talk with your child's doctor. Some side effects can be decreased by taking a smaller dose of medicine, by stopping the medicine, by changing to another medicine, or by adding another medicine.

Many people who take olanzapine gain weight. Children seem to have more problems with this than adults. The weight gain may be from increased appetite and from ways that the medicine changes how the body processes food. Olanzapine may also change the way that the body handles glucose (sugar) and cause high blood sugar levels (*hyperglycemia*). People who take olanzapine, especially those who gain a lot of weight, are at increased risk of developing *diabetes* and of having increased fats (*lipids—cholesterol and triglycerides*) in their blood. Over time, both diabetes and increased fats in the blood may lead to heart disease, stroke, and other complications. The FDA has put warnings on all atypical agents about the increased risks of hyperglycemia, diabetes, and increased blood cholesterol and triglycerides when taking one of these medicines and has recommended that olanzapine generally be considered as a treatment only after trying other atypical antipsychotics first because of apparent increased risk of elevated blood sugar and fats. It is much easier to prevent weight gain than to lose weight later. When your child first starts taking olanzapine, it is a good idea to be sure that he or she eats a well-balanced diet without "junk food" and with healthy snacks like fruits and vegetables, not sweets or fried foods. He or she should drink water or skim milk, not pop, sodas, soft drinks, or sugary juices. Regular exercise is important for maintaining a healthy weight (and may also help with sleep).

The medicine may increase the level of *prolactin*, a natural hormone made in the part of the brain called the *pituitary*. This may cause side effects such as breast tenderness or swelling or production of milk in both boys and girls. It also may interfere with sexual functioning in teenage boys and with regular menstrual cycles (periods) in teenage girls. A blood test can measure the level of prolactin. If these side effects do not go away and are troublesome, talk with your child's doctor about substituting another medicine for olanzapine.

One very rare side effect that may not go away is *tardive dyskinesia* (or TD). Patients with tardive dyskinesia have involuntary movements (movements that they cannot help making) of the body, especially the mouth and tongue. The patient may look as though he or she is making faces over and over again. Jerky movements of the arms, legs, or body may occur. There may be fine, wormlike, or sudden repeated movements of the tongue, or the person may appear to be chewing something or smacking or puckering his or her lips. The fingers may look as though they are rolling something. If you notice any unusual movements, be sure to tell the doctor. The doctor may use the AIMS test to look for these movements.

Neuroleptic malignant syndrome is a very rare side effect that can lead to death. The symptoms are severe muscle stiffness, high fever, increased heart rate and blood pressure, irregular heartbeat (pulse), and sweating. It may lead to unconsciousness. If you suspect this, **call 911 or go to an emergency room right away.**

The Zyprexa Relprevv long-acting injection has rarely been associated with marked sedation and acute confusion and disorientation within 3 hours of getting the shot.

Sometimes this medicine can cause a *dystonic reaction*. This is a sudden stiffening of the muscles, most often in the jaw, neck, tongue, face, or shoulders. If this happens, and your child is not having trouble breathing, you may give a dose of diphenhydramine (Benadryl). Follow the dose instructions on the package for your child's age. This should relax the muscles in a few minutes. Then call your doctor to tell him or her what happened. If the muscles do not relax, take your child to the emergency department.

Some Interactions With Other Medicines or Food

Please note that the following are only the most likely interactions with other medicines or food.

Olanzapine may be taken with or without food.

Fluvoxamine (Luvox), fluoxetine (Prozac), and some antibiotics such as erythromycin or ciprofloxacin can increase the levels of olanzapine and increase the risk of side effects.

Carbamazepine (Tegretol) and oxcarbazepine (Trileptal) can decrease the levels of olanzapine so that it does not work as well.

Heart problems are rare with olanzapine but are more common if other medicines that affect the heart are being taken also. Be sure to tell all your child's doctors and your pharmacist about all medications your child is taking.

It is better to limit drinks with caffeine (coffee, tea, soft drinks) because caffeine works in the opposite way from this medicine, and the positive effects might be decreased.

What Could Happen if This Medicine Is Stopped Suddenly?

Involuntary movements, or *withdrawal dyskinesias*, may appear within 1–4 weeks of lowering the dose or stopping the medicine. Usually these go away, but they can last for days to months. If olanzapine is stopped suddenly, emotional disturbance (such as irritability, nervousness, moodiness, or oppositional behavior) or physical problems (such as stomachache, loss of appetite, nausea, vomiting, diarrhea, sweating, indigestion, trouble sleeping, trembling, or shaking) may appear. These problems usually last only a few days to a few weeks. If they happen, you should tell your child's doctor. The medicine dose may need to be lowered more slowly (tapered). Always check with the doctor before stopping a medicine.

How Long Will This Medicine Be Needed?

How long your child will need to take this medicine depends partly on the reason that it was prescribed. Some problems last for only a few months, whereas others last much longer. It is important to ask the doctor whether medicine is still needed, especially with medicines as powerful as this one. Every few months, you should discuss with your child's doctor the reasons for using olanzapine and whether the medicine may be stopped or the dose lowered.

What Else Should I Know About This Medicine?

There are other medicines that are used for the same kinds of problems. If your child is having bad side effects or the medicine does not seem to be working, ask the doctor if another medicine might work as well or better and have fewer side effects for your child. Each person reacts differently to medicines.

It is not a good idea to split or crush the tablets, because their coating can be very sharp when broken.

When giving Zydis, peel off the foil on both sides; do not push the tablet through the foil. The disk should be placed in the mouth right away and allowed to melt before swallowing.

Pharmacies sometimes confuse Zyprexa with Zyrtec (an antihistamine). If your child's prescription is new or the pills look different, be sure to check with the pharmacist.

Taking this medicine could make overheating or heatstroke more likely. Have your child decrease activity in hot weather, stay out of the sun, and drink water to prevent this.

Notes

Use this space to take notes or to write down questions you want to ask the doctor.

_____

_____

_____

_____

_____

_____

_____

_____

_____

_____

_____

Medication Information for Parents and Teachers

Omega-3 Fatty Acids—Epanova, Lovaza

General Information About Medication

Each child and adolescent is different. No one has exactly the same combination of medical and psychological problems. It is a good idea to talk with the doctor or nurse about the reasons a medicine is being used. It is very important to keep all appointments and to be in touch by telephone if you have concerns. It is important to communicate with the doctor, nurse, or therapist. An *advanced practice nurse* (APN) has additional education and training after becoming a registered nurse (RN). Your child's medication may be prescribed by a medical doctor (MD or DO) or an APN. In addition, a *physician assistant* (PA) working with a physician may prescribe certain medications. In this information sheet, "doctor" includes medical doctors as well as APNs and PAs who prescribe medication. Often a nurse (RN) will be part of the team and answer questions and give information.

It is very important that the medicine be taken exactly as the doctor instructs. However, once in a while, everyone forgets to give a medicine on time. It is a good idea to ask the doctor or nurse what to do if this happens. Do not stop or change a medicine without asking the doctor or nurse first.

If the medicine seems to stop working, it may be because it is not being taken regularly. The youth may be "cheeking" or hiding the medicine or forgetting to take it (especially at school). The doses may be too far apart or a different dose or medicine may be needed. Something at school, at home, or in the neighborhood may be upsetting the youth, or he or she may need special help for learning disabilities or tutoring. Please discuss your concerns with the doctor. **Do not just increase the dose.** It is also very important not to decrease the dose or stop the medicine without talking to the doctor first. The problem being treated may come back, or there could be uncomfortable or even dangerous results.

All medicines should be kept in a safe place, out of the reach of children, and should be supervised by an adult. If someone takes too much of a medicine, call the doctor, the poison control center, or a hospital emergency room.

Each medicine has a "generic" or chemical name. Just like laundry detergents or paper towels, some medicines are sold by more than one company under different brand names. The same medicine may be available under a generic name and several brand names. The generic medications are usually less expensive than the brand name ones. The generic medications have the same chemical formula, but they may or may not be exactly the same strength as the brand-name medications. Also, some brands of pills contain dye or other things that can cause allergic reactions. It is a good idea to talk to the doctor and the pharmacist about whether it is important to use a specific brand of medicine.

Any medicine can cause an allergic reaction. Examples are hives, itching, rashes, swelling, and trouble breathing. Even a tiny amount of a medicine can cause a reaction in patients who are allergic to that medicine. Be *sure* to talk to the doctor before restarting a medicine that has caused an allergic reaction and tell the doctor about any reactions to medicine that your child has had before.

Taking more than one medicine at the same time may cause more side effects or cause one of the medicines to not work as well. Always ask the doctor, nurse, or pharmacist before adding another medicine, either prescription or bought without a prescription in a store or on the Internet. Be sure

383

that each doctor knows about *all* of the medicines your child is taking. Also tell the doctor about any vitamins, herbal medicines, or supplements your child may be taking. Some of these may have side effects alone or when taken with this medication. It is a very good idea to keep a list with you of the names and doses of all medicines that your child is taking.

Everyone taking medicine should have a physical examination at least once a year.

If you think that your child may be using drugs or alcohol, please tell the doctor right away.

Pregnancy requires special care in the use of medicine. Some medicines can cause birth defects if taken by a pregnant mother. **Please tell the doctor immediately if you suspect the teenager is at risk of becoming pregnant.** The doctor may wish to discuss sexual behavior and/or birth control with your daughter.

Printed information like this applies to children and adolescents in general. If you have questions about the medicine, or if you notice changes or anything unusual, please ask the doctor or nurse. As scientific research advances, knowledge increases and advice changes. Even experts do not always agree. Many medicines have not been "approved" by the U.S. Food and Drug Administration (FDA) for use in children or use for particular problems. For this reason, use of the medicine for a problem or age group often is not listed in the *Physicians' Desk Reference*. This does not necessarily mean that the medicine is dangerous or does not work, only that the company that makes the medicine has not received permission to advertise the medicine for use in children. Companies often do not apply for this permission because it is expensive to do the tests needed to apply for approval for use in children. Once a medication is approved by the FDA for any purpose, a doctor is allowed to prescribe it according to research and clinical experience.

Note to Teachers

It is a good idea to talk with the parent(s) about the reason(s) that a medication is being used. If the parent(s) sign consent to release information, it is often helpful for you to talk with the doctor. If the parent(s) give permission, the doctor may ask you to fill out rating forms about your experience with the student's behavior, feelings, academic performance, and medication side effects. This information is very useful in selecting and monitoring medication treatment. If you have observations that you think are important, do not hesitate to share these with the student's parent(s) and treating clinicians (with parental consent).

It is very important that the medicine be taken exactly as the doctor instructs. However, everyone forgets to give a medicine on time once in a while. It is a good idea to ask the parent(s) in advance what to do if this happens. Do not stop or change the time you are giving a medicine at school without parental permission. If a medication is to be taken with food, but lunchtime or snack time changes, be sure to notify the parent(s) so appropriate adjustments can be made.

All medicines should be kept in a secure place and should be supervised by an adult. If someone takes too much of a medicine, follow your school procedure for an urgent medical problem.

Taking medicine is a private matter and is best managed discreetly and confidentially. It is important to be sensitive to the student's feelings about taking medicine.

If you suspect that the student is using drugs or alcohol, please tell the parent(s) or a school counselor right away.

Please tell the parent(s) or school nurse if you suspect medication side effects.

Modifications of the classroom environment or assignments may be useful in addition to medication. The student may need to be evaluated for additional help or a 504 plan or an Individualized Education Plan for learning problems or emotional or behavioral issues.

Any expression of suicidal thoughts or feelings or self-harm by a child or adolescent is a signal of distress and should be taken seriously. These behaviors should not be dismissed as "attention seeking." School procedures for safety issues should be followed.

What Are Omega-3 Fatty Acids?

The main *essential fatty acids* in the human diet are called *omega-3* and *omega-6*. Foods that provide omega-3 fatty acids include fish oil and certain plant and nut oils. Omega-6 fatty acids can be found in palm, soybean, rapeseed, and sunflower oils. Most people in the United States get plenty of omega-6 fatty acids but not enough omega-3. Increasing the amount of fatty fish (like salmon) or plants like flaxseed or walnuts can increase omega-3 fatty acids in the diet. Taking omega-3 supplements can also do this. Fish oil contains two omega-3 fatty acids called *docosahexaenoic acid (DHA)* and *eicosapentaenoic acid (EPA)*. Some nuts, seeds, and vegetable oils contain *alpha-linolenic acid (ALA)*, which may be converted to DHA and EPA in the body.

Omega-3 fatty acids are also available as prescription medicines, such as Epanova and Lovaza.

How Can This Medicine Help?

Omega-3 fatty acids are thought to be good for health in many ways, including a lower risk of heart disease and improvement in cholesterol levels. Omega-3 fatty acids have been shown to slightly improve attention-deficit/hyperactivity disorder (ADHD) symptoms of inattention and hyperactivity. They are not as effective as prescription ADHD medications (such as stimulants and others), but they can be helpful. It is safe to give omega-3 fatty acids along with traditional ADHD medications to possibly improve their effect. Omega-3 fatty acids may also improve depression symptoms in adults, either when taken alone or when taken as an adjunctive (helper) treatment with an antidepressant medication. It may take as long as 3 months to see improvement when taking an omega-3 fatty acid supplement.

How Does This Medicine Work?

Omega-3 fatty acids are thought to work as *anti-inflammatory* agents by changing cell membrane properties. Inflammatory processes in the brain may contribute to mental health disorders.

How Long Does This Medicine Last?

Omega-3 fatty acids are generally taken once a day.

How Will the Doctor Monitor This Medicine?

The doctor will review your child's medical history and physical examination before starting omega-3 fatty acids. The doctor may order some blood or urine tests to be sure your child does not have a hidden medical condition. The doctor or nurse may measure your child's pulse and blood pressure before starting omega-3 fatty acids.

After the medicine is started, the doctor will want to have regular appointments with you and your child to see how the medicine is working, to see if a dose change is needed, to watch for side effects, to see if omega-3 fatty acids are still needed, and to see if any other treatment is needed. The doctor or nurse may check your child's height, weight, pulse, and blood pressure or order tests.

What Side Effects Can This Medicine Have?

Any medicine can have side effects, including an allergy to the medicine. Because each patient is different, the doctor will monitor the youth closely, especially when the medicine is started. The doctor will work with you to increase the positive effects and decrease the negative effects of the medicine. Please tell the doctor if any of the listed side effects appear or if you think that the medicine is causing any other problems. Not all of the rare or unusual side effects are listed.

Allergic Reaction

Tell the doctor in a day or two (if possible, before the next dose of medicine):

- Hives
- Itching
- Rash

Get *immediate* medical care:

- Trouble breathing or chest tightness
- Swelling of lips, tongue, or throat

Other Side Effects

Omega-3 fatty acids have few or no side effects at standard doses. The fish oil capsules can cause a fishy taste in the mouth or increased burping. Some people have an upset stomach or diarrhea. Taking the pills with meals may help with this problem.

Omega-3 fatty acids may very rarely increase bleeding in people with blood clotting disorders. If your child has a clotting or bleeding disorder, discuss this with your doctor.

Some Interactions With Other Medicines

Please note that the following are only the most likely interactions with other medicines or food.

Omega-3 fatty acids may increase the effect of warfarin (Coumadin) and increase the risk of bleeding.

What Could Happen if This Medicine Is Stopped Suddenly?

No problems should occur if omega-3 fatty acids are stopped suddenly.

How Long Will This Medicine Be Needed?

Omega-3 fatty acids may be helpful for as long as the condition they are treating is present. There is no time limit on how long they can be taken.

What Else Should I Know About This Medicine?

Omega-3 fatty acids are often taken as dietary supplements and come in a lot of different forms and different brands. Studies of omega-3 fatty acids in children used doses over a wide range but generally from 500 mg up to 1,500 mg per day. In treating ADHD, the most helpful of the fatty acids may be eicosapentaenoic acid (EPA). Doses of EPA above 500 mg may be better than lower doses. Supplements like omega-3 fatty acids that are bought over the counter or on the Internet do not have as many quality controls as prescription medications. Products labeled USP are more likely to contain exactly what their label says.

Notes

Use this space to take notes or to write down questions you want to ask the doctor.

_____

_____

_____

_____

_____

_____

_____

_____

_____

_____

chanical errors sometimes occur, we recommend that readers follow the advice of a physician who is directly involved in their care or the care of a member of their family.

From Dulcan MK, Ballard R (editors): *Helping Parents and Teachers Understand Medications for Behavioral and Emotional Problems: A Resource Book of Medication Information Handouts*, Fourth Edition. Washington, DC, American Psychiatric Publishing, 2015

Medication Information for Parents and Teachers

Oxcarbazepine—Trileptal, Oxtellar XR

General Information About Medication

Each child and adolescent is different. No one has exactly the same combination of medical and psychological problems. It is a good idea to talk with the doctor or nurse about the reasons a medicine is being used. It is very important to keep all appointments and to be in touch by telephone if you have concerns. It is important to communicate with the doctor, nurse, or therapist. An *advanced practice nurse* (APN) has additional education and training after becoming a registered nurse (RN). Your child's medication may be prescribed by a medical doctor (MD or DO) or an APN. In addition, a *physician assistant* (PA) working with a physician may prescribe certain medications. In this information sheet, "doctor" includes medical doctors as well as APNs and PAs who prescribe medication. Often a nurse (RN) will be part of the team and answer questions and give information.

It is very important that the medicine be taken exactly as the doctor instructs. However, once in a while, everyone forgets to give a medicine on time. It is a good idea to ask the doctor or nurse what to do if this happens. Do not stop or change a medicine without asking the doctor or nurse first.

If the medicine seems to stop working, it may be because it is not being taken regularly. The youth may be "cheeking" or hiding the medicine or forgetting to take it (especially at school). The doses may be too far apart or a different dose or medicine may be needed. Something at school, at home, or in the neighborhood may be upsetting the youth, or he or she may need special help for learning disabilities or tutoring. Please discuss your concerns with the doctor. **Do not just increase the dose.** It is also very important not to decrease the dose or stop the medicine without talking to the doctor first. The problem being treated may come back, or there could be uncomfortable or even dangerous results.

All medicines should be kept in a safe place, out of the reach of children, and should be supervised by an adult. If someone takes too much of a medicine, call the doctor, the poison control center, or a hospital emergency room.

Each medicine has a "generic" or chemical name. Just like laundry detergents or paper towels, some medicines are sold by more than one company under different brand names. The same medicine may be available under a generic name and several brand names. The generic medications are usually less expensive than the brand name ones. The generic medications have the same chemical formula, but they may or may not be exactly the same strength as the brand-name medications. Also, some brands of pills contain dye or other things that can cause allergic reactions. It is a good idea to talk to the doctor and the pharmacist about whether it is important to use a specific brand of medicine.

Any medicine can cause an allergic reaction. Examples are hives, itching, rashes, swelling, and trouble breathing. Even a tiny amount of a medicine can cause a reaction in patients who are allergic to that medicine. Be *sure* to talk to the doctor before restarting a medicine that has caused an allergic reaction and tell the doctor about any reactions to medicine that your child has had before.

Taking more than one medicine at the same time may cause more side effects or cause one of the medicines to not work as well. Always ask the doctor, nurse, or pharmacist before adding another

389

medicine, either prescription or bought without a prescription in a store or on the Internet. **Be sure that each doctor knows about *all* of the medicines your child is taking. Also tell the doctor about any vitamins, herbal medicines, or supplements your child may be taking.** Some of these may have side effects alone or when taken with this medication. It is a very good idea to keep a list with you of the names and doses of all medicines that your child is taking.

Everyone taking medicine should have a physical examination at least once a year.

If you think that your child may be using drugs or alcohol, please tell the doctor right away.

Pregnancy requires special care in the use of medicine. Some medicines can cause birth defects if taken by a pregnant mother. **Please tell the doctor immediately if you suspect the teenager is at risk of becoming pregnant.** The doctor may wish to discuss sexual behavior and/or birth control with your daughter.

Printed information like this applies to children and adolescents in general. If you have questions about the medicine, or if you notice changes or anything unusual, please ask the doctor or nurse. As scientific research advances, knowledge increases and advice changes. Even experts do not always agree. Many medicines have not been "approved" by the U.S. Food and Drug Administration (FDA) for use in children or use for particular problems. For this reason, use of the medicine for a problem or age group often is not listed in the *Physicians' Desk Reference.* This does not necessarily mean that the medicine is dangerous or does not work, only that the company that makes the medicine has not received permission to advertise the medicine for use in children. Companies often do not apply for this permission because it is expensive to do the tests needed to apply for approval for use in children. Once a medication is approved by the FDA for any purpose, a doctor is allowed to prescribe it according to research and clinical experience.

Note to Teachers

It is a good idea to talk with the parent(s) about the reason(s) that a medication is being used. If the parent(s) sign consent to release information, it is often helpful for you to talk with the doctor. If the parent(s) give permission, the doctor may ask you to fill out rating forms about your experience with the student's behavior, feelings, academic performance, and medication side effects. This information is very useful in selecting and monitoring medication treatment. If you have observations that you think are important, do not hesitate to share these with the student's parent(s) and treating clinicians (with parental consent).

It is very important that the medicine be taken exactly as the doctor instructs. However, everyone forgets to give a medicine on time once in a while. It is a good idea to ask the parent(s) in advance what to do if this happens. Do not stop or change the time you are giving a medicine at school without parental permission. If a medication is to be taken with food, but lunchtime or snack time changes, be sure to notify the parent(s) so appropriate adjustments can be made.

All medicines should be kept in a secure place and should be supervised by an adult. If someone takes too much of a medicine, follow your school procedure for an urgent medical problem.

Taking medicine is a private matter and is best managed discreetly and confidentially. It is important to be sensitive to the student's feelings about taking medicine.

If you suspect that the student is using drugs or alcohol, please tell the parent(s) or a school counselor right away.

Please tell the parent(s) or school nurse if you suspect medication side effects.

Modifications of the classroom environment or assignments may be useful in addition to medication. The student may need to be evaluated for additional help or a 504 plan or an Individualized Education Plan for learning problems or emotional or behavioral issues.

Any expression of suicidal thoughts or feelings or self-harm by a child or adolescent is a signal of distress and should be taken seriously. These behaviors should not be dismissed as "attention seeking." School procedures for safety issues should be followed.

What Is Oxcarbazepine (Trileptal, Oxtellar XR)?

Oxcarbazepine was first used to treat seizures (fits, convulsions), so it is sometimes called an *anticonvulsant* or *antiepileptic*. Now it is also used for behavioral problems or bipolar disorder whether or not the patient has seizures. It also may be used when the patient has a history of severe mood changes, sometimes called *mood swings*. When used for emotional or behavioral symptoms, this medicine is more commonly called a *mood stabilizer*.

Oxcarbazepine comes in brand name Trileptal tablets and liquid and brand name Oxtellar XR extended-release tablets.

How Can This Medicine Help?

Oxcarbazepine can reduce aggression, anger, and severe mood swings. It also can treat mania.

How Does This Medicine Work?

Oxcarbazepine is thought to work by stabilizing a part of the brain cell (the cell membrane or envelope) and decreasing the spread of abnormal electrical impulses in the brain cells.

How Long Does This Medicine Last?

Trileptal needs to be taken twice a day. Oxtellar XR may be taken only once a day.

How Will the Doctor Monitor This Medicine?

The doctor will review your child's medical history and physical examination before starting oxcarbazepine. The doctor may order blood or urine tests to be sure your child does not have a hidden kidney condition that would make it unsafe to use this medicine. The doctor or nurse will measure your child's height, weight, pulse, and blood pressure before starting oxcarbazepine.

After the medicine is started, the doctor will want to have regular appointments with you and your child to see how the medicine is working, to see if a dose change is needed, to watch for side effects, to see if oxcarbazepine is still needed, and to see if any other treatment is needed. The doctor or nurse may check your child's height, weight, pulse, and blood pressure. The doctor will need to order blood tests every month or so to make sure that the medicine is at the right dose and to check for side effects, such as a decreased level of sodium in the blood. Blood should be drawn first thing in the morning, 10–12 hours after the evening dose and before the morning dose. Many things can change the levels of oxcarbazepine, so tests may be needed every week when the dose of this or other medicines is being changed.

What Side Effects Can This Medicine Have?

Any medicine can have side effects, including an allergy to the medicine. Because each patient is different, the doctor will monitor the youth closely, especially when the medicine is started. The doctor will work with you to increase the positive effects and decrease the negative effects of the medicine. Please tell the doctor if any of the listed side effects appear or if you think that the medicine is causing any other problems. Not all of the rare or unusual side effects are listed.

Side effects are most common after starting the medicine or after a dose increase. Many side effects can be avoided or lessened by starting with a very low dose and increasing it slowly—ask the doctor.

Allergic Reaction

Tell the doctor in a day or two (if possible, before the next dose of medicine):

- Hives
- Itching
- Rash

Stop the medicine and get *immediate* medical care:

- Trouble breathing or chest tightness
- Swelling of lips, tongue, or throat

General Side Effects

Tell the doctor within a week or two:

- Acne
- Alopecia (hair loss)

The following side effects are more common when first starting the medicine:

- Daytime sleepiness—Do not allow your child to drive, ride a bicycle or motorcycle, or operate machinery if this happens.
- Dizziness
- Nausea or upset stomach—Have your child take the medicine with food.
- Headaches

The following side effects are more common at higher doses:

- Double or blurred vision
- Jerky, side-to-side eye movements (nystagmus)
- Clumsiness or decreased coordination

Side Effects Requiring Prompt Medical Attention

Call the doctor within a day or two:

- Problems with attention or concentration
- New or increased anxiety or nervousness
- New or increased moodiness
- Slowing of movements and/or speech

Very Rare, but Possibly Dangerous, Side Effects

Call the doctor *immediately*:

- Worsening or new suicidal thoughts or behaviors
- Agitation
- Confusion
- Skin rash with fever
- Feeling sick or unusually tired
- Loss of appetite
- Persistent nausea
- Vomiting
- Yellowing of the skin or eyes
- Headaches that do not go away
- Dark urine or pale bowel movements
- Swelling of the legs or eyes
- Greatly increased thirst
- Greatly increased or decreased urination (peeing)

Some Interactions With Other Medicines or Food

Please note that the following are only the most likely interactions with other medicines or food.

Caffeine may increase side effects.

Oxcarbazepine interacts with many other medicines. Taking it with another medicine may make one or both not work as well or may cause more side effects. Be sure that each doctor knows about *all* the medicines your child is taking.

Oxcarbazepine may decrease the blood levels of birth control pills (oral contraceptives) so that they do not work as well—this may lead to accidental pregnancy. An alternative form of birth control may be needed.

Carbamazepine (Tegretol) and divalproex (Depakote) may lower the blood levels of oxcarbazepine and make it not work as well.

What Could Happen if This Medicine Is Stopped Suddenly?

Stopping oxcarbazepine suddenly may cause uncomfortable withdrawal symptoms. If the person is taking oxcarbazepine for epilepsy (seizures), stopping the medicine suddenly could lead to an increase in very dangerous seizures (convulsions).

How Long Will This Medicine Be Needed?

The length of time a person needs to take oxcarbazepine depends on what problem is being treated. For example, someone with an impulse control disorder usually takes the medicine only until behavioral therapy begins to work. Someone with bipolar disorder may need to take the medicine for many years. Please ask the doctor about the length of treatment needed.

What Else Should I Know About This Medicine?

Oxcarbazepine increases the risk of sunburn. Be sure that your child wears sunscreen or protective clothing or stays out of the sun.

Taking oxcarbazepine with food may decrease stomach upset.

Oxcarbazepine is processed by the kidneys. Great caution should be used in patients with kidney problems.

Keep the medicine in a safe place under close supervision. An overdose can be very dangerous to small children. Keep the pill container tightly closed and in a dry place, away from bathrooms, showers, and humidifiers.

Notes

Use this space to take notes or to write down questions you want to ask the doctor.

_____

_____

_____

_____

_____

_____

_____

———————————————————————————

———————————————————————————

———————————————————————————

———————————————————————————

———————————————————————————

From Dulcan MK, Ballard R (editors): *Helping Parents and Teachers Understand Medications for Behavioral and Emotional Problems: A Resource Book of Medication Information Handouts*, Fourth Edition. Washington, DC, American Psychiatric Publishing, 2015

Medication Information for Parents and Teachers

Paliperidone—Invega

General Information About Medication

Each child and adolescent is different. No one has exactly the same combination of medical and psychological problems. It is a good idea to talk with the doctor or nurse about the reasons a medicine is being used. It is very important to keep all appointments and to be in touch by telephone if you have concerns. It is important to communicate with the doctor, nurse, or therapist. An *advanced practice nurse* (APN) has additional education and training after becoming a registered nurse (RN). Your child's medication may be prescribed by a medical doctor (MD or DO) or an APN. In addition, a *physician assistant* (PA) working with a physician may prescribe certain medications. In this information sheet, "doctor" includes medical doctors as well as APNs and PAs who prescribe medication. Often a nurse (RN) will be part of the team and answer questions and give information.

It is very important that the medicine be taken exactly as the doctor instructs. However, once in a while, everyone forgets to give a medicine on time. It is a good idea to ask the doctor or nurse what to do if this happens. Do not stop or change a medicine without asking the doctor or nurse first.

If the medicine seems to stop working, it may be because it is not being taken regularly. The youth may be "cheeking" or hiding the medicine or forgetting to take it (especially at school). The doses may be too far apart or a different dose or medicine may be needed. Something at school, at home, or in the neighborhood may be upsetting the youth, or he or she may need special help for learning disabilities or tutoring. Please discuss your concerns with the doctor. **Do not just increase the dose.** It is also very important not to decrease the dose or stop the medicine without talking to the doctor first. The problem being treated may come back, or there could be uncomfortable or even dangerous results.

All medicines should be kept in a safe place, out of the reach of children, and should be supervised by an adult. If someone takes too much of a medicine, call the doctor, the poison control center, or a hospital emergency room.

Each medicine has a "generic" or chemical name. Just like laundry detergents or paper towels, some medicines are sold by more than one company under different brand names. The same medicine may be available under a generic name and several brand names. The generic medications are usually less expensive than the brand name ones. The generic medications have the same chemical formula, but they may or may not be exactly the same strength as the brand-name medications. Also, some brands of pills contain dye or other things that can cause allergic reactions. It is a good idea to talk to the doctor and the pharmacist about whether it is important to use a specific brand of medicine.

Any medicine can cause an allergic reaction. Examples are hives, itching, rashes, swelling, and trouble breathing. Even a tiny amount of a medicine can cause a reaction in patients who are allergic to that medicine. Be *sure* to talk to the doctor before restarting a medicine that has caused an allergic reaction and tell the doctor about any reactions to medicine that your child has had before.

Taking more than one medicine at the same time may cause more side effects or cause one of the medicines to not work as well. Always ask the doctor, nurse, or pharmacist before adding another medicine, either prescription or bought without a prescription in a store or on the Internet. Be sure

that each doctor knows about *all* of the medicines your child is taking. Also tell the doctor about any vitamins, herbal medicines, or supplements your child may be taking. Some of these may have side effects alone or when taken with this medication. It is a very good idea to keep a list with you of the names and doses of all medicines that your child is taking.

Everyone taking medicine should have a physical examination at least once a year.

If you think that your child may be using drugs or alcohol, please tell the doctor right away.

Pregnancy requires special care in the use of medicine. Some medicines can cause birth defects if taken by a pregnant mother. **Please tell the doctor immediately if you suspect the teenager is at risk of becoming pregnant.** The doctor may wish to discuss sexual behavior and/or birth control with your daughter.

Printed information like this applies to children and adolescents in general. If you have questions about the medicine, or if you notice changes or anything unusual, please ask the doctor or nurse. As scientific research advances, knowledge increases and advice changes. Even experts do not always agree. Many medicines have not been "approved" by the U.S. Food and Drug Administration (FDA) for use in children or use for particular problems. For this reason, use of the medicine for a problem or age group often is not listed in the *Physicians' Desk Reference*. This does not necessarily mean that the medicine is dangerous or does not work, only that the company that makes the medicine has not received permission to advertise the medicine for use in children. Companies often do not apply for this permission because it is expensive to do the tests needed to apply for approval for use in children. Once a medication is approved by the FDA for any purpose, a doctor is allowed to prescribe it according to research and clinical experience.

Note to Teachers

It is a good idea to talk with the parent(s) about the reason(s) that a medication is being used. If the parent(s) sign consent to release information, it is often helpful for you to talk with the doctor. If the parent(s) give permission, the doctor may ask you to fill out rating forms about your experience with the student's behavior, feelings, academic performance, and medication side effects. This information is very useful in selecting and monitoring medication treatment. If you have observations that you think are important, do not hesitate to share these with the student's parent(s) and treating clinicians (with parental consent).

It is very important that the medicine be taken exactly as the doctor instructs. However, everyone forgets to give a medicine on time once in a while. It is a good idea to ask the parent(s) in advance what to do if this happens. Do not stop or change the time you are giving a medicine at school without parental permission. If a medication is to be taken with food, but lunchtime or snack time changes, be sure to notify the parent(s) so appropriate adjustments can be made.

All medicines should be kept in a secure place and should be supervised by an adult. If someone takes too much of a medicine, follow your school procedure for an urgent medical problem.

Taking medicine is a private matter and is best managed discreetly and confidentially. It is important to be sensitive to the student's feelings about taking medicine.

If you suspect that the student is using drugs or alcohol, please tell the parent(s) or a school counselor right away.

Please tell the parent(s) or school nurse if you suspect medication side effects.

Modifications of the classroom environment or assignments may be useful in addition to medication. The student may need to be evaluated for additional help or a 504 plan or an Individualized Education Plan for learning problems or emotional or behavioral issues.

Any expression of suicidal thoughts or feelings or self-harm by a child or adolescent is a signal of distress and should be taken seriously. These behaviors should not be dismissed as "attention seeking." School procedures for safety issues should be followed.

What Is Paliperidone (Invega)?

This medicine is called an *atypical* or *second-generation antipsychotic*. It is sometimes called an *atypical psychotropic agent* or simply an *atypical*. It comes in brand name Invega long-acting tablets and Invega Sustenna, a long-acting injection (shot).

How Can This Medicine Help?

Paliperidone is used to treat psychosis, such as in schizophrenia, mania, or very severe depression. It can reduce *positive symptoms* such as hallucinations (hearing voices or seeing things that are not there); delusions (troubling beliefs that other people do not share); agitation; and very unusual thinking, speech, and behavior. It is also used to lessen the *negative symptoms* of schizophrenia, such as lack of interest in doing things (apathy), lack of motivation, social withdrawal, and lack of energy.

Paliperidone may be used as a *mood stabilizer* in patients with bipolar disorder or severe mood swings. It can reduce mania and may be able to help maintain a stable mood.

Sometimes paliperidone is used to reduce severe aggression or very serious behavioral problems in young people with conduct disorder, intellectual disability, or autism spectrum disorder.

Paliperidone may be used for behavior problems after a head injury.

This medicine is very powerful and is used to treat very serious problems or symptoms that other medicines do not help. Be patient; the positive effects of this medicine may not appear for 2–3 weeks.

How Does This Medicine Work?

Cells in the brain communicate using chemicals called *neurotransmitters*. Too much or too little of these substances in parts of the brain can cause problems. Paliperidone works by blocking the action of two of these neurotransmitters—*dopamine and serotonin*—in certain areas of the brain.

How Long Does This Medicine Last?

Paliperidone is usually taken once a day. Invega Sustenna lasts for 4 weeks, but when it is first started, it must be given in two doses 1 week apart.

How Will the Doctor Monitor This Medicine?

The doctor will review your child's medical history and physical examination before starting paliperidone. The doctor may order blood or urine tests to be sure your child does not have a hidden medical condition that would make it unsafe to use this medicine. The doctor or nurse may measure your child's pulse and blood pressure before starting paliperidone. The doctor may order other tests, such as baseline tests for blood sugar and cholesterol or an ECG (electrocardiogram or heart rhythm test).

Be sure to tell the doctor if anyone in the family has diabetes, high blood pressure, high cholesterol, or heart disease.

Before your child starts taking paliperidone and every so often afterward, a test such as the Abnormal Involuntary Movement Scale (AIMS) may be used to check your child's tongue, legs, and arms for unusual movements that could be caused by the medicine.

After the medicine is started, the doctor will want to have regular appointments with you and your child to see how the medicine is working, to see if a dose change is needed, to watch for side effects, to see if paliperidone is still needed, and to see if any other treatment is needed. The doctor or nurse will check your child's height, weight, pulse, and blood pressure and watch for abnormal movements. Sometimes blood tests are needed to watch for diabetes or increased cholesterol.

What Side Effects Can This Medicine Have?

Any medicine can have side effects, including an allergy to the medicine. Because each patient is different, the doctor will monitor the youth closely, especially when the medicine is started. The doctor will work with you to increase the positive effects and decrease the negative effects of the medicine. Please tell the doctor if any of the listed side effects appear or if you think that the medicine is causing any other problems. Not all of the rare or unusual side effects are listed.

Side effects are most common after starting the medicine or after a dose increase. Many side effects can be avoided or lessened by starting with a very low dose and increasing it slowly—ask the doctor.

Allergic Reaction

Tell the doctor in a day or two (if possible, before the next dose of medicine):

- Hives
- Itching
- Rash

Stop the medicine and get *immediate* medical care:

- Trouble breathing or chest tightness
- Swelling of lips, tongue, or throat

Common, but Not Usually Serious, Side Effects

Discuss the following side effects with your child's doctor when convenient. These side effects often can be helped by lowering the dose of medicine, changing the times medicine is taken, or adding another medicine.

- Daytime sleepiness or tiredness—Do not allow your child to drive, ride a bicycle or motorcycle, or operate machinery if this happens. This problem may be lessened by taking the medicine at bedtime.
- Dry mouth—Have your child try using sugar-free gum or candy.
- Constipation—Encourage your child to drink more fluids and eat high-fiber foods; if necessary, the doctor may recommend a fiber medicine such as Benefiber or a stool softener such as Colace or mineral oil.
- Dizziness—This side effect is worse when the child stands up quickly, especially when getting out of bed in the morning; try having the child stand up slowly.
- Increased appetite

- Weight gain—Seek nutritional counseling; provide your child with low-calorie snacks and encourage regular exercise.
- Increased risk of sunburn—Have your child wear sunscreen or protective clothing or stay out of the sun.
- Nausea
- Vomiting
- Insomnia (trouble sleeping)

Less Common, but Not Usually Serious, Side Effects

Discuss the following side effects with your child's doctor when convenient. These side effects often can be helped by lowering the dose of medicine, changing the times medicine is taken, or adding another medicine.

- Drooling
- Increased restlessness or inability to sit still
- Shaking of hands and fingers
- Decreased or slowed movement and decreased facial expressions
- Decreased sexual interest or ability
- Changes in menstrual cycle
- Increase in breast size or discharge from the breasts (in both boys and girls)—This may go away with time.

Less Common, but Potentially Serious, Side Effects

Call the doctor *immediately*:

- Stiffness of the tongue, jaw, neck, back, or legs
- Seizure (fit, convulsion)—This is more common in people with a history of seizures or head injury.
- Increased thirst, frequent urination (having to go to the bathroom often), lethargy, tiredness, dizziness, and blurred vision—These could be signs of diabetes, especially if your child is overweight or there is a family history of diabetes. **Talk to a doctor within a day.**

Very Rare, but Serious, Side Effects

- Extreme stiffness or lack of movement, very high fever, mental confusion, irregular pulse rate, or eye pain—**This is a medical emergency. Go to an emergency room right away.**
- Sudden stiffness and inability to breathe or swallow—**Go to an emergency room or call 911.** Tell the paramedics, nurses, and doctors that the patient is taking paliperidone. Other medicines can be used to treat this problem quickly.

What Else Should I Know About Side Effects?

Most side effects lessen over time. If they are troublesome, talk with your child's doctor. Some side effects can be decreased by taking a smaller dose of medicine, by stopping the medicine, by changing to another medicine, or by adding another medicine.

Many young people who take paliperidone gain weight. The weight gain may be from increased appetite and also from ways that the medicine changes how the body processes food. Paliperidone may also change the way that the body handles glucose (sugar) and cause high levels of blood sugar (*hyperglycemia*). People who take paliperidone, especially those who gain a lot of weight, might be at increased risk of developing *diabetes* and of having increased fats (*lipids—cholesterol and triglycerides*) in their blood. Over time, both diabetes and increased fats in the blood may lead to heart disease, stroke, and other complications. The FDA has put warnings on all atypical agents about the increased risks of hyperglycemia, diabetes, and increased blood cholesterol and triglycerides when taking one of these medicines. It is much easier to prevent weight gain than to lose weight later. When your child first starts taking paliperidone, it is a good idea to be sure that he or she eats a well-balanced diet without "junk food" and with healthy snacks like fruits and vegetables, not sweets or fried foods. He or she should drink water or skim milk, not pop, sodas, soft drinks, or sugary juices. Regular exercise is important for maintaining a healthy weight (and may also help with sleep).

The medicine may increase the level of *prolactin*, a natural hormone made in the part of the brain called the *pituitary*. This may cause side effects such as breast tenderness or swelling or production of milk in both boys and girls. It also may interfere with sexual functioning in teenage boys and with regular menstrual cycles (periods) in teenage girls. A blood test can measure the level of prolactin. If these side effects do not go away and are troublesome, talk with your child's doctor about substituting another medicine for paliperidone.

One very rare side effect that may not go away is *tardive dyskinesia* (or TD). Patients with tardive dyskinesia have involuntary movements (movements that they cannot help making) of the body, especially the mouth and tongue. The patient may look as though he or she is making faces over and over again. Jerky movements of the arms, legs, or body may occur. There may be fine, wormlike, or sudden repeated movements of the tongue, or the person may appear to be chewing something or smacking or puckering his or her lips. The fingers may look as though they are rolling something. If you notice any unusual movements, be sure to tell the doctor. The doctor may use the AIMS test to look for these movements.

Neuroleptic malignant syndrome is a very rare side effect that can lead to death. The symptoms are severe muscle stiffness, high fever, increased heart rate and blood pressure, irregular heartbeat (pulse), and sweating. It may lead to unconsciousness. If you suspect this, **call 911 or go to an emergency room right away.**

Sometimes this medicine can cause a *dystonic reaction*. This is a sudden stiffening of the muscles, most often in the jaw, neck, tongue, face, or shoulders. If this happens, and your child is not having trouble breathing, you may give a dose of diphenhydramine (Benadryl). Follow the dose instructions on the package for your child's age. This should relax the muscles in a few minutes. Then call your doctor to tell him or her what happened. If the muscles do not relax, take your child to the emergency department.

Some Interactions With Other Medicines or Food

Please note that the following are only the most likely interactions with other medicines or food.

Paliperidone may be taken with or without food.

Carbamazepine (Tegretol) can decrease the levels of paliperidone so that it does not work as well.

Heart problems are more common if other medicines that affect the heart are being taken as well. Be sure to tell all your child's doctors and your pharmacist about all medications your child is taking.

It is better to limit drinks with caffeine (coffee, tea, soft drinks) because caffeine works in the opposite way from this medicine, and the positive effects might be decreased

What Could Happen if This Medicine Is Stopped Suddenly?

Involuntary movements, or *withdrawal dyskinesias*, may appear within 1–4 weeks of lowering the dose or stopping the medicine. Usually these go away, but they can last for days to months. If this medicine is stopped suddenly, emotional disturbance (such as irritability, nervousness, moodiness, or oppositional behavior) or physical problems (such as stomachache, loss of appetite, nausea, vomiting, diarrhea, sweating, indigestion, trouble sleeping, trembling, or shaking) may appear. These problems usually last only a few days to a few weeks. If they happen, you should tell your child's doctor. The medicine dose may need to be lowered more slowly (tapered). Always check with the doctor before stopping a medicine.

How Long Will This Medicine Be Needed?

How long your child will need to take this medicine depends partly on the reason that it was prescribed. Some problems last for only a few months, whereas others last much longer. It is important to ask the doctor whether medicine is still needed, especially with medicines as powerful as this one. Every few months, you should discuss with your child's doctor the reasons for using the medicine and whether the medicine may be stopped or the dose lowered.

What Else Should I Know About This Medicine?

There are other medicines that are used for the same kinds of problems. If your child is having bad side effects or the medicine does not seem to be working, ask the doctor if another medicine might work as well or better and have fewer side effects for your child. Each person reacts differently to medicines.

Taking this medicine could make overheating or heatstroke more likely. Have your child decrease activity in hot weather, stay out of the sun, and drink water to prevent this.

Notes

Use this space to take notes or to write down questions you want to ask the doctor.

_____

_____

_____

_____

_____

_____

_____

_____

_____

_____

_____

_____

Medication Information for Parents and Teachers

Paroxetine—Paxil, Pexeva, Brisdelle, Paxil CR

General Information About Medication

Each child and adolescent is different. No one has exactly the same combination of medical and psychological problems. It is a good idea to talk with the doctor or nurse about the reasons a medicine is being used. It is very important to keep all appointments and to be in touch by telephone if you have concerns. It is important to communicate with the doctor, nurse, or therapist. An *advanced practice nurse* (APN) has additional education and training after becoming a registered nurse (RN). Your child's medication may be prescribed by a medical doctor (MD or DO) or an APN. In addition, a *physician assistant* (PA) working with a physician may prescribe certain medications. In this information sheet, "doctor" includes medical doctors as well as APNs and PAs who prescribe medication. Often a nurse (RN) will be part of the team and answer questions and give information.

It is very important that the medicine be taken exactly as the doctor instructs. However, once in a while, everyone forgets to give a medicine on time. It is a good idea to ask the doctor or nurse what to do if this happens. Do not stop or change a medicine without asking the doctor or nurse first.

If the medicine seems to stop working, it may be because it is not being taken regularly. The youth may be "cheeking" or hiding the medicine or forgetting to take it (especially at school). The doses may be too far apart or a different dose or medicine may be needed. Something at school, at home, or in the neighborhood may be upsetting the youth, or he or she may need special help for learning disabilities or tutoring. Please discuss your concerns with the doctor. **Do not just increase the dose.** It is also very important not to decrease the dose or stop the medicine without talking to the doctor first. The problem being treated may come back, or there could be uncomfortable or even dangerous results.

All medicines should be kept in a safe place, out of the reach of children, and should be supervised by an adult. If someone takes too much of a medicine, call the doctor, the poison control center, or a hospital emergency room.

Each medicine has a "generic" or chemical name. Just like laundry detergents or paper towels, some medicines are sold by more than one company under different brand names. The same medicine may be available under a generic name and several brand names. The generic medications are usually less expensive than the brand name ones. The generic medications have the same chemical formula, but they may or may not be exactly the same strength as the brand-name medications. Also, some brands of pills contain dye or other things that can cause allergic reactions. It is a good idea to talk to the doctor and the pharmacist about whether it is important to use a specific brand of medicine.

Any medicine can cause an allergic reaction. Examples are hives, itching, rashes, swelling, and trouble breathing. Even a tiny amount of a medicine can cause a reaction in patients who are allergic to that medicine. Be *sure* to talk to the doctor before restarting a medicine that has caused an allergic reaction and tell the doctor about any reactions to medicine that your child has had before.

Taking more than one medicine at the same time may cause more side effects or cause one of the medicines to not work as well. Always ask the doctor, nurse, or pharmacist before adding another medicine, either prescription or bought without a prescription in a store or on the Internet. Be sure that each doctor knows about *all* of the medicines your child is taking. Also tell the doctor about any vitamins, herbal medicines, or supplements your child may be taking. Some of these may have side effects alone or when taken with this medication. It is a very good idea to keep a list with you of the names and doses of all medicines that your child is taking.

Everyone taking medicine should have a physical examination at least once a year.

If you think that your child may be using drugs or alcohol, please tell the doctor right away.

Pregnancy requires special care in the use of medicine. Some medicines can cause birth defects if taken by a pregnant mother. **Please tell the doctor immediately if you suspect the teenager is at risk of becoming pregnant.** The doctor may wish to discuss sexual behavior and/or birth control with your daughter.

Printed information like this applies to children and adolescents in general. If you have questions about the medicine, or if you notice changes or anything unusual, please ask the doctor or nurse. As scientific research advances, knowledge increases and advice changes. Even experts do not always agree. Many medicines have not been "approved" by the U.S. Food and Drug Administration (FDA) for use in children or use for particular problems. For this reason, use of the medicine for a problem or age group often is not listed in the *Physicians' Desk Reference*. This does not necessarily mean that the medicine is dangerous or does not work, only that the company that makes the medicine has not received permission to advertise the medicine for use in children. Companies often do not apply for this permission because it is expensive to do the tests needed to apply for approval for use in children. Once a medication is approved by the FDA for any purpose, a doctor is allowed to prescribe it according to research and clinical experience.

Note to Teachers

It is a good idea to talk with the parent(s) about the reason(s) that a medication is being used. If the parent(s) sign consent to release information, it is often helpful for you to talk with the doctor. If the parent(s) give permission, the doctor may ask you to fill out rating forms about your experience with the student's behavior, feelings, academic performance, and medication side effects. This information is very useful in selecting and monitoring medication treatment. If you have observations that you think are important, do not hesitate to share these with the student's parent(s) and treating clinicians (with parental consent).

It is very important that the medicine be taken exactly as the doctor instructs. However, everyone forgets to give a medicine on time once in a while. It is a good idea to ask the parent(s) in advance what to do if this happens. Do not stop or change the time you are giving a medicine at school without parental permission. If a medication is to be taken with food, but lunchtime or snack time changes, be sure to notify the parent(s) so appropriate adjustments can be made.

All medicines should be kept in a secure place and should be supervised by an adult. If someone takes too much of a medicine, follow your school procedure for an urgent medical problem.

Taking medicine is a private matter and is best managed discreetly and confidentially. It is important to be sensitive to the student's feelings about taking medicine.

If you suspect that the student is using drugs or alcohol, please tell the parent(s) or a school counselor right away.

Please tell the parent(s) or school nurse if you suspect medication side effects.

Modifications of the classroom environment or assignments may be useful in addition to medication. The student may need to be evaluated for additional help or a 504 plan or an Individualized Education Plan for learning problems or emotional or behavioral issues.

Any expression of suicidal thoughts or feelings or self-harm by a child or adolescent is a signal of distress and should be taken seriously. These behaviors should not be dismissed as "attention seeking." School procedures for safety issues should be followed.

What Is Paroxetine (Paxil, Pexeva, Bridelle, Paxil CR)?

Paroxetine (brand name Paxil) is an antidepressant known as a *selective serotonin reuptake inhibitor* (SSRI). It comes in generic and brand name Paxil and Pexeva tablets and Paxil CR and generic extended-release forms. It also comes in brand name Paxil liquid form. The controlled-release tablets do not last longer, but the medicine is released more slowly, and this may lessen side effects. It also comes in Brisdelle brand capsules, which are used for "hot flashes" in women after menopause.

How Can This Medicine Help?

Paroxetine is used to treat depression and anxiety disorders such as obsessive-compulsive disorder (OCD), posttraumatic stress disorder (PTSD), panic disorder, separation anxiety disorder, selective mutism, social anxiety disorder, and generalized anxiety disorder.

How Does This Medicine Work?

Paroxetine increases the amount of a *neurotransmitter* called *serotonin* in certain parts of the brain. People with emotional and behavioral problems, such as depression and anxiety, may have low levels of serotonin in certain parts of the brain. SSRIs such as paroxetine help by increasing the action of brain serotonin to more normal levels.

How Long Does This Medicine Last?

Paroxetine can be taken only once a day for most people.

How Will the Doctor Monitor This Medicine?

The doctor will review your child's medical history and physical examination before starting paroxetine. The doctor may order some blood or urine tests to be sure your child does not have a hidden medical condition that would make it unsafe to use this medicine. Extra care is needed when using SSRIs in youth with seizures (epilepsy); heart, liver, or kidney problems; or diabetes. The doctor or nurse may measure your child's pulse, blood pressure, and weight before starting the medicine.

Be sure to tell the doctor if your child or anyone in the family has bipolar disorder or has tried to kill himself or herself.

After the medicine is started, the doctor will want to have regular appointments with you and your child to see how the medicine is working, to see if a dose change is needed, to watch for side effects, to see if paroxetine is still needed, and to see if any other treatment is needed. The doctor or nurse may check your child's height, weight, pulse, and blood pressure.

Before using medicine and at times afterward, the doctor may ask your child to fill out a rating scale about depression or anxiety to help see how your child is doing.

What Side Effects Can This Medicine Have?

Any medicine can have side effects, including an allergy to the medicine. Because each patient is different, the doctor will monitor the youth closely, especially when the medicine is started. The doctor will work with you to increase the positive effects and decrease the negative effects of the medicine. Please tell the doctor if any of the listed side effects appear or if you think that the medicine is causing any other problems. Not all of the rare or unusual side effects are listed.

Side effects are most common after starting the medicine or after a dose increase. Many side effects can be avoided or lessened by starting with a very low dose and increasing it slowly—ask the doctor.

Allergic Reaction

Tell the doctor in a day or two (if possible, before the next dose of medicine):

- Hives
- Itching
- Rash

Stop the medicine and get *immediate* medical care:

- Trouble breathing or chest tightness
- Swelling of lips, tongue, or throat

Common Side Effects

Tell the doctor within a week or two, or sooner if the problems are getting worse:

- Nausea, upset stomach, vomiting
- Diarrhea or excessive gas
- Dry mouth—Have your child try using sugar-free gum or candy.
- Constipation—Encourage your child to drink more fluids and eat high-fiber foods; if necessary, the doctor may recommend a fiber medicine such as Benefiber or a stool softener such as Colace or mineral oil.
- Headache
- Anxiety or nervousness
- Insomnia (trouble sleeping)
- Restlessness, increased activity level
- Daytime sleepiness or tiredness—Do not allow your child to drive, ride a bicycle or motorcycle, or operate machinery if this side effect is present.
- Dizziness—This side effect is worse when the child stands up quickly, especially when getting out of bed in the morning; try having the child stand up slowly.

- Tremor (shakiness)
- Excessive sweating
- Apathy, lack of interest in school or friends—This may happen after an initial good response to treatment.
- Decreased sexual interest, trouble with sexual functioning
- Weight gain
- Weight loss

Less Common, but More Serious, Side Effects

Call the doctor within a day or two:

- Significant suicidal thoughts or self-injurious behavior
- Increased activity, rapid speech, feeling "speeded up," decreased need for sleep, being very excited or irritable (cranky), agitation, acting out of character
- Bleeding, such as bruising or nosebleeds, or bleeding with surgery

Serious Side Effects

Call the doctor *immediately* or go to the nearest emergency room:

- Seizure (fit, convulsion)
- Stiffness, high fever, confusion, tremors (shaking)
- Overheating or heatstroke—Prevent by decreasing activity in hot weather, staying out of the sun, and drinking water.

Serotonin Syndrome

A very serious side effect called *serotonin syndrome* can happen when certain kinds of medicines (including SSRI antidepressants, clomipramine, and other medicines, such as triptans for migraine headaches, buspirone, linezolid, tramadol, or St. John's wort) are taken by the same person. Very rarely, serotonin syndrome can happen at high doses of just one medicine. The early signs are restlessness, confusion, shaking, skin turning red, sweating, muscle stiffness, sweating, and jerking of muscles. If you see these symptoms, stop the medicine and send or take the youth to an emergency room right away.

Some Interactions With Other Medicines or Food

Please note that the following are only the most likely interactions with other medicines or food.

Paroxetine interacts with many other prescription and over-the-counter medicines, including some antibiotics and other psychiatric medicines. It is especially important to tell the doctor and pharmacist about all of the medicines your child is taking or has taken in the past few months, including over-the-counter and herbal medicines. Sometimes one medicine can increase or decrease the blood level of another medicine, so that different doses are needed. Erythromycin and similar antibiotics, as well as antifungal agents such as ketoconazole, may increase levels of paroxetine and increase side effects. Paroxetine may increase the heart side effects of pimozide (Orap), so those two medicines should not be taken by the same person. Tryptophan or the herbal medicine St. John's Wort also increases serotonin and can cause serious side effects if taken with paroxetine. Taking paroxetine with aspirin, nonsteroidal anti-inflammatory drugs (NSAIDs; medications including ibuprofen or naproxen), or anticoagulant medications (including warfarin) increases risk of abnormal bleeding.

It can be *very dangerous* to take an SSRI at the same time as or even within a month of taking another type of medicine called a *monoamine oxidase inhibitor* (MAOI), such as selegiline (Eldepryl), phenelzine (Nardil), tranylcypromine (Parnate), or isocarboxazid (Marplan).

Paroxetine can be taken with or without food.

Caffeine may increase side effects.

What Could Happen if This Medicine Is Stopped Suddenly?

No known serious medical effects occur if paroxetine is stopped suddenly, but there may be uncomfortable feelings, which should be avoided if possible. Your child might have trouble sleeping, nervousness, irritability, dizziness, and flu-like symptoms. Ask the doctor before stopping paroxetine or if these symptoms happen while the dose is being decreased.

How Long Will This Medicine Be Needed?

Paroxetine may take up to 1–2 months to reach its full effect. If your child has a good response to paroxetine, it is a good idea to continue the medicine for at least 6–12 months. It is important to review this with your doctor.

What Else Should I Know About This Medicine?

The controlled-release capsules must be swallowed whole and must not be crushed, broken, or chewed.

In youth who have bipolar disorder or who may be at risk for bipolar disorder, any antidepressant medicine may increase the risk of hypomania or mania (excitement, agitation, increased activity, decreased sleep).

In hot weather, make sure your child drinks enough water or other liquids and does not get overheated.

Sometimes, after a person has improved while taking paroxetine, he or she loses interest in school or friends or just stops trying. Please tell your child's doctor if this happens—it may be a side effect of the medicine. A lower dose or a different medicine may be needed.

Store the medicine away from sunlight, heat, moisture, and humidity.

Black Box Antidepressant Warning

In 2004, an advisory committee to the FDA decided that there might be an increased risk of suicidal behavior for some youth taking medicines called *antidepressants*. In the research studies that the committee reviewed, about 3%–4% of youth with depression who took an antidepressant medicine—and 1%–2% of youth with depression who took a placebo (pill without active medicine)—talked about suicidal thoughts (thinking about killing themselves or wishing they were dead) or did something to harm themselves. This means that almost twice as many youth who were taking an antidepressant to treat their depression talked about suicide or had suicidal behavior compared with youth with depression who were taking inactive medicine. There were *no* completed suicides in any of these research studies, which included more than 4,000 children and adolescents.

For youth being treated for anxiety, there was no difference in suicidal talking or behavior between those taking antidepressant medication and those taking placebo.

The FDA told drug companies to add a *black box warning* label to all antidepressant medicines. Because of this label, a doctor (or advanced practice nurse) prescribing one of these medicines has to warn youth and their families that there might be more suicidal thoughts and actions in youth taking these medicines.

On the other hand, in places where more youth are taking the newer antidepressant medicines, the number of adolescents who commit suicide has gotten smaller. Also, thinking about or attempting suicide is more common in surveys of teenagers in the community than it is in depressed youth treated in research studies with antidepressant medicine.

If a youth is being treated with this medicine and is doing well, then no changes are needed as a result of this warning. Increased suicidal talk or action is most likely to happen in the first few months of treatment with a medicine. If your child has recently started this medicine or is about to start, then you and your doctor (or advanced practice nurse) should watch for any changes in behavior. People who are depressed often have suicidal thoughts or actions. It is hard to know whether suicidal thoughts or actions in depressed people are caused by the depression itself or by the medicine. Also, as their depression is getting better, some people talk more about the suicidal thoughts that they had before but did not talk about. As young people get better from depression, they might be at higher risk of doing something about suicidal thoughts that they have had for some time, because they have more energy.

What Should a Parent Do?

1. Be honest with your child about possible risks and benefits of medicine.
2. Talk to your child about whether he or she is having any suicidal thoughts, and tell your child to come to you if he or she is having such thoughts.
3. You, your child, and your child's doctor or nurse should develop a safety plan. Pick adults whom your child can tell if he or she is thinking about suicide.
4. Be sure to tell your child's doctor, nurse, or therapist if you suspect that your child is using alcohol or drugs or if something has happened that might make your child feel worse, such as a family separation, breaking up with a boyfriend or girlfriend, someone close dying or attempting suicide, physical or sexual abuse, or failure in school.
5. Be sure that there are no guns in the home and that all medicines (including over-the-counter medicines like Tylenol) are closely supervised by an adult and kept in a safe place.
6. Watch for new or worse thoughts of suicide, self-harm, depression, anxiety (nerves), feeling very agitated or restless, being angry or aggressive, having more trouble sleeping, or anything else that you see for the first time, seems worse, or worries your child or you. If these appear, contact a mental health professional **right away.** Do not just stop or change the dose of the medicine on your own. If the problems are serious, and you cannot reach one of your clinicians, call a 24-hour psychiatry emergency telephone number or take your child to an emergency room.

Youth taking antidepressant medicine should be watched carefully by their parent(s), clinician(s) (doctor, advanced practice nurse, nurse, therapist), and other concerned adults for the first weeks of treatment. It is a good idea to have regular contact with the doctor, APN, nurse, or therapist for the first months to check for feelings of depression or sadness, thoughts of killing or harming himself or herself, and any problems with the medication. If you have questions, be sure to ask the doctor, APN, nurse, or therapist.

For more information, see http://www.parentsmedguide.org/.

Notes

Use this space to take notes or to write down questions you want to ask the doctor.

_____

_____

_____

_____

_____

_____

_____

_____

_____

_____

_____

_____

_____

_____

From Dulcan MK, Ballard R (editors): _Helping Parents and Teachers Understand Medications for Behavioral and Emotional Problems: A Resource Book of Medication Information Handouts_, Fourth Edition. Washington, DC, American Psychiatric Publishing, 2015

Perphenazine

General Information About Medication

Each child and adolescent is different. No one has exactly the same combination of medical and psychological problems. It is a good idea to talk with the doctor or nurse about the reasons a medicine is being used. It is very important to keep all appointments and to be in touch by telephone if you have concerns. It is important to communicate with the doctor, nurse, or therapist. An *advanced practice nurse* (APN) has additional education and training after becoming a registered nurse (RN). Your child's medication may be prescribed by a medical doctor (MD or DO) or an APN. In addition, a *physician assistant* (PA) working with a physician may prescribe certain medications. In this information sheet, "doctor" includes medical doctors as well as APNs and PAs who prescribe medication. Often a nurse (RN) will be part of the team and answer questions and give information.

It is very important that the medicine be taken exactly as the doctor instructs. However, once in a while, everyone forgets to give a medicine on time. It is a good idea to ask the doctor or nurse what to do if this happens. Do not stop or change a medicine without asking the doctor or nurse first.

If the medicine seems to stop working, it may be because it is not being taken regularly. The youth may be "cheeking" or hiding the medicine or forgetting to take it (especially at school). The doses may be too far apart or a different dose or medicine may be needed. Something at school, at home, or in the neighborhood may be upsetting the youth, or he or she may need special help for learning disabilities or tutoring. Please discuss your concerns with the doctor. **Do not just increase the dose.** It is also very important not to decrease the dose or stop the medicine without talking to the doctor first. The problem being treated may come back, or there could be uncomfortable or even dangerous results.

All medicines should be kept in a safe place, out of the reach of children, and should be supervised by an adult. If someone takes too much of a medicine, call the doctor, the poison control center, or a hospital emergency room.

Each medicine has a "generic" or chemical name. Just like laundry detergents or paper towels, some medicines are sold by more than one company under different brand names. The same medicine may be available under a generic name and several brand names. The generic medications are usually less expensive than the brand name ones. The generic medications have the same chemical formula, but they may or may not be exactly the same strength as the brand-name medications. Also, some brands of pills contain dye or other things that can cause allergic reactions. It is a good idea to talk to the doctor and the pharmacist about whether it is important to use a specific brand of medicine.

Any medicine can cause an allergic reaction. Examples are hives, itching, rashes, swelling, and trouble breathing. Even a tiny amount of a medicine can cause a reaction in patients who are allergic to that medicine. Be *sure* to talk to the doctor before restarting a medicine that has caused an allergic reaction and tell the doctor about any reactions to medicine that your child has had before.

Taking more than one medicine at the same time may cause more side effects or cause one of the medicines to not work as well. Always ask the doctor, nurse, or pharmacist before adding another

413

medicine, either prescription or bought without a prescription in a store or on the Internet. Be sure that each doctor knows about *all* of the medicines your child is taking. Also tell the doctor about any vitamins, herbal medicines, or supplements your child may be taking. Some of these may have side effects alone or when taken with this medication. It is a very good idea to keep a list with you of the names and doses of all medicines that your child is taking.

Everyone taking medicine should have a physical examination at least once a year.

If you think that your child may be using drugs or alcohol, please tell the doctor right away.

Pregnancy requires special care in the use of medicine. Some medicines can cause birth defects if taken by a pregnant mother. **Please tell the doctor immediately if you suspect the teenager is at risk of becoming pregnant.** The doctor may wish to discuss sexual behavior and/or birth control with your daughter.

Printed information like this applies to children and adolescents in general. If you have questions about the medicine, or if you notice changes or anything unusual, please ask the doctor or nurse. As scientific research advances, knowledge increases and advice changes. Even experts do not always agree. Many medicines have not been "approved" by the U.S. Food and Drug Administration (FDA) for use in children or use for particular problems. For this reason, use of the medicine for a problem or age group often is not listed in the *Physicians' Desk Reference*. This does not necessarily mean that the medicine is dangerous or does not work, only that the company that makes the medicine has not received permission to advertise the medicine for use in children. Companies often do not apply for this permission because it is expensive to do the tests needed to apply for approval for use in children. Once a medication is approved by the FDA for any purpose, a doctor is allowed to prescribe it according to research and clinical experience.

Note to Teachers

It is a good idea to talk with the parent(s) about the reason(s) that a medication is being used. If the parent(s) sign consent to release information, it is often helpful for you to talk with the doctor. If the parent(s) give permission, the doctor may ask you to fill out rating forms about your experience with the student's behavior, feelings, academic performance, and medication side effects. This information is very useful in selecting and monitoring medication treatment. If you have observations that you think are important, do not hesitate to share these with the student's parent(s) and treating clinicians (with parental consent).

It is very important that the medicine be taken exactly as the doctor instructs. However, everyone forgets to give a medicine on time once in a while. It is a good idea to ask the parent(s) in advance what to do if this happens. Do not stop or change the time you are giving a medicine at school without parental permission. If a medication is to be taken with food, but lunchtime or snack time changes, be sure to notify the parent(s) so appropriate adjustments can be made.

All medicines should be kept in a secure place and should be supervised by an adult. If someone takes too much of a medicine, follow your school procedure for an urgent medical problem.

Taking medicine is a private matter and is best managed discreetly and confidentially. It is important to be sensitive to the student's feelings about taking medicine.

If you suspect that the student is using drugs or alcohol, please tell the parent(s) or a school counselor right away.

Please tell the parent(s) or school nurse if you suspect medication side effects.

Modifications of the classroom environment or assignments may be useful in addition to medication. The student may need to be evaluated for additional help or a 504 plan or an Individualized Education Plan for learning problems or emotional or behavioral issues.

Any expression of suicidal thoughts or feelings or self-harm by a child or adolescent is a signal of distress and should be taken seriously. These behaviors should not be dismissed as "attention seeking." School procedures for safety issues should be followed.

What Is Perphenazine?

Perphenazine is sometimes called a *typical*, *conventional*, or *first-generation antipsychotic* medicine. It is also called a *neuroleptic* or *phenothiazine*. It used to be called a *major tranquilizer*. It comes in generic tablets and liquid. It used to come in brand name Trilafon, so sometimes it is called that.

How Can This Medicine Help?

Perphenazine is used to treat psychosis, such as in schizophrenia, mania, or very severe depression. It can reduce hallucinations (hearing voices or seeing things that are not there) and delusions (troubling beliefs that other people do not share). Perphenazine can help the patient be less upset and agitated. It can improve the patient's ability to think clearly.

Sometimes perphenazine is used to decrease severe aggression or very serious behavioral problems in young people with conduct disorder, intellectual disability, or autism spectrum disorder.

This medicine is very powerful and should be used to treat very serious problems or symptoms that other medicines do not help. Be patient; the positive effects of this medicine may not appear for 2–3 weeks.

How Does This Medicine Work?

Cells in the brain *(neurons)* communicate using chemicals called *neurotransmitters*. Too much or too little of these substances in certain parts of the brain can cause problems. Perphenazine reduces the activity of one of these neurotransmitters, *dopamine*. Blocking the effect of dopamine in certain parts of the brain reduces what have been called *positive symptoms* of psychosis: delusions; hallucinations; disorganized and unusual thinking, speaking, and behavior; excessive activity (agitation); and lack of activity (catatonia). Blocking dopamine can also reduce tics. Reducing dopamine action in other parts of the brain may lead to the side effects of this medicine.

How Long Does This Medicine Last?

Perphenazine usually may be taken only once a day, unless divided doses are used to lessen side effects.

How Will the Doctor Monitor This Medicine?

The doctor will review your child's medical history and physical examination before starting perphenazine. The doctor may order some blood or urine tests to be sure your child does not have a hidden medical condition. The doctor or nurse may measure your child's pulse and blood pressure before starting perphenazine.

Before starting perphenazine and every so often afterward, a test such as the AIMS (Abnormal Involuntary Movement Scale) may be used to check your child's tongue, legs, and arms for unusual movements that could be caused by the medicine.

After the medicine is started, the doctor will want to have regular appointments with you and your child to see how the medicine is working, to see if a dose change is needed, to watch for side effects, to see if per-

415

phenazine is still needed, and to see if any other treatment is needed. The doctor or nurse may check your child's height, weight, pulse, and blood pressure and watch for abnormal movements.

What Side Effects Can This Medicine Have?

Any medicine can have side effects, including an allergy to the medicine. Because each patient is different, the doctor will monitor the youth closely, especially when the medicine is started. The doctor will work with you to increase the positive effects and decrease the negative effects of the medicine. Please tell the doctor if any of the listed side effects appear or if you think that the medicine is causing any other problems. Not all of the rare or unusual side effects are listed.

Side effects are most common after starting the medicine or after a dose increase. Many side effects can be avoided or lessened by starting with a very low dose and increasing it slowly—ask the doctor.

Allergic Reaction

Tell the doctor in a day or two (if possible, before the next dose of medicine):

- Hives
- Itching
- Rash

Stop the medicine and get *immediate* medical care:

- Trouble breathing or chest tightness
- Swelling of lips, tongue, or throat

Common, but Not Usually Serious, Side Effects

Discuss the following side effects with your child's doctor within a week or two. They often can be helped by lowering the dose of medicine, changing the times medicine is taken, or adding another medicine.

- Dry mouth—Have your child try using sugar-free gum or candy.
- Constipation—Encourage your child to drink more fluids and eat high-fiber foods; if necessary, the doctor may recommend a fiber medicine such as Benefiber or a stool softener such as Colace or mineral oil.
- Increased risk of sunburn—Have your child wear sunscreen or protective clothing or stay out of the sun.
- Mild trouble urinating
- Blurred vision
- Weight gain—Seek nutritional counseling; provide your child with low-calorie snacks and encourage regular exercise.
- Sadness, irritability, nervousness, clinginess, not wanting to go to school
- Restlessness or inability to sit still
- Shaking of hands and fingers

Less Common, but Not Usually Serious, Side Effects

Discuss the following side effects with your child's doctor within a week or two. They often can be helped by lowering the dose of medicine, changing the times medicine is taken, or adding another medicine.

- Daytime sleepiness or tiredness—Do not allow your child to drive, ride a bicycle or motorcycle, or operate machinery if this happens. This problem may be lessened by taking the medicine at bedtime.
- Dizziness—This side effect is worse when the child stands up quickly, especially when getting out of bed in the morning; try having the child stand up slowly.
- Decreased or slowed movement and decreased facial expressions
- Drooling
- Decreased sexual interest or ability
- Changes in menstrual cycle
- Increase in breast size or discharge from the breasts (in both boys and girls)—This may go away with time.

Less Common, but Potentially Serious, Side Effects

Call the doctor or go to an emergency room *right away:*

- Stiffness of the tongue, jaw, neck, back, or legs
- Overheating or heatstroke—Prevent by decreasing activity in hot weather, staying out of the sun, and drinking water.
- Seizure (fit, convulsion)—This is more likely in people with a history of seizures or head injury.
- Severe confusion

Rare, but Serious, Side Effects

- Extreme stiffness or lack of movement, very high fever, mental confusion, irregular pulse rate, or eye pain—**This is a medical emergency. Go to an emergency room right away.**
- Sudden stiffness and inability to breathe or swallow—**Go to an emergency room or call 911.** Tell the paramedics, nurses, and doctors that the patient is taking perphenazine. Other medicines can be used to treat this problem fast.
- Increased thirst, frequent urination, lethargy, tiredness, dizziness—These could be signs of diabetes (especially if your child is overweight or there is a family history of diabetes). **Talk to a doctor within a day.**

What Else Should I Know About Side Effects?

Most side effects lessen over time. If they are troublesome, talk with your child's doctor. Some side effects can be decreased by taking a smaller dose of medicine, by stopping the medicine, by changing to another medicine, or by adding another medicine.

One side effect that may not go away is *tardive dyskinesia* (or TD). Patients with tardive dyskinesia have involuntary movements of the body, especially the mouth and tongue. The patient may look as though he or she is making faces over and over again. Jerky movements of the arms, legs, or body may occur. There may be fine, wormlike, or sudden repeated movements of the tongue, or the person may appear to be chewing something or smacking or puckering his or her lips. The fingers may look as though they are rolling something. If you notice any unusual movements, be sure to tell the doctor. The doctor may use the AIMS test to look for these movements.

The medicine may increase the level of *prolactin*, a natural hormone made in the part of the brain called the *pituitary*. This may cause side effects such as breast tenderness or swelling or production of milk in both boys and girls. It also may interfere with sexual functioning in teenage boys and with regular menstrual cycles (periods) in teenage girls. A blood test can measure the level of prolactin. If these side effects do not go away and are troublesome, talk with your child's doctor about substituting another medicine for perphenazine.

Heart problems are rare with perphenazine but are more common if other medicines are being taken also. Be sure to tell all your child's doctors and your pharmacist about all medications your child is taking.

Neuroleptic malignant syndrome is a very rare side effect that can lead to death. The symptoms are severe muscle stiffness, high fever, increased heart rate and blood pressure, irregular heartbeat (pulse), and sweating. It may lead to unconsciousness. If you suspect this, **call 911 or go to an emergency room right away.**

Sometimes this medicine can cause a *dystonic reaction*. This is a sudden stiffening of the muscles, most often in the jaw, neck, tongue, face, or shoulders. If this happens, and your child is not having trouble breathing, you may give a dose of diphenhydramine (Benadryl). Follow the dose instructions on the package for your child's age. This should relax the muscles in a few minutes. Then call your doctor to tell him or her what happened. If the muscles do not relax, take your child to the emergency department.

Some Interactions With Other Medicines or Food

Please note that the following are only the most likely interactions with other medicines or food.

Perphenazine may be taken with or without food. If the medicine causes stomach upset, taking it with food may help.

It is better to limit drinks with caffeine (coffee, tea, soft drinks) because caffeine works in the opposite way from this medicine, and the positive effects might be decreased.

What Could Happen if This Medicine Is Stopped Suddenly?

Involuntary movements, or *withdrawal dyskinesias*, may appear within 1–4 weeks of lowering the dose or stopping the medicine. Usually these go away, but they can last for days to months. If perphenazine is stopped suddenly, emotional problems such as irritability, nervousness, moodiness; behavior problems; or physical problems such as stomachache, loss of appetite, nausea, vomiting, diarrhea, sweating, indigestion, trouble sleeping, trembling, or shaking may appear. These problems usually last only a few days to a few weeks. If they happen, tell your child's doctor. The medicine dose may need to be lowered more slowly (tapered). Always check with the doctor before stopping a medicine.

How Long Will This Medicine Be Needed?

How long your child will need to be on perphenazine depends partly on the reason that it was prescribed. Some problems last for only a few months, whereas others last much longer. Sometimes perphenazine is used for only a short time until other medicines or behavioral treatments start to work. Some people need to take perphenazine for years. It is especially important with medicines as powerful as this one to ask the doctor whether it is still needed. Every few months, you should discuss with your child's doctor the reasons for using perphenazine and whether it is time for a trial of lowering the dose.

What Else Should I Know About This Medicine?

There are many other medicines that are used for the same kinds of problems. If your child is having bad side effects or the medicine does not seem to be working, ask the doctor if another medicine in this group might work as well or better and have fewer side effects for your child.

Be sure to tell the doctor if there is anyone in your family who died suddenly or had a heart problem.

Notes

Use this space to take notes or to write down questions you want to ask the doctor.

_____

_____

_____

_____

_____

_____

_____

_____

_____

From Dulcan MK, Ballard R (editors): _Helping Parents and Teachers Understand Medications for Behavioral and Emotional Problems: A Resource Book of Medication Information Handouts,_ Fourth Edition. Washington, DC, American Psychiatric Publishing, 2015

Medication Information
for Parents and Teachers

Pimozide—Orap

General Information About Medication

Each child and adolescent is different. No one has exactly the same combination of medical and psychological problems. It is a good idea to talk with the doctor or nurse about the reasons a medicine is being used. It is very important to keep all appointments and to be in touch by telephone if you have concerns. It is important to communicate with the doctor, nurse, or therapist. An *advanced practice nurse* (APN) has additional education and training after becoming a registered nurse (RN). Your child's medication may be prescribed by a medical doctor (MD or DO) or an APN. In addition, a *physician assistant* (PA) working with a physician may prescribe certain medications. In this information sheet, "doctor" includes medical doctors as well as APNs and PAs who prescribe medication. Often a nurse (RN) will be part of the team and answer questions and give information.

It is very important that the medicine be taken exactly as the doctor instructs. However, once in a while, everyone forgets to give a medicine on time. It is a good idea to ask the doctor or nurse what to do if this happens. Do not stop or change a medicine without asking the doctor or nurse first.

If the medicine seems to stop working, it may be because it is not being taken regularly. The youth may be "cheeking" or hiding the medicine or forgetting to take it (especially at school). The doses may be too far apart or a different dose or medicine may be needed. Something at school, at home, or in the neighborhood may be upsetting the youth, or he or she may need special help for learning disabilities or tutoring. Please discuss your concerns with the doctor. **Do not just increase the dose.** It is also very important not to decrease the dose or stop the medicine without talking to the doctor first. The problem being treated may come back, or there could be uncomfortable or even dangerous results.

All medicines should be kept in a safe place, out of the reach of children, and should be supervised by an adult. If someone takes too much of a medicine, call the doctor, the poison control center, or a hospital emergency room.

Each medicine has a "generic" or chemical name. Just like laundry detergents or paper towels, some medicines are sold by more than one company under different brand names. The same medicine may be available under a generic name and several brand names. The generic medications are usually less expensive than the brand name ones. The generic medications have the same chemical formula, but they may or may not be exactly the same strength as the brand-name medications. Also, some brands of pills contain dye or other things that can cause allergic reactions. It is a good idea to talk to the doctor and the pharmacist about whether it is important to use a specific brand of medicine.

Any medicine can cause an allergic reaction. Examples are hives, itching, rashes, swelling, and trouble breathing. Even a tiny amount of a medicine can cause a reaction in patients who are allergic to that medicine. Be *sure* to talk to the doctor before restarting a medicine that has caused an allergic reaction and tell the doctor about any reactions to medicine that your child has had before.

Taking more than one medicine at the same time may cause more side effects or cause one of the medicines to not work as well. Always ask the doctor, nurse, or pharmacist before adding another

medicine, either prescription or bought without a prescription in a store or on the Internet. Be sure that each doctor knows about *all* of the medicines your child is taking. Also tell the doctor about any vitamins, herbal medicines, or supplements your child may be taking. Some of these may have side effects alone or when taken with this medication. It is a very good idea to keep a list with you of the names and doses of all medicines that your child is taking.

Everyone taking medicine should have a physical examination at least once a year.

If you think that your child may be using drugs or alcohol, please tell the doctor right away.

Pregnancy requires special care in the use of medicine. Some medicines can cause birth defects if taken by a pregnant mother. **Please tell the doctor immediately if you suspect the teenager is at risk of becoming pregnant.** The doctor may wish to discuss sexual behavior and/or birth control with your daughter.

Printed information like this applies to children and adolescents in general. If you have questions about the medicine, or if you notice changes or anything unusual, please ask the doctor or nurse. As scientific research advances, knowledge increases and advice changes. Even experts do not always agree. Many medicines have not been "approved" by the U.S. Food and Drug Administration (FDA) for use in children or use for particular problems. For this reason, use of the medicine for a problem or age group often is not listed in the *Physicians' Desk Reference*. This does not necessarily mean that the medicine is dangerous or does not work, only that the company that makes the medicine has not received permission to advertise the medicine for use in children. Companies often do not apply for this permission because it is expensive to do the tests needed to apply for approval for use in children. Once a medication is approved by the FDA for any purpose, a doctor is allowed to prescribe it according to research and clinical experience.

Note to Teachers

It is a good idea to talk with the parent(s) about the reason(s) that a medication is being used. If the parent(s) sign consent to release information, it is often helpful for you to talk with the doctor. If the parent(s) give permission, the doctor may ask you to fill out rating forms about your experience with the student's behavior, feelings, academic performance, and medication side effects. This information is very useful in selecting and monitoring medication treatment. If you have observations that you think are important, do not hesitate to share these with the student's parent(s) and treating clinicians (with parental consent).

It is very important that the medicine be taken exactly as the doctor instructs. However, everyone forgets to give a medicine on time once in a while. It is a good idea to ask the parent(s) in advance what to do if this happens. Do not stop or change the time you are giving a medicine at school without parental permission. If a medication is to be taken with food, but lunchtime or snack time changes, be sure to notify the parent(s) so appropriate adjustments can be made.

All medicines should be kept in a secure place and should be supervised by an adult. If someone takes too much of a medicine, follow your school procedure for an urgent medical problem.

Taking medicine is a private matter and is best managed discreetly and confidentially. It is important to be sensitive to the student's feelings about taking medicine.

If you suspect that the student is using drugs or alcohol, please tell the parent(s) or a school counselor right away.

Please tell the parent(s) or school nurse if you suspect medication side effects.

Modifications of the classroom environment or assignments may be useful in addition to medication. The student may need to be evaluated for additional help or a 504 plan or an Individualized Education Plan for learning problems or emotional or behavioral issues.

Any expression of suicidal thoughts or feelings or self-harm by a child or adolescent is a signal of distress and should be taken seriously. These behaviors should not be dismissed as "attention seeking." School procedures for safety issues should be followed.

What Is Pimozide (Orap)?

Pimozide is sometimes called a *typical* or *first-generation antipsychotic* medicine. It is also called a *neuroleptic*. It comes only in brand name Orap tablets.

How Can This Medicine Help?

Pimozide is used to decrease motor and vocal tics (fast, repeated movements or sounds) and behavioral problems in people with Tourette's disorder.

This medicine is very powerful and should be used to treat very serious problems or symptoms that other medicines do not help. Be patient; the positive effects of these medicines may not appear for 2–3 weeks.

How Does This Medicine Work?

Cells in the brain *(neurons)* communicate using chemicals called *neurotransmitters*. Too much or too little of these substances in certain parts of the brain can cause problems. Pimozide reduces the activity of one of these neurotransmitters, *dopamine*. Blocking the effect of dopamine in certain parts of the brain can also reduce tics. Reducing dopamine action in other parts of the brain may lead to the side effects of this medicine.

How Long Does This Medicine Last?

Pimozide usually is taken several times a day.

How Will the Doctor Monitor This Medicine?

The doctor will review your child's medical history and physical examination before starting pimozide. The doctor may order some blood or urine tests to be sure your child does not have a hidden medical condition. The doctor or nurse may measure your child's pulse and blood pressure before starting pimozide. An ECG (electrocardiogram or heart rhythm test) will be done before and after starting the medicine and after dose changes. Blood tests for potassium or for genetic ability to process this medicine also may be done.

Be sure to tell the doctor if anyone in the family is hearing impaired or has had heart problems or died suddenly.

Before your child starts taking pimozide and every so often afterward, a test such as the AIMS (Abnormal Involuntary Movement Scale) may be used to check your child's tongue, legs, and arms for unusual movements that could be caused by the medicine.

After the medicine is started, the doctor will want to have regular appointments with you and your child to see how the medicine is working, to see if a dose change is needed, to watch for side effects, to see if pimozide is still needed, and to see if any other treatment is needed. The doctor or nurse may check your child's height, weight, pulse, and blood pressure and watch for abnormal movements. Sometimes an ECG may be needed.

What Side Effects Can This Medicine Have?

Any medicine can have side effects, including an allergy to the medicine. Because each patient is different, the doctor will monitor the youth closely, especially when the medicine is started. The doctor will work with you to increase the positive effects and decrease the negative effects of the medicine. Please tell the doctor if any of the listed side effects appear or if you think that the medicine is causing any other problems. Not all of the rare or unusual side effects are listed.

Side effects are most common after starting the medicine or after a dose increase. Many side effects can be avoided or lessened by starting with a very low dose and increasing it slowly—ask the doctor.

Allergic Reaction

Tell the doctor in a day or two (if possible, before the next dose of medicine):

- Hives
- Itching
- Rash

Stop the medicine and get *immediate* medical care:

- Trouble breathing or chest tightness
- Swelling of lips, tongue, or throat

Common, but Not Usually Serious, Side Effects

Discuss the following side effects with your child's doctor within a week or two. They often can be helped by lowering the dose of medicine, changing the times medicine is taken, or adding another medicine.

- Dry mouth—Have your child try using sugar-free gum or candy.
- Constipation—Encourage your child to drink more fluids and eat high-fiber foods; if necessary, the doctor may recommend a fiber medicine such as Benefiber or a stool softener such as Colace or mineral oil.
- Mild trouble urinating
- Blurred vision
- Increased risk of sunburn—Have your child wear sunscreen or protective clothing or stay out of the sun.
- Weight gain—Seek nutritional counseling; provide your child with low-calorie snacks and encourage regular exercise.
- Sadness, irritability, nervousness, clinginess, not wanting to go to school
- Increased restlessness or inability to sit still
- Shaking of hands and fingers

Less Common, but Not Usually Serious, Side Effects

Discuss the following side effects with your child's doctor within a week or two. They often can be helped by lowering the dose of medicine, changing the times medicine is taken, or adding another medicine.

- Daytime sleepiness or tiredness—Do not allow your child to drive, ride a bicycle or motorcycle, or operate machinery if this happens.

- Dizziness—This side effect is worse when the child stands up quickly, especially when getting out of bed in the morning; try having the child stand up slowly.
- Drooling
- Decreased or slowed movement and decreased facial expressions
- Decreased sexual interest or ability
- Changes in menstrual cycle
- Increase in breast size or discharge from the breasts (in both boys and girls)—This may go away with time.

Less Common, but Potentially Serious, Side Effects

Call the doctor or go to an emergency room *right away*:

- Stiffness of the tongue, jaw, neck, back, or legs
- Overheating or heatstroke—Prevent by decreasing activity in hot weather, staying out of the sun, and drinking water.
- Seizure (fit, convulsion)—This is more likely in people with a history of seizures or head injury.
- Severe confusion
- Very fast or irregular heartbeat

Rare, but Serious, Side Effects

- Extreme stiffness or lack of movement, very high fever, mental confusion, irregular pulse rate, or eye pain—**This is a medical emergency. Go to an emergency room right away.**
- Sudden stiffness and inability to breathe or swallow—**Go to an emergency room or call 911.** Tell the paramedics, nurses, and doctors that the patient is taking pimozide. Other medicines can be used to treat this problem fast.
- Increased thirst, frequent urination, lethargy, tiredness, dizziness—These could be signs of diabetes (especially if your child is overweight or there is a family history of diabetes). **Talk to a doctor within a day.**

What Else Should I Know About Side Effects?

Most side effects lessen over time. If they are troublesome, talk with your child's doctor. Some side effects can be decreased by taking a smaller dose of medicine, by stopping the medicine, by changing to another medicine, or by adding another medicine.

One side effect that may not go away is *tardive dyskinesia* (or TD). Patients with tardive dyskinesia have involuntary movements of the body, especially the mouth and tongue. The patient may look as though he or she is making faces over and over again. Jerky movements of the arms, legs, or body may occur. There may be fine, wormlike, or sudden repeated movements of the tongue, or the person may appear to be chewing something or smacking or puckering his or her lips. The fingers may look as though they are rolling something. If you notice any unusual movements, be sure to tell the doctor. The doctor may use the AIMS test to look for these movements.

Heart problems are more common if other medicines are being taken also. Be sure to tell all your child's doctors and your pharmacist about all medications your child is taking.

Neuroleptic malignant syndrome is a very rare side effect that can lead to death. The symptoms are severe muscle stiffness, high fever, increased heart rate and blood pressure, irregular heartbeat (pulse), and sweating. It may lead to unconsciousness. If you suspect this, **call 911 or go to an emergency room right away.**

Sometimes this medicine can cause a *dystonic reaction*. This is a sudden stiffening of the muscles, most often in the jaw, neck, tongue, face, or shoulders. If this happens, and your child is not having trouble breathing, you may give a dose of diphenhydramine (Benadryl). Follow the dose instructions on the package for your child's age. This should relax the muscles in a few minutes. Then call your doctor to tell him or her what happened. If the muscles do not relax, take your child to the emergency department.

Some Interactions With Other Medicines or Food

Please note that the following are only the most likely interactions with other medicines or food.

Pimozide blood levels may become dangerously high with increased side effects in the heart if the medicine is taken with grapefruit juice, fluoxetine (Prozac), paroxetine (Paxil), sertraline (Zoloft), or some antibiotics (such as erythromycin and others) and antifungal medicines (such as ketoconazole and others). It can interact with many other medications. Be sure to tell your child's doctor about any medications your child is taking while on pimozide.

Pimozide may be taken with or without food.

It is better to limit drinks with caffeine (coffee, tea, soft drinks) because caffeine works in the opposite way from this medicine, and the positive effects might be decreased.

What Could Happen if This Medicine Is Stopped Suddenly?

Involuntary movements, or *withdrawal dyskinesias*, may appear within 1–4 weeks of lowering the dose or stopping the medicine. Usually these go away, but they can last for days to months. If pimozide is stopped suddenly, emotional problems such as irritability, nervousness, moodiness; behavior problems; or physical problems such as stomachache, loss of appetite, nausea, vomiting, diarrhea, sweating, indigestion, trouble sleeping, trembling, or shaking may appear. These problems usually last only a few days to a few weeks. If they happen, tell your child's doctor. The medicine dose may need to be lowered more slowly (tapered). Always check with the doctor before stopping a medicine.

How Long Will This Medicine Be Needed?

How long your child will need to be on pimozide depends on how severe the tics are and whether they start to go away as your child grows up. It is especially important with medicines as powerful as this one to ask the doctor whether it is still needed. Every few months, you should discuss with your child's doctor the reasons for using pimozide and whether it is time for a trial of lowering the dose.

What Else Should I Know About This Medicine?

There are newer medicines that are used for the same kinds of problems. If your child is having bad side effects or the medicine does not seem to be working, ask the doctor if another medicine might work as well or better and have fewer side effects for your child.

Notes

Use this space to take notes or to write down questions you want to ask the doctor.

_____

_____

_____

_____

_____

_____

_____

_____

_____

_____

_____

_____

_____

From Dulcan MK, Ballard R (editors): _Helping Parents and Teachers Understand Medications for Behavioral and Emotional Problems: A Resource Book of Medication Information Handouts_, Fourth Edition. Washington, DC, American Psychiatric Publishing, 2015

Pindolol

General Information About Medication

Each child and adolescent is different. No one has exactly the same combination of medical and psychological problems. It is a good idea to talk with the doctor or nurse about the reasons a medicine is being used. It is very important to keep all appointments and to be in touch by telephone if you have concerns. It is important to communicate with the doctor, nurse, or therapist. An *advanced practice nurse* (APN) has additional education and training after becoming a registered nurse (RN). Your child's medication may be prescribed by a medical doctor (MD or DO) or an APN. In addition, a *physician assistant* (PA) working with a physician may prescribe certain medications. In this information sheet, "doctor" includes medical doctors as well as APNs and PAs who prescribe medication. Often a nurse (RN) will be part of the team and answer questions and give information.

It is very important that the medicine be taken exactly as the doctor instructs. However, once in a while, everyone forgets to give a medicine on time. It is a good idea to ask the doctor or nurse what to do if this happens. Do not stop or change a medicine without asking the doctor or nurse first.

If the medicine seems to stop working, it may be because it is not being taken regularly. The youth may be "cheeking" or hiding the medicine or forgetting to take it (especially at school). The doses may be too far apart or a different dose or medicine may be needed. Something at school, at home, or in the neighborhood may be upsetting the youth, or he or she may need special help for learning disabilities or tutoring. Please discuss your concerns with the doctor. **Do not just increase the dose.** It is also very important not to decrease the dose or stop the medicine without talking to the doctor first. The problem being treated may come back, or there could be uncomfortable or even dangerous results.

All medicines should be kept in a safe place, out of the reach of children, and should be supervised by an adult. If someone takes too much of a medicine, call the doctor, the poison control center, or a hospital emergency room.

Each medicine has a "generic" or chemical name. Just like laundry detergents or paper towels, some medicines are sold by more than one company under different brand names. The same medicine may be available under a generic name and several brand names. The generic medications are usually less expensive than the brand name ones. The generic medications have the same chemical formula, but they may or may not be exactly the same strength as the brand-name medications. Also, some brands of pills contain dye or other things that can cause allergic reactions. It is a good idea to talk to the doctor and the pharmacist about whether it is important to use a specific brand of medicine.

Any medicine can cause an allergic reaction. Examples are hives, itching, rashes, swelling, and trouble breathing. Even a tiny amount of a medicine can cause a reaction in patients who are allergic to that medicine. Be *sure* to talk to the doctor before restarting a medicine that has caused an allergic reaction and tell the doctor about any reactions to medicine that your child has had before.

Taking more than one medicine at the same time may cause more side effects or cause one of the medicines to not work as well. Always ask the doctor, nurse, or pharmacist before adding another

429

medicine, either prescription or bought without a prescription in a store or on the Internet. Be sure that each doctor knows about *all* of the medicines your child is taking. Also tell the doctor about any vitamins, herbal medicines, or supplements your child may be taking. Some of these may have side effects alone or when taken with this medication. It is a very good idea to keep a list with you of the names and doses of all medicines that your child is taking.

Everyone taking medicine should have a physical examination at least once a year.

If you think that your child may be using drugs or alcohol, please tell the doctor right away.

Pregnancy requires special care in the use of medicine. Some medicines can cause birth defects if taken by a pregnant mother. **Please tell the doctor immediately if you suspect the teenager is at risk of becoming pregnant.** The doctor may wish to discuss sexual behavior and/or birth control with your daughter.

Printed information like this applies to children and adolescents in general. If you have questions about the medicine, or if you notice changes or anything unusual, please ask the doctor or nurse. As scientific research advances, knowledge increases and advice changes. Even experts do not always agree. Many medicines have not been "approved" by the U.S. Food and Drug Administration (FDA) for use in children or use for particular problems. For this reason, use of the medicine for a problem or age group often is not listed in the *Physicians' Desk Reference*. This does not necessarily mean that the medicine is dangerous or does not work, only that the company that makes the medicine has not received permission to advertise the medicine for use in children. Companies often do not apply for this permission because it is expensive to do the tests needed to apply for approval for use in children. Once a medication is approved by the FDA for any purpose, a doctor is allowed to prescribe it according to research and clinical experience.

Note to Teachers

It is a good idea to talk with the parent(s) about the reason(s) that a medication is being used. If the parent(s) sign consent to release information, it is often helpful for you to talk with the doctor. If the parent(s) give permission, the doctor may ask you to fill out rating forms about your experience with the student's behavior, feelings, academic performance, and medication side effects. This information is very useful in selecting and monitoring medication treatment. If you have observations that you think are important, do not hesitate to share these with the student's parent(s) and treating clinicians (with parental consent).

It is very important that the medicine be taken exactly as the doctor instructs. However, everyone forgets to give a medicine on time once in a while. It is a good idea to ask the parent(s) in advance what to do if this happens. Do not stop or change the time you are giving a medicine at school without parental permission. If a medication is to be taken with food, but lunchtime or snack time changes, be sure to notify the parent(s) so appropriate adjustments can be made.

All medicines should be kept in a secure place and should be supervised by an adult. If someone takes too much of a medicine, follow your school procedure for an urgent medical problem.

Taking medicine is a private matter and is best managed discreetly and confidentially. It is important to be sensitive to the student's feelings about taking medicine.

If you suspect that the student is using drugs or alcohol, please tell the parent(s) or a school counselor right away.

Please tell the parent(s) or school nurse if you suspect medication side effects.

Modifications of the classroom environment or assignments may be useful in addition to medication. The student may need to be evaluated for additional help or a 504 plan or an Individualized Education Plan for learning problems or emotional or behavioral issues.

Any expression of suicidal thoughts or feelings or self-harm by a child or adolescent is a signal of distress and should be taken seriously. These behaviors should not be dismissed as "attention seeking." School procedures for safety issues should be followed.

What Is Pindolol?

Pindolol is called a *beta-blocker*. It was first used to treat high blood pressure and irregular heartbeat. A newer use is the treatment of emotional and behavioral problems. In adults, it has been used together with an anti-depressant medicine (selective serotonin reuptake inhibitors) for depression that has not gotten better with treatment or together with other medicines for bipolar disorder that is difficult to treat. It is also sometimes used to treat *akathisia*, which is a side effect of some antipsychotic medications. It is used for migraine head-aches and a number of other medical conditions. It comes in generic tablets.

How Can This Medicine Help?

Pindolol can decrease aggressive or violent behavior in children and adolescents. It may be particularly useful for patients who have developmental delays or autism spectrum disorder. In addition, pindolol may reduce the aggression and anger that sometimes follow brain injuries. It may reduce some symptoms of anxiety (nervousness) and help children and adolescents who have experienced very frightening events and have posttraumatic stress disorder (PTSD). Pindolol may reduce the severe restlessness resulting from other medicines.

Your child may need to continue taking pindolol for at least 4 weeks before the doctor is able to decide whether the medicine is working.

How Does This Medicine Work?

When pindolol is prescribed for patients with anxiety, aggression, or other behavioral problems, these medicines stop the effect of certain chemicals on nerves in the body and possibly in the brain that are causing the symptoms. For example, pindolol can decrease the physical anxiety symptoms of shaking, sweating, and fast heartbeat. When used for treatment-resistant mood disorders, pindolol affects the functions of *serotonin*, one of the *neurotransmitters* (chemicals that the brain makes for cells to communicate).

How Will the Doctor Monitor This Medicine?

The doctor will review your child's medical history and physical examination before starting pindolol. Extreme caution is needed for children and adolescents with asthma, heart disease, diabetes, kidney disease, or thyroid disease. Please be sure to tell the doctor if your child or anyone in the family has one of these problems. The doctor may order some blood or urine tests to be sure your child does not have a hidden medical condition that would make it unsafe to use this medicine. The doctor or nurse will measure your child's height, weight, pulse, and blood pressure before starting pindolol. The doctor may order an ECG (electrocardiogram or heart rhythm test) before starting pindolol.

After the medicine is started, the doctor will want to have regular appointments with you and your child to see how the medicine is working, to see if a dose change is needed, to watch for side effects, to see if pindolol is still needed, and to see if any other treatment is needed. The doctor or nurse will measure pulse rate and blood pressure at each visit, particularly as the dose is increased. Sometimes these measurements are taken while the patient is both sitting or lying down and standing up. If either pulse rate or blood pressure drops too low, a pill may not be given at that time or the regular dose may be decreased.

What Side Effects Can This Medicine Have?

Any medicine can have side effects, including an allergy to the medicine. Because each patient is different, the doctor will monitor the youth closely, especially when the medicine is started. The doctor will work with you to increase the positive effects and decrease the negative effects of the medicine. Please tell the doctor if any of the listed side effects appear or if you think that the medicine is causing any other problems. Not all of the rare or unusual side effects are listed.

Side effects are most common after starting the medicine or after a dose increase. Many side effects can be avoided or lessened by starting with a very low dose and increasing it slowly—ask the doctor.

Allergic Reaction

Tell the doctor in a day or two (if possible, before the next dose of medicine):

- Hives
- Itching
- Rash

Stop the medicine and get *immediate* medical care:

- Trouble breathing or chest tightness
- Swelling of lips, tongue, or throat

Occasional Side Effects

Tell the doctor within a week or two:

- Tingling, numbness, cold, or pain in the fingers or toes (Raynaud's phenomenon)
- Tiredness or weakness, especially with exercise
- Slow heartbeat
- Low blood pressure
- Dizziness or light-headedness—This side effect is worse when the child stands up quickly, especially when getting out of bed in the morning; try having the child stand up slowly.
- Cough

Uncommon Side Effects

Call the doctor within a day or two:

- Sadness or irritability lasting more than a few days
- Nausea
- Trouble sleeping or nightmares
- Diarrhea
- Muscle cramps
- Swelling of the face, fingers, or feet

Serious Side Effects

Call the doctor *immediately:*

- Wheezing or shortness of breath
- Chest pain or discomfort
- Fast heartbeat
- Fainting
- Hallucinations (hearing voices or seeing things that are not there)

Some Interactions With Other Medicines or Food

Please note that the following are only the most likely interactions with other medicines or food.

Giving pindolol with food will decrease side effects.

Pindolol interacts with many other medicines. Be sure to tell the doctor about all medicines being taken. A doctor may use pindolol in combination with other medicines to treat a behavioral problem. Talk with your doctor and pharmacist about possible medicine interactions.

What Could Happen if This Medicine Is Stopped Suddenly?

Stopping pindolol suddenly may cause a fast or irregular heartbeat, high blood pressure, or severe emotional problems. Pindolol should be decreased slowly over at least 2 weeks under a doctor's supervision. It is especially important not to miss doses of this medicine, because withdrawal problems may occur. **Be sure not to let the prescription run out!**

How Long Will This Medicine Be Needed?

The length of time pindolol will be needed depends on how well the medicine works for your child, whether any side effects occur, and what condition is being treated. Sometimes medicine is needed for a short time to treat a particular problem. Occasionally a person may require treatment lasting for several months or may need to start the medicine again if symptoms return.

What Else Should I Know About This Medicine?

People with diabetes should be very careful if taking pindolol because it can hide symptoms of low blood sugar.

Notes

Use this space to take notes or to write down questions you want to ask the doctor.

_____

_____

_____

_____

_____

_____

_____

_____

_____

_____

_____

_____

_____

_____

From Dulcan MK, Ballard R (editors): _Helping Parents and Teachers Understand Medications for Behavioral and Emotional Problems: A Resource Book of Medication Information Handouts_, Fourth Edition. Washington, DC, American Psychiatric Publishing, 2015

Prazosin—Minipress

General Information About Medication

Each child and adolescent is different. No one has exactly the same combination of medical and psychological problems. It is a good idea to talk with the doctor or nurse about the reasons a medicine is being used. It is very important to keep all appointments and to be in touch by telephone if you have concerns. It is important to communicate with the doctor, nurse, or therapist. An *advanced practice nurse* (APN) has additional education and training after becoming a registered nurse (RN). Your child's medication may be prescribed by a medical doctor (MD or DO) or an APN. In addition, a *physician assistant* (PA) working with a physician may prescribe certain medications. In this information sheet, "doctor" includes medical doctors as well as APNs and PAs who prescribe medication. Often a nurse (RN) will be part of the team and answer questions and give information.

It is very important that the medicine be taken exactly as the doctor instructs. However, once in a while, everyone forgets to give a medicine on time. It is a good idea to ask the doctor or nurse what to do if this happens. Do not stop or change a medicine without asking the doctor or nurse first.

If the medicine seems to stop working, it may be because it is not being taken regularly. The youth may be "cheeking" or hiding the medicine or forgetting to take it (especially at school). The doses may be too far apart or a different dose or medicine may be needed. Something at school, at home, or in the neighborhood may be upsetting the youth, or he or she may need special help for learning disabilities or tutoring. Please discuss your concerns with the doctor. **Do not just increase the dose.** It is also very important not to decrease the dose or stop the medicine without talking to the doctor first. The problem being treated may come back, or there could be uncomfortable or even dangerous results.

All medicines should be kept in a safe place, out of the reach of children, and should be supervised by an adult. If someone takes too much of a medicine, call the doctor, the poison control center, or a hospital emergency room.

Each medicine has a "generic" or chemical name. Just like laundry detergents or paper towels, some medicines are sold by more than one company under different brand names. The same medicine may be available under a generic name and several brand names. The generic medications are usually less expensive than the brand name ones. The generic medications have the same chemical formula, but they may or may not be exactly the same strength as the brand-name medications. Also, some brands of pills contain dye or other things that can cause allergic reactions. It is a good idea to talk to the doctor and the pharmacist about whether it is important to use a specific brand of medicine.

Any medicine can cause an allergic reaction. Examples are hives, itching, rashes, swelling, and trouble breathing. Even a tiny amount of a medicine can cause a reaction in patients who are allergic to that medicine. Be *sure* to talk to the doctor before restarting a medicine that has caused an allergic reaction and tell the doctor about any reactions to medicine that your child has had before.

Taking more than one medicine at the same time may cause more side effects or cause one of the medicines to not work as well. Always ask the doctor, nurse, or pharmacist before adding another

medicine, either prescription or bought without a prescription in a store or on the Internet. Be sure that each doctor knows about *all* of the medicines your child is taking. Also tell the doctor about any vitamins, herbal medicines, or supplements your child may be taking. Some of these may have side effects alone or when taken with this medication. It is a very good idea to keep a list with you of the names and doses of all medicines that your child is taking.

Everyone taking medicine should have a physical examination at least once a year.

If you think that your child may be using drugs or alcohol, please tell the doctor right away.

Pregnancy requires special care in the use of medicine. Some medicines can cause birth defects if taken by a pregnant mother. **Please tell the doctor immediately if you suspect the teenager is at risk of becoming pregnant.** The doctor may wish to discuss sexual behavior and/or birth control with your daughter.

Printed information like this applies to children and adolescents in general. If you have questions about the medicine, or if you notice changes or anything unusual, please ask the doctor or nurse. As scientific research advances, knowledge increases and advice changes. Even experts do not always agree. Many medicines have not been "approved" by the U.S. Food and Drug Administration (FDA) for use in children or use for particular problems. For this reason, use of the medicine for a problem or age group often is not listed in the *Physicians' Desk Reference*. This does not necessarily mean that the medicine is dangerous or does not work, only that the company that makes the medicine has not received permission to advertise the medicine for use in children. Companies often do not apply for this permission because it is expensive to do the tests needed to apply for approval for use in children. Once a medication is approved by the FDA for any purpose, a doctor is allowed to prescribe it according to research and clinical experience.

Note to Teachers

It is a good idea to talk with the parent(s) about the reason(s) that a medication is being used. If the parent(s) sign consent to release information, it is often helpful for you to talk with the doctor. If the parent(s) give permission, the doctor may ask you to fill out rating forms about your experience with the student's behavior, feelings, academic performance, and medication side effects. This information is very useful in selecting and monitoring medication treatment. If you have observations that you think are important, do not hesitate to share these with the student's parent(s) and treating clinicians (with parental consent).

It is very important that the medicine be taken exactly as the doctor instructs. However, everyone forgets to give a medicine on time once in a while. It is a good idea to ask the parent(s) in advance what to do if this happens. Do not stop or change the time you are giving a medicine at school without parental permission. If a medication is to be taken with food, but lunchtime or snack time changes, be sure to notify the parent(s) so appropriate adjustments can be made.

All medicines should be kept in a secure place and should be supervised by an adult. If someone takes too much of a medicine, follow your school procedure for an urgent medical problem.

Taking medicine is a private matter and is best managed discreetly and confidentially. It is important to be sensitive to the student's feelings about taking medicine.

If you suspect that the student is using drugs or alcohol, please tell the parent(s) or a school counselor right away.

Please tell the parent(s) or school nurse if you suspect medication side effects.

Modifications of the classroom environment or assignments may be useful in addition to medication. The student may need to be evaluated for additional help or a 504 plan or an Individualized Education Plan for learning problems or emotional or behavioral issues.

Any expression of suicidal thoughts or feelings or self-harm by a child or adolescent is a signal of distress and should be taken seriously. These behaviors should not be dismissed as "attention seeking." School procedures for safety issues should be followed.

What Is Prazosin (Minipress)?

Prazosin was first used to treat high blood pressure, so it is sometimes called an *antihypertensive*. It is also called an *alpha 1 blocker*. It may be used to treat urinary problems associated with prostate enlargement and stiffness associated with Raynaud's disease. A newer use for prazosin is the treatment of sleep-related and other problems in people with posttraumatic stress disorder (PTSD). It comes as brand name Minipress and generic tablets.

How Can This Medicine Help?

Prazosin may help with falling asleep and staying asleep in people with PTSD, who have experienced very frightening events. It can help decrease intrusive thoughts, lessen hyperarousal, and decrease nightmares.

The positive effects of prazosin may be observed right away, but sometimes your child may need to take prazosin for a longer period of time before the full benefit of the medication is seen. Sometimes the dose needs to be increased to see a benefit. Once the medicine is at the right dose, it may take up to 2 weeks before the doctor is able to decide whether the medicine is working.

How Does This Medicine Work?

Prazosin works by decreasing the level of excitement in parts of the brain. It blocks the action of certain nerve impulses. It affects the levels of *norepinephrine*, one of the *neurotransmitters*—a chemical that the brain makes for nerve cells to communicate with each other. Norepinephrine is released by the body during times of stress and/or anxiety. It is believed that blocking the effects of norepinephrine in the brain can help decrease symptoms such as nightmares and sleep problems in people who have PTSD. Prazosin is chemically different from sedatives or tranquilizers, even though it may make your child sleepy when he or she first starts taking it.

How Long Does This Medicine Last?

Prazosin is usually started before bedtime. It reaches its highest levels in the body between 1 and 3 hours after it is taken and is broken down in the body after that time. Sometimes an additional morning dose is needed.

How Will the Doctor Monitor This Medicine?

The doctor will review your child's medical history and physical examination before starting prazosin. The doctor may order some blood or urine tests to be sure your child does not have a hidden medical condition that would make it unsafe to use this medicine. Be sure to tell the doctor if your child or anyone in the family has high blood pressure, heart disease, or diabetes. The doctor or nurse may measure your child's pulse and blood pressure before starting prazosin. The doctor may also want to obtain an electrocardiogram (ECG or heart rhythm test) before starting the medicine.

After the medicine is started, the doctor will want to have regular appointments with you and your child to see how the medicine is working, to see if a dose change is needed, and to watch for side effects. The doctor will also want to evaluate whether prazosin is still needed and to see if any other treatment is needed. The doctor or nurse will check your child's height, weight, pulse, and blood pressure.

What Side Effects Can This Medicine Have?

Any medicine can have side effects, including an allergy to the medicine. Because each patient is different, the doctor will monitor the youth closely, especially when the medicine is started. The doctor will work with you to increase the positive effects and decrease the negative effects of the medicine. Please tell the doctor if any of the listed side effects appear or if you think that the medicine is causing any other problems. Not all of the rare or unusual side effects are listed.

Side effects are most common after starting the medicine or after a dose increase. Many side effects can be avoided or lessened by starting with a very low dose and increasing it slowly—ask the doctor.

Allergic Reaction

Tell the doctor in a day or two (if possible, before the next dose of medicine):

- Hives
- Itching
- Rash

Stop the medicine and get *immediate* medical care:

- Trouble breathing or chest tightness
- Swelling of lips, tongue, or throat

Common, but Usually Mild, Side Effects

The following side effects are more common at first or as the dose is increased. If they do not go away after a week or two, contact the doctor:

- Dizziness or light-headedness—This side effect is generally worse when the child stands up quickly, especially when getting out of bed in the morning. Try having the child stand up slowly.
- Daytime sleepiness—Usually worse in the first 2–4 weeks. Do not allow your child to drive a car, ride a bicycle or motorcycle, or operate machinery if this happens.
- Fatigue or tiredness
- Low blood pressure—Rarely a serious problem as this medication only weakly affects blood pressure
- Headache
- Stomachache, nausea
- Slow pulse rate (heartbeat)

Less Common Side Effects

Tell the doctor within a day or two:

- Nasal congestion
- Dry mouth

- Increased blood sugar (mainly in persons with diabetes)
- Diarrhea or constipation
- Mood changes such as depression or irritability
- Bed-wetting or frequent urination
- Vivid and intense dreams right before falling asleep or waking up
- Confusion
- Blurred vision
- Muscle cramping
- Hair loss

Less Common, but Serious, Side Effects

Call the doctor *immediately*:

- Severe or increased dizziness or light-headedness
- Fainting

Very Rare, but Serious, Side Effects

Call the doctor *immediately* or go to the emergency room:

- Irregular heartbeat
- Trouble breathing
- Decreased frequency of urination; rapid, puffy swelling of the body (especially legs and feet); sudden headache with nausea and vomiting—These could be signs of kidney failure.
- Erection of the penis lasting more than 1 hour—This may be painful and could cause permanent damage.

Some Interactions With Other Medicines or Food

Please note that the following are only the most likely interactions with other medicines or food.

Talk to your doctor about any other medications your child may be taking that also affect blood pressure before starting this medication.

Because this medication is cleared from the body through the liver, the dose of prazosin may need to be adjusted in children with liver disease.

Increased sleepiness can occur in combination with medications used for anxiety (sedatives or tranquilizers), sleep (hypnotics), allergy or colds (antihistamines), or psychosis or seizures (anticonvulsants).

Prazosin can be taken with or without food.

What Could Happen if This Medicine Is Stopped Suddenly?

Do not stop this medication suddenly without talking to your doctor. Some problems may worsen if the medication is stopped suddenly, including

- Increase in blood pressure and/or heartbeat
- Worsening of nightmares
- Trouble sleeping
- Nervousness or anxiety

Because of these effects, it is important not to stop prazosin suddenly. Prazosin should be decreased slowly (tapered) as directed by the doctor. It is also important to avoid missing a dose of prazosin because withdrawal symptoms such as heart or blood pressure problems can occur. **Be sure not to let the prescription run out!**

How Long Will This Medicine Be Needed?

There is no way to know how long your child will need to take prazosin. The length of time will largely depend on how well the medicine works for him or her, whether there are side effects, and what condition is being treated. Sometimes medicine is needed for a short time to treat a particular problem. Occasionally a person may require treatment lasting for several months or may need to start the medicine again if symptoms return.

What Else Should I Know About This Medicine?

If your child is sleepy from prazosin, do not allow him or her to drive or operate machinery until you are sure that he or she can perform these tasks safely.

Prazosin may be confused with prednisone. Be sure to check the medicine when you get it from the pharmacy.

Notes

Use this space to take notes or to write down questions you want to ask the doctor.

_____

_____

_____

_____

_____

_____

_____

Propranolol—Inderal

General Information About Medication

Each child and adolescent is different. No one has exactly the same combination of medical and psychological problems. It is a good idea to talk with the doctor or nurse about the reasons a medicine is being used. It is very important to keep all appointments and to be in touch by telephone if you have concerns. It is important to communicate with the doctor, nurse, or therapist. An *advanced practice nurse* (APN) has additional education and training after becoming a registered nurse (RN). Your child's medication may be prescribed by a medical doctor (MD or DO) or an APN. In addition, a *physician assistant* (PA) working with a physician may prescribe certain medications. In this information sheet, "doctor" includes medical doctors as well as APNs and PAs who prescribe medication. Often a nurse (RN) will be part of the team and answer questions and give information.

It is very important that the medicine be taken exactly as the doctor instructs. However, once in a while, everyone forgets to give a medicine on time. It is a good idea to ask the doctor or nurse what to do if this happens. Do not stop or change a medicine without asking the doctor or nurse first.

If the medicine seems to stop working, it may be because it is not being taken regularly. The youth may be "cheeking" or hiding the medicine or forgetting to take it (especially at school). The doses may be too far apart or a different dose or medicine may be needed. Something at school, at home, or in the neighborhood may be upsetting the youth, or he or she may need special help for learning disabilities or tutoring. Please discuss your concerns with the doctor. **Do not just increase the dose.** It is also very important not to decrease the dose or stop the medicine without talking to the doctor first. The problem being treated may come back, or there could be uncomfortable or even dangerous results.

All medicines should be kept in a safe place, out of the reach of children, and should be supervised by an adult. If someone takes too much of a medicine, call the doctor, the poison control center, or a hospital emergency room.

Each medicine has a "generic" or chemical name. Just like laundry detergents or paper towels, some medicines are sold by more than one company under different brand names. The same medicine may be available under a generic name and several brand names. The generic medications are usually less expensive than the brand name ones. The generic medications have the same chemical formula, but they may or may not be exactly the same strength as the brand-name medications. Also, some brands of pills contain dye or other things that can cause allergic reactions. It is a good idea to talk to the doctor and the pharmacist about whether it is important to use a specific brand of medicine.

Any medicine can cause an allergic reaction. Examples are hives, itching, rashes, swelling, and trouble breathing. Even a tiny amount of a medicine can cause a reaction in patients who are allergic to that medicine. Be *sure* to talk to the doctor before restarting a medicine that has caused an allergic reaction and tell the doctor about any reactions to medicine that your child has had before.

Taking more than one medicine at the same time may cause more side effects or cause one of the medicines to not work as well. Always ask the doctor, nurse, or pharmacist before adding another

medicine, either prescription or bought without a prescription in a store or on the Internet. Be sure that each doctor knows about *all* **of the medicines your child is taking. Also tell the doctor about any vitamins, herbal medicines, or supplements your child may be taking.** Some of these may have side effects alone or when taken with this medication. It is a very good idea to keep a list with you of the names and doses of all medicines that your child is taking.

Everyone taking medicine should have a physical examination at least once a year.

If you think that your child may be using drugs or alcohol, please tell the doctor right away.

Pregnancy requires special care in the use of medicine. Some medicines can cause birth defects if taken by a pregnant mother. **Please tell the doctor immediately if you suspect the teenager is at risk of becoming pregnant.** The doctor may wish to discuss sexual behavior and/or birth control with your daughter.

Printed information like this applies to children and adolescents in general. If you have questions about the medicine, or if you notice changes or anything unusual, please ask the doctor or nurse. As scientific research advances, knowledge increases and advice changes. Even experts do not always agree. Many medicines have not been "approved" by the U.S. Food and Drug Administration (FDA) for use in children or use for particular problems. For this reason, use of the medicine for a problem or age group often is not listed in the *Physicians' Desk Reference*. This does not necessarily mean that the medicine is dangerous or does not work, only that the company that makes the medicine has not received permission to advertise the medicine for use in children. Companies often do not apply for this permission because it is expensive to do the tests needed to apply for approval for use in children. Once a medication is approved by the FDA for any purpose, a doctor is allowed to prescribe it according to research and clinical experience.

Note to Teachers

It is a good idea to talk with the parent(s) about the reason(s) that a medication is being used. If the parent(s) sign consent to release information, it is often helpful for you to talk with the doctor. If the parent(s) give permission, the doctor may ask you to fill out rating forms about your experience with the student's behavior, feelings, academic performance, and medication side effects. This information is very useful in selecting and monitoring medication treatment. If you have observations that you think are important, do not hesitate to share these with the student's parent(s) and treating clinicians (with parental consent).

It is very important that the medicine be taken exactly as the doctor instructs. However, everyone forgets to give a medicine on time once in a while. It is a good idea to ask the parent(s) in advance what to do if this happens. Do not stop or change the time you are giving a medicine at school without parental permission. If a medication is to be taken with food, but lunchtime or snack time changes, be sure to notify the parent(s) so appropriate adjustments can be made.

All medicines should be kept in a secure place and should be supervised by an adult. If someone takes too much of a medicine, follow your school procedure for an urgent medical problem.

Taking medicine is a private matter and is best managed discreetly and confidentially. It is important to be sensitive to the student's feelings about taking medicine.

If you suspect that the student is using drugs or alcohol, please tell the parent(s) or a school counselor right away.

Please tell the parent(s) or school nurse if you suspect medication side effects.

Modifications of the classroom environment or assignments may be useful in addition to medication. The student may need to be evaluated for additional help or a 504 plan or an Individualized Education Plan for learning problems or emotional or behavioral issues.

Any expression of suicidal thoughts or feelings or self-harm by a child or adolescent is a signal of distress and should be taken seriously. These behaviors should not be dismissed as "attention seeking." School procedures for safety issues should be followed.

What Is Propranolol (Inderal)?

Propranolol is called a *beta-blocker*. It was first used to treat high blood pressure and irregular heartbeat. A newer use is the treatment of emotional and behavioral problems. It is also sometimes used to treat *akathisia*, which is a side effect of some antipsychotic medications, or to reduce tremor (shaking) in people taking lithium. It is used for migraine headaches and a number of other medical conditions.

Propranolol comes in generic propranolol and brand name Inderal tablets and liquid, Inderal LA sustained-release capsules, and InnoPranXL extended-release capsules.

How Can This Medicine Help?

Propranolol can decrease aggressive or violent behavior in children and adolescents. It may be particularly useful for patients who have developmental delays or autism spectrum disorder. In addition, propranolol may reduce the aggression and anger that sometimes follow brain injuries. It may reduce some symptoms of anxiety (nervousness) and help children and adolescents who have experienced very frightening events and have posttraumatic stress disorder (PTSD). Propranolol may reduce the severe restlessness or shaking resulting from other medicines.

Your child may need to continue taking propranolol for at least 4 weeks before the doctor is able to decide whether the medicine is working.

How Does This Medicine Work?

When propranolol is prescribed for patients with anxiety, aggression, or other behavioral problems, it stops the effects of certain chemicals on nerves in the body and possibly in the brain that are causing the symptoms. For example, propranolol can decrease the physical anxiety symptoms of shaking, sweating, and fast heartbeat.

How Long Does This Medicine Last?

Propranolol is usually taken three times a day.

How Will the Doctor Monitor This Medicine?

The doctor will review your child's medical history and physical examination before starting propranolol. Extreme caution is needed for children and adolescents with asthma, heart disease, diabetes, kidney disease, or thyroid disease. Please be sure to tell the doctor if your child or anyone in the family has one of these problems. The doctor may order some blood or urine tests to be sure your child does not have a hidden medical condition that would make it unsafe to use this medicine. The doctor or nurse will measure your child's height, weight, pulse, and blood pressure before starting propranolol. The doctor may order an electrocardiogram (ECG or heart rhythm test) before starting propranolol.

After the medicine is started, the doctor will want to have regular appointments with you and your child to see how the medicine is working, to see if a dose change is needed, to watch for side effects, to see if propranolol is still needed, and to see if any other treatment is needed. The doctor or nurse will measure pulse rate and blood pressure at each visit, particularly as the dose is increased. Sometimes these measurements are taken while the patient is both sitting or lying down and standing up. If either pulse rate or blood pressure drops too low, a pill may not be given at that time or the regular dose may be decreased.

What Side Effects Can This Medicine Have?

Any medicine can have side effects, including an allergy to the medicine. Because each patient is different, the doctor will monitor the youth closely, especially when the medicine is started. The doctor will work with you to increase the positive effects and decrease the negative effects of the medicine. Please tell the doctor if any of the listed side effects appear or if you think that the medicine is causing any other problems. Not all of the rare or unusual side effects are listed.

Side effects are most common after starting the medicine or after a dose increase. Many side effects can be avoided or lessened by starting with a very low dose and increasing it slowly—ask the doctor.

Allergic Reaction

Tell the doctor in a day or two (if possible, before the next dose of medicine):

- Hives
- Itching
- Rash

Stop the medicine and get *immediate* medical care:

- Trouble breathing or chest tightness
- Swelling of lips, tongue, or throat

Occasional Side Effects

Tell the doctor within a week or two:

- Tingling, numbness, cold, or pain in the fingers or toes (Raynaud's phenomenon)
- Tiredness or weakness, especially with exercise
- Slow heartbeat
- Low blood pressure
- Dizziness—This side effect is worse when the child stands up quickly, especially when getting out of bed in the morning; try having the child stand up slowly.
- Cough

Uncommon Side Effects

Call the doctor within a day or two:

- Sadness or irritability lasting more than a few days
- Nausea

446

- Trouble sleeping or nightmares
- Diarrhea
- Muscle cramps
- Swelling of the face, fingers, or feet

Serious Side Effects

Call the doctor *immediately*:

- Wheezing or shortness of breath
- Chest pain or discomfort
- Fast heartbeat
- Fainting
- Hallucinations (hearing voices or seeing things that are not there)

Some Interactions With Other Medicines or Food

Please note that the following are only the most likely interactions with other medicines or food.

Giving propranolol with food will decrease side effects. The extended-release capsule should be taken the same way each time, either always with food or always without food.

Propranolol interacts with many other medicines. Be sure to tell the doctor about all medicines being taken. A doctor may use propranolol in combination with other medicines to treat a behavioral problem. The blood level of certain drugs (such as chlorpromazine [Thorazine]) increases when taken with beta-blockers. Talk with your doctor and pharmacist about possible medicine interactions.

What Could Happen if This Medicine Is Stopped Suddenly?

Stopping propranolol suddenly may cause a fast or irregular heartbeat, high blood pressure, or severe emotional problems. Propranolol should be decreased slowly over at least 2 weeks under a doctor's supervision. It is especially important not to miss doses of this medicine, because withdrawal problems may occur. **Be sure not to let the prescription run out!**

How Long Will This Medicine Be Needed?

The length of time propranolol will be needed depends on how well the medicine works for your child, whether any side effects occur, and what condition is being treated. Sometimes medicine is needed for a short time to treat a particular problem. Occasionally a person may require treatment lasting for several months or may need to start the medicine again if symptoms return.

What Else Should I Know About This Medicine?

The extended-release capsule should not be chewed or crushed; it should always be swallowed whole.

The oral solution should be mixed with water, fruit juice, or food such as applesauce before giving.

Inderal may be confused with Adderall. Be sure to check the medicine when you get it from the pharmacy.

People with diabetes should be very careful if taking propranolol because it can hide symptoms of low blood sugar.

Notes

Use this space to take notes or to write down questions you want to ask the doctor.

_____

_____

_____

_____

_____

_____

_____

_____

_____

_____

_____

_____

_____

lication and consistent with standards set by the U.S. Food and Drug Administration and the general medical community and accepted child psychiatric practice. The information on this medication sheet does not cover all the possible uses, precautions, side effects, or interactions of this drug. For a complete listing of side effects, see the manufacturer's package insert, which can be obtained from your physician or pharmacist. As medical research and practice advance, therapeutic standards may change. For this reason and because human and mechanical errors sometimes occur, we recommend that readers follow the advice of a physician who is directly involved in their care or the care of a member of their family.

From Dulcan MK, Ballard R (editors): *Helping Parents and Teachers Understand Medications for Behavioral and Emotional Problems: A Resource Book of Medication Information Handouts*, Fourth Edition. Washington, DC, American Psychiatric Publishing, 2015

Medication Information for Parents and Teachers

Quetiapine—Seroquel

General Information About Medication

Each child and adolescent is different. No one has exactly the same combination of medical and psychological problems. It is a good idea to talk with the doctor or nurse about the reasons a medicine is being used. It is very important to keep all appointments and to be in touch by telephone if you have concerns. It is important to communicate with the doctor, nurse, or therapist. An *advanced practice nurse* (APN) has additional education and training after becoming a registered nurse (RN). Your child's medication may be prescribed by a medical doctor (MD or DO) or an APN. In addition, a *physician assistant* (PA) working with a physician may prescribe certain medications. In this information sheet, "doctor" includes medical doctors as well as APNs and PAs who prescribe medication. Often a nurse (RN) will be part of the team and answer questions and give information.

It is very important that the medicine be taken exactly as the doctor instructs. However, once in a while, everyone forgets to give a medicine on time. It is a good idea to ask the doctor or nurse what to do if this happens. Do not stop or change a medicine without asking the doctor or nurse first.

If the medicine seems to stop working, it may be because it is not being taken regularly. The youth may be "cheeking" or hiding the medicine or forgetting to take it (especially at school). The doses may be too far apart or a different dose or medicine may be needed. Something at school, at home, or in the neighborhood may be upsetting the youth, or he or she may need special help for learning disabilities or tutoring. Please discuss your concerns with the doctor. **Do not just increase the dose.** It is also very important not to decrease the dose or stop the medicine without talking to the doctor first. The problem being treated may come back, or there could be uncomfortable or even dangerous results.

All medicines should be kept in a safe place, out of the reach of children, and should be supervised by an adult. If someone takes too much of a medicine, call the doctor, the poison control center, or a hospital emergency room.

Each medicine has a "generic" or chemical name. Just like laundry detergents or paper towels, some medicines are sold by more than one company under different brand names. The same medicine may be available under a generic name and several brand names. The generic medications are usually less expensive than the brand name ones. The generic medications have the same chemical formula, but they may or may not be exactly the same strength as the brand-name medications. Also, some brands of pills contain dye or other things that can cause allergic reactions. It is a good idea to talk to the doctor and the pharmacist about whether it is important to use a specific brand of medicine.

Any medicine can cause an allergic reaction. Examples are hives, itching, rashes, swelling, and trouble breathing. Even a tiny amount of a medicine can cause a reaction in patients who are allergic to that medicine. Be *sure* to talk to the doctor before restarting a medicine that has caused an allergic reaction and tell the doctor about any reactions to medicine that your child has had before.

Taking more than one medicine at the same time may cause more side effects or cause one of the medicines to not work as well. Always ask the doctor, nurse, or pharmacist before adding another

451

medicine, either prescription or bought without a prescription in a store or on the Internet. Be sure that each doctor knows about *all* of the medicines your child is taking. Also tell the doctor about any vitamins, herbal medicines, or supplements your child may be taking. Some of these may have side effects alone or when taken with this medication. It is a very good idea to keep a list with you of the names and doses of all medicines that your child is taking.

Everyone taking medicine should have a physical examination at least once a year.

If you think that your child may be using drugs or alcohol, please tell the doctor right away.

Pregnancy requires special care in the use of medicine. Some medicines can cause birth defects if taken by a pregnant mother. **Please tell the doctor immediately if you suspect the teenager is at risk of becoming pregnant.** The doctor may wish to discuss sexual behavior and/or birth control with your daughter.

Printed information like this applies to children and adolescents in general. If you have questions about the medicine, or if you notice changes or anything unusual, please ask the doctor or nurse. As scientific research advances, knowledge increases and advice changes. Even experts do not always agree. Many medicines have not been "approved" by the U.S. Food and Drug Administration (FDA) for use in children or use for particular problems. For this reason, use of the medicine for a problem or age group often is not listed in the *Physicians' Desk Reference.* This does not necessarily mean that the medicine is dangerous or does not work, only that the company that makes the medicine has not received permission to advertise the medicine for use in children. Companies often do not apply for this permission because it is expensive to do the tests needed to apply for approval for use in children. Once a medication is approved by the FDA for any purpose, a doctor is allowed to prescribe it according to research and clinical experience.

Note to Teachers

It is a good idea to talk with the parent(s) about the reason(s) that a medication is being used. If the parent(s) sign consent to release information, it is often helpful for you to talk with the doctor. If the parent(s) give permission, the doctor may ask you to fill out rating forms about your experience with the student's behavior, feelings, academic performance, and medication side effects. This information is very useful in selecting and monitoring medication treatment. If you have observations that you think are important, do not hesitate to share these with the student's parent(s) and treating clinicians (with parental consent).

It is very important that the medicine be taken exactly as the doctor instructs. However, everyone forgets to give a medicine on time once in a while. It is a good idea to ask the parent(s) in advance what to do if this happens. Do not stop or change the time you are giving a medicine at school without parental permission. If a medication is to be taken with food, but lunchtime or snack time changes, be sure to notify the parent(s) so appropriate adjustments can be made.

All medicines should be kept in a secure place and should be supervised by an adult. If someone takes too much of a medicine, follow your school procedure for an urgent medical problem.

Taking medicine is a private matter and is best managed discreetly and confidentially. It is important to be sensitive to the student's feelings about taking medicine.

If you suspect that the student is using drugs or alcohol, please tell the parent(s) or a school counselor right away.

Please tell the parent(s) or school nurse if you suspect medication side effects.

Modifications of the classroom environment or assignments may be useful in addition to medication. The student may need to be evaluated for additional help or a 504 plan or an Individualized Education Plan for learning problems or emotional or behavioral issues.

Any expression of suicidal thoughts or feelings or self-harm by a child or adolescent is a signal of distress and should be taken seriously. These behaviors should not be dismissed as "attention seeking." School procedures for safety issues should be followed.

What Is Quetiapine (Seroquel)?

This medicine is called an *atypical* or *second-generation antipsychotic*. It is sometimes called an *atypical psychotropic agent* or simply an *atypical*. It comes in brand name Seroquel and generic tablets and brand name Seroquel XR extended-release tablets.

How Can This Medicine Help?

Quetiapine is used to treat psychosis, such as in schizophrenia, mania, or very severe depression. It can reduce *positive symptoms* such as hallucinations (hearing voices or seeing things that are not there); delusions (troubling beliefs that other people do not share); agitation; and very unusual thinking, speech, and behavior. It is also used to lessen the *negative symptoms* of schizophrenia, such as lack of interest in doing things (apathy), lack of motivation, social withdrawal, and lack of energy.

Quetiapine may be used as a *mood stabilizer* in patients with bipolar disorder or severe mood swings. It can reduce mania and may be able to help maintain a stable mood over the long term. Quetiapine has been shown to be effective in treating the depressive phase of bipolar disorder in adults.

Sometimes quetiapine is used to reduce severe aggression or very serious behavioral problems in young people with conduct disorder, intellectual disability, or autism spectrum disorder.

Quetiapine may be used for behavior problems that arise after a head injury.

This medicine is very powerful and is used to treat very serious problems or symptoms that other medicines do not help. Be patient; the positive effects of this medicine may not appear for 2–3 weeks.

How Does This Medicine Work?

Cells in the brain communicate using chemicals called *neurotransmitters*. Too much or too little of these substances in parts of the brain can cause problems. Quetiapine works by blocking the action of two of these neurotransmitters, *dopamine* and *serotonin*, in certain areas of the brain.

How Long Does This Medicine Last?

Quetiapine is usually taken two or three times a day. Seroquel XR is usually taken once daily.

How Will the Doctor Monitor This Medicine?

The doctor will review your child's medical history and physical examination before starting quetiapine. The doctor may order some blood or urine tests to be sure your child does not have a hidden medical condition that would make it unsafe to use this medicine. The doctor or nurse may measure your child's pulse and blood pressure before starting quetiapine. The doctor may order other tests, such as baseline tests for blood sugar and cholesterol.

Be sure to tell the doctor if anyone in the family has diabetes, high blood pressure, high cholesterol, heart disease, or thyroid problems.

Before starting quetiapine and every so often afterward, a test such as the AIMS (Abnormal Involuntary Movement Scale) may be used to check your child's tongue, legs, and arms for unusual movements that could be caused by the medicine.

After the medicine is started, the doctor will want to have regular appointments with you and your child to see how the medicine is working, to see if a dose change is needed, to watch for side effects, to see if quetiapine is still needed, and to see if any other treatment is needed. The doctor or nurse may check your child's height, weight, pulse, and blood pressure and watch for abnormal movements. Sometimes blood tests are needed to watch for diabetes or increased cholesterol.

What Side Effects Can This Medicine Have?

Any medicine can have side effects, including an allergy to the medicine. Because each patient is different, the doctor will monitor the youth closely, especially when the medicine is started. The doctor will work with you to increase the positive effects and decrease the negative effects of the medicine. Please tell the doctor if any of the listed side effects appear or if you think that the medicine is causing any other problems. Not all of the rare or unusual side effects are listed.

Side effects are most common after starting the medicine or after a dose increase. Many side effects can be avoided or lessened by starting with a very low dose and increasing it slowly—ask the doctor.

Allergic Reaction

Tell the doctor in a day or two (if possible, before the next dose of medicine):

- Hives
- Itching
- Rash

Stop the medicine and get *immediate* medical care:

- Trouble breathing or chest tightness
- Swelling of lips, tongue, or throat

Common, but Not Usually Serious, Side Effects

Discuss the following side effects with your child's doctor when convenient. These side effects often can be helped by lowering the dose of medicine, changing the times medicine is taken, or adding another medicine.

- Daytime sleepiness or tiredness—Do not allow your child to drive, ride a bicycle or motorcycle, or operate machinery if this happens. This problem may be lessened by taking the medicine at bedtime.
- Dry mouth—Have your child try using sugar-free gum or candy.
- Constipation—Encourage your child to drink more fluids and eat high-fiber foods; if necessary, the doctor may recommend a fiber medicine such as Benefiber or a stool softener such as Colace or mineral oil.
- Dizziness—This side effect is worse when the child stands up quickly, especially when getting out of bed in the morning; try having the child stand up slowly.
- Increased appetite

454

- Weight gain—Seek nutritional counseling; provide your child with low-calorie snacks and encourage regular exercise.

Less Common, but Not Usually Serious, Side Effects

Discuss the following side effects with your child's doctor when convenient. These side effects often can be helped by lowering the dose of medicine, changing the times medicine is taken, or adding another medicine.

- Increased restlessness or inability to sit still
- Shaking of hands and fingers
- Decreased or slowed movement and decreased facial expressions

Less Common, but Potentially Serious, Side Effects

Call the doctor *immediately*:

- Stiffness of the tongue, jaw, neck, back, or legs
- Seizure (fit, convulsion)—This is more common in people with a history of seizures or head injury.
- Increased thirst, frequent urination (having to go to the bathroom often), lethargy, tiredness, dizziness, and blurred vision—These could be signs of diabetes (especially if your child is overweight or there is a family history of diabetes). **Talk to a doctor within a day.**

Very Rare, but Serious, Side Effects

- Extreme stiffness or lack of movement, very high fever, mental confusion, irregular pulse rate, or eye pain—**This is a medical emergency. Go to an emergency room right away.**
- Sudden stiffness and inability to breathe or swallow—**Go to an emergency room or call 911.** Tell the paramedics, nurses, and doctors that the patient is taking quetiapine. Other medicines can be used to treat this problem fast.
- Illness, yellowing of eyes or skin, stomach pain—This may mean damage to the liver. **Call the doctor within a day or two.**

What Else Should I Know About Side Effects?

Most side effects lessen over time. If they are troublesome, talk with your child's doctor. Some side effects can be decreased by taking a smaller dose of medicine, by stopping the medicine, by changing to another medicine, or by adding another medicine.

Many people who take quetiapine gain weight. Children seem to have more problems with this than adults. The weight gain may be from increased appetite and from ways that the medicine changes how the body processes food. Quetiapine may also change the way that the body handles glucose (sugar) and cause high blood sugar levels (*hyperglycemia*). People who take quetiapine, especially those who gain a lot of weight, are at increased risk of developing *diabetes* and of having increased fats (*lipids—cholesterol and triglycerides*) in their blood. Over time, both diabetes and increased fats in the blood may lead to heart disease, stroke, and other complications. The FDA has put warnings on all atypical agents about the increased risks of hyperglycemia, diabetes, and increased blood cholesterol and triglycerides when taking one of these medicines. It is much easier to prevent weight gain than to lose weight later. When your child first starts taking quetiapine, it is a good idea to be sure that he or she eats a well-balanced diet without "junk food" and with healthy snacks like fruits and vegetables, not sweets or fried foods. He or she should drink water or skim milk, not pop, sodas, soft drinks, or sugary juices. Regular exercise is important for maintaining a healthy weight (and may also help with sleep).

One very rare side effect that may not go away is *tardive dyskinesia* (or TD). Patients with tardive dyskinesia have involuntary movements (movements that they cannot help making) of the body, especially the mouth and tongue. The patient may look as though he or she is making faces over and over again. Jerky movements of the arms, legs, or body may occur. There may be fine, wormlike, or sudden repeated movements of the tongue, or the person may appear to be chewing something or smacking or puckering his or her lips. The fingers may look as though they are rolling something. If you notice any unusual movements, be sure to tell the doctor. The doctor may use the AIMS test to look for these movements.

Neuroleptic malignant syndrome is a very rare side effect that can lead to death. The symptoms are severe muscle stiffness, high fever, increased heart rate and blood pressure, irregular heartbeat (pulse), and sweating. It may lead to unconsciousness. If you suspect this, **call 911 or go to an emergency room right away.**

Sometimes this medicine can cause a *dystonic reaction*. This is a sudden stiffening of the muscles, most often in the jaw, neck, tongue, face, or shoulders. If this happens, and your child is not having trouble breathing, you may give a dose of diphenhydramine (Benadryl). Follow the dose instructions on the package for your child's age. This should relax the muscles in a few minutes. Then call your doctor to tell him or her what happened. If the muscles do not relax, take your child to the emergency department.

Some Interactions With Other Medicines or Food

Please note that the following are only the most likely interactions with other medicines or food.

Quetiapine may be taken with or without food.

Carbamazepine (Tegretol) and phenytoin (Dilantin) may decrease levels of quetiapine, making it not work as well.

It is better to limit drinks with caffeine (coffee, tea, soft drinks) because caffeine works in the opposite way from this medicine, and the positive effects might be decreased.

What Could Happen if This Medicine Is Stopped Suddenly?

Involuntary movements, or *withdrawal dyskinesias*, may appear within 1–4 weeks of lowering the dose or stopping the medicine. Usually these go away, but they can last for days to months. If quetiapine is stopped suddenly, emotional disturbance (such as irritability, nervousness, moodiness, or oppositional behavior) or physical problems (such as stomachache, loss of appetite, nausea, vomiting, diarrhea, sweating, indigestion, trouble sleeping, trembling, or shaking) may appear. These problems usually last only a few days to a few weeks. If they happen, you should tell your child's doctor. The medicine dose may need to be lowered more slowly (tapered). Always check with the doctor before stopping a medicine.

How Long Will This Medicine Be Needed?

How long your child will need to take this medicine depends partly on the reason that it was prescribed. Some problems last for only a few months, whereas others last much longer. It is important to ask the doctor whether medicine is still needed, especially with medicines as powerful as this one. Every few months, you should discuss with your child's doctor the reasons for using quetiapine and whether it may be stopped or the dose lowered.

What Else Should I Know About This Medicine?

There are other medicines that are used for the same kinds of problems. If your child is having bad side effects or the medicine does not seem to be working, ask the doctor if another medicine might work as well or better and have fewer side effects for your child. Each person reacts differently to medicines.

Taking this medicine could make overheating or heatstroke more likely. Have your child decrease activity in hot weather, stay out of the sun, and drink water to prevent this.

Black Box Antidepressant Warning

In 2004, an advisory committee to the FDA decided that there might be an increased risk of suicidal behavior for some youth taking medicines called *antidepressants*. In the research studies that the committee reviewed, about 3%–4% of youth with depression who took an antidepressant medicine—and 1%–2% of youth with depression who took a placebo (pill without active medicine)—talked about suicidal thoughts (thinking about killing themselves or wishing they were dead) or did something to harm themselves. This means that almost twice as many youth who were taking an antidepressant to treat their depression talked about suicide or had suicidal behavior compared with youth with depression who were taking inactive medicine. There were *no* completed suicides in any of these research studies, which included more than 4,000 children and adolescents. For youth being treated for anxiety, there was no difference in suicidal talking or behavior between those taking antidepressant medication and those taking placebo.

The FDA told drug companies to add a *black box warning* label to all antidepressant medicines. Because of this label, a doctor (or advanced practice nurse) prescribing one of these medicines has to warn youth and their families that there might be more suicidal thoughts and actions in youth taking these medicines.

On the other hand, in places where more youth are taking the newer antidepressant medicines, the number of adolescents who commit suicide has gotten smaller. Also, thinking about or attempting suicide is more common in surveys of teenagers in the community than it is in depressed youth treated in research studies with antidepressant medicine.

If a youth is being treated with this medicine and is doing well, then no changes are needed as a result of this warning. Increased suicidal talk or action is most likely to happen in the first few months of treatment with a medicine. If your child has recently started this medicine or is about to start, then you and your doctor (or advanced practice nurse) should watch for any changes in behavior. People who are depressed often have suicidal thoughts or actions. It is hard to know whether suicidal thoughts or actions in depressed people are caused by the depression itself or by the medicine. Also, as their depression is getting better, some people talk more about the suicidal thoughts that they had before but did not talk about. As young people get better from depression, they might be at higher risk of doing something about suicidal thoughts that they have had for some time, because they have more energy.

What Should a Parent Do?

1. Be honest with your child about possible risks and benefits of medicine.
2. Talk to your child about whether he or she is having any suicidal thoughts, and tell your child to come to you if he or she is having such thoughts.
3. You, your child, and your child's doctor or nurse should develop a safety plan. Pick adults whom your child can tell if he or she is thinking about suicide.

4. Be sure to tell your child's doctor, nurse, or therapist if you suspect that your child is using alcohol or drugs or if something has happened that might make your child feel worse, such as a family separation, breaking up with a boyfriend or girlfriend, someone close dying or attempting suicide, physical or sexual abuse, or failure in school.

5. Be sure that there are no guns in the home and that all medicines (including over-the-counter medicines like Tylenol) are closely supervised by an adult and kept in a safe place.

6. Watch for new or worse thoughts of suicide, self-harm, depression, anxiety (nerves), feeling very agitated or restless, being angry or aggressive, having more trouble sleeping, or anything else that you see for the first time, seems worse, or worries your child or you. If these appear, contact a mental health professional **right away.** Do not just stop or change the dose of the medicine on your own. If the problems are serious, and you cannot reach one of your clinicians, call a 24-hour psychiatry emergency telephone number or take your child to an emergency room.

Youth taking antidepressant medicine should be watched carefully by their parent(s), clinician(s) (doctor, advanced practice nurse, nurse, therapist), and other concerned adults for the first weeks of treatment. It is a good idea to have regular contact with the doctor, APN, nurse, or therapist for the first months to check for feelings of depression or sadness, thoughts of killing or harming himself or herself, and any problems with the medication. If you have questions, be sure to ask the doctor, APN, nurse, or therapist.

For more information, see http://www.parentsmedguide.org/.

Notes

Use this space to take notes or to write down questions you want to ask the doctor.

_____

_____

_____

_____

_____

_____

_____

_____

_____

_____

From Dulcan MK, Ballard R (editors): *Helping Parents and Teachers Understand Medications for Behavioral and Emotional Problems: A Resource Book of Medication Information Handouts,* Fourth Edition. Washington, DC, American Psychiatric Publishing, 2015

Ramelteon—Rozerem

General Information About Medication

Each child and adolescent is different. No one has exactly the same combination of medical and psychological problems. It is a good idea to talk with the doctor or nurse about the reasons a medicine is being used. It is very important to keep all appointments and to be in touch by telephone if you have concerns. It is important to communicate with the doctor, nurse, or therapist. An *advanced practice nurse* (APN) has additional education and training after becoming a registered nurse (RN). Your child's medication may be prescribed by a medical doctor (MD or DO) or an APN. In addition, a *physician assistant* (PA) working with a physician may prescribe certain medications. In this information sheet, "doctor" includes medical doctors as well as APNs and PAs who prescribe medication. Often a nurse (RN) will be part of the team and answer questions and give information.

It is very important that the medicine be taken exactly as the doctor instructs. However, once in a while, everyone forgets to give a medicine on time. It is a good idea to ask the doctor or nurse what to do if this happens. Do not stop or change a medicine without asking the doctor or nurse first.

If the medicine seems to stop working, it may be because it is not being taken regularly. The youth may be "cheeking" or hiding the medicine or forgetting to take it (especially at school). The doses may be too far apart or a different dose or medicine may be needed. Something at school, at home, or in the neighborhood may be upsetting the youth, or he or she may need special help for learning disabilities or tutoring. Please discuss your concerns with the doctor. **Do not just increase the dose.** It is also very important not to decrease the dose or stop the medicine without talking to the doctor first. The problem being treated may come back, or there could be uncomfortable or even dangerous results.

All medicines should be kept in a safe place, out of the reach of children, and should be supervised by an adult. If someone takes too much of a medicine, call the doctor, the poison control center, or a hospital emergency room.

Each medicine has a "generic" or chemical name. Just like laundry detergents or paper towels, some medicines are sold by more than one company under different brand names. The same medicine may be available under a generic name and several brand names. The generic medications are usually less expensive than the brand name ones. The generic medications have the same chemical formula, but they may or may not be exactly the same strength as the brand-name medications. Also, some brands of pills contain dye or other things that can cause allergic reactions. It is a good idea to talk to the doctor and the pharmacist about whether it is important to use a specific brand of medicine.

Any medicine can cause an allergic reaction. Examples are hives, itching, rashes, swelling, and trouble breathing. Even a tiny amount of a medicine can cause a reaction in patients who are allergic to that medicine. Be *sure* to talk to the doctor before restarting a medicine that has caused an allergic reaction and tell the doctor about any reactions to medicine that your child has had before.

Taking more than one medicine at the same time may cause more side effects or cause one of the medicines to not work as well. Always ask the doctor, nurse, or pharmacist before adding another

medicine, either prescription or bought without a prescription in a store or on the Internet. Be sure that each doctor knows about *all* of the medicines your child is taking. Also tell the doctor about any vitamins, herbal medicines, or supplements your child may be taking. Some of these may have side effects alone or when taken with this medication. It is a very good idea to keep a list with you of the names and doses of all medicines that your child is taking.

Everyone taking medicine should have a physical examination at least once a year.

If you think that your child may be using drugs or alcohol, please tell the doctor right away.

Pregnancy requires special care in the use of medicine. Some medicines can cause birth defects if taken by a pregnant mother. **Please tell the doctor immediately if you suspect the teenager is at risk of becoming pregnant.** The doctor may wish to discuss sexual behavior and/or birth control with your daughter.

Printed information like this applies to children and adolescents in general. If you have questions about the medicine, or if you notice changes or anything unusual, please ask the doctor or nurse. As scientific research advances, knowledge increases and advice changes. Even experts do not always agree. Many medicines have not been "approved" by the U.S. Food and Drug Administration (FDA) for use in children or use for particular problems. For this reason, use of the medicine for a problem or age group often is not listed in the *Physicians' Desk Reference*. This does not necessarily mean that the medicine is dangerous or does not work, only that the company that makes the medicine has not received permission to advertise the medicine for use in children. Companies often do not apply for this permission because it is expensive to do the tests needed to apply for approval for use in children. Once a medication is approved by the FDA for any purpose, a doctor is allowed to prescribe it according to research and clinical experience.

Note to Teachers

It is a good idea to talk with the parent(s) about the reason(s) that a medication is being used. If the parent(s) sign consent to release information, it is often helpful for you to talk with the doctor. If the parent(s) give permission, the doctor may ask you to fill out rating forms about your experience with the student's behavior, feelings, academic performance, and medication side effects. This information is very useful in selecting and monitoring medication treatment. If you have observations that you think are important, do not hesitate to share these with the student's parent(s) and treating clinicians (with parental consent).

It is very important that the medicine be taken exactly as the doctor instructs. However, everyone forgets to give a medicine on time once in a while. It is a good idea to ask the parent(s) in advance what to do if this happens. Do not stop or change the time you are giving a medicine at school without parental permission. If a medication is to be taken with food, but lunchtime or snack time changes, be sure to notify the parent(s) so appropriate adjustments can be made.

All medicines should be kept in a secure place and should be supervised by an adult. If someone takes too much of a medicine, follow your school procedure for an urgent medical problem.

Taking medicine is a private matter and is best managed discreetly and confidentially. It is important to be sensitive to the student's feelings about taking medicine.

If you suspect that the student is using drugs or alcohol, please tell the parent(s) or a school counselor right away.

Please tell the parent(s) or school nurse if you suspect medication side effects.

Modifications of the classroom environment or assignments may be useful in addition to medication. The student may need to be evaluated for additional help or a 504 plan or an Individualized Education Plan for learning problems or emotional or behavioral issues.

Any expression of suicidal thoughts or feelings or self-harm by a child or adolescent is a signal of distress and should be taken seriously. These behaviors should not be dismissed as "attention seeking." School procedures for safety issues should be followed.

What Is Ramelteon (Rozerem)?

Ramelteon is a *hypnotic* or *sedative-hypnotic* medicine. It is *not* a *benzodiazepine*. It comes in Rozerem brand name tablets.

How Can This Medicine Help?

Ramelteon is used to treat insomnia (problems falling asleep or staying asleep).

How Does This Medicine Work?

Ramelteon works in the same way as a natural substance called *melatonin* that is produced by the body. It helps regulate the sleep-wake cycle (circadian rhythm).

How Long Does This Medicine Last?

Ramelteon is taken before bedtime and starts working within an hour.

How Will the Doctor Monitor This Medicine?

The doctor will review your child's medical history and physical examination before starting ramelteon. Be sure to tell the doctor if your child has liver disease.

After the medicine is started, the doctor will want to have regular appointments with you and your child to see how the medicine is working, to see if a dose change is needed, to watch for side effects, to see if ramelteon is still needed, and to see if any other treatment is needed.

What Side Effects Can This Medicine Have?

Any medicine can have side effects, including an allergy to the medicine. Because each patient is different, the doctor will monitor the youth closely, especially when the medicine is started. The doctor will work with you to increase the positive effects and decrease the negative effects of the medicine. Please tell the doctor if any of the listed side effects appear or if you think that the medicine is causing any other problems. Not all of the rare or unusual side effects are listed.

Side effects are most common after starting the medicine or after a dose increase. Many side effects can be avoided or lessened by starting with a very low dose and increasing it slowly—ask the doctor.

Allergic Reaction

Tell the doctor in a day or two (if possible, before the next dose of medicine):

- Hives
- Itching
- Rash

Stop the medicine and get *immediate* medical care:

- Trouble breathing or chest tightness
- Swelling of lips, tongue, or throat

Common Side Effects

Tell the doctor within a week or two:

- Daytime sleepiness—Do not allow your child to drive a car, ride a bicycle or motorcycle, or operate machinery if this happens.
- Dizziness, feeling "spacey," or decreased coordination
- Low energy or tiredness
- Headache

Less Common Side Effects

Tell the doctor within a week or two:

- More trouble sleeping
- Nausea
- Diarrhea

Rare, but Potentially Serious, Side Effects

Tell the doctor within a week or two:

- Missed menstrual periods
- Fluid discharge from the breasts

Rare, but Serious, Side Effects

Stop the medicine and call the doctor right away:

- Depression
- Thoughts of harming oneself

Some Interactions With Other Medicines or Food

Please note that the following are only the most likely interactions with other medicines or food.

Caffeine may cause trouble sleeping and make ramelteon less effective. If caffeine is eliminated, less ramelteon may be needed, or ramelteon may not be needed at all.

Do not take ramelteon with or immediately after a high-fat meal because fat can affect how well this drug works.

Do not take ramelteon with fluvoxamine (Luvox).

It is important not to use other sedatives, tranquilizers, or sleeping pills or antihistamines (such as Benadryl) when taking ramelteon because of increased side effects.

What Could Happen if This Medicine Is Stopped Suddenly?

There are no known medical withdrawal effects, but the sleep problem may come back.

How Long Will This Medicine Be Needed?

Ramelteon is usually prescribed for a short time, but some people may need to take it for longer. A behavioral program, such as regular soothing routines at bedtime and increased exercise in the daytime, should be used along with the medicine to improve sleep. Finding developmentally appropriate bedtimes and wake times and sticking to them is very important. These strategies should be continued after the medicine is stopped or when the medicine is used only occasionally.

What Else Should I Know About This Medicine?

People who take ramelteon must not drink alcohol. Severe sleepiness or even loss of consciousness may result.

People with sleep apnea (breathing stops while they are asleep) should not take ramelteon. Tell the doctor if your child snores very loudly, which may be a symptom of sleep apnea.

Notes

Use this space to take notes or to write down questions you want to ask the doctor.

_____

_____

_____

_____

_____

_____

_____

_____

_____

_____

From Dulcan MK, Ballard R (editors): *Helping Parents and Teachers Understand Medications for Behavioral and Emotional Problems: A Resource Book of Medication Information Handouts,* Fourth Edition. Washington, DC, American Psychiatric Publishing, 2015

Medication Information for Parents and Teachers

Risperidone—Risperdal

General Information About Medication

Each child and adolescent is different. No one has exactly the same combination of medical and psychological problems. It is a good idea to talk with the doctor or nurse about the reasons a medicine is being used. It is very important to keep all appointments and to be in touch by telephone if you have concerns. It is important to communicate with the doctor, nurse, or therapist. An *advanced practice nurse* (APN) has additional education and training after becoming a registered nurse (RN). Your child's medication may be prescribed by a medical doctor (MD or DO) or an APN. In addition, a *physician assistant* (PA) working with a physician may prescribe certain medications. In this information sheet, "doctor" includes medical doctors as well as APNs and PAs who prescribe medication. Often a nurse (RN) will be part of the team and answer questions and give information.

It is very important that the medicine be taken exactly as the doctor instructs. However, once in a while, everyone forgets to give a medicine on time. It is a good idea to ask the doctor or nurse what to do if this happens. Do not stop or change a medicine without asking the doctor or nurse first.

If the medicine seems to stop working, it may be because it is not being taken regularly. The youth may be "cheeking" or hiding the medicine or forgetting to take it (especially at school). The doses may be too far apart or a different dose or medicine may be needed. Something at school, at home, or in the neighborhood may be upsetting the youth, or he or she may need special help for learning disabilities or tutoring. Please discuss your concerns with the doctor. **Do not just increase the dose.** It is also very important not to decrease the dose or stop the medicine without talking to the doctor first. The problem being treated may come back, or there could be uncomfortable or even dangerous results.

All medicines should be kept in a safe place, out of the reach of children, and should be supervised by an adult. If someone takes too much of a medicine, call the doctor, the poison control center, or a hospital emergency room.

Each medicine has a "generic" or chemical name. Just like laundry detergents or paper towels, some medicines are sold by more than one company under different brand names. The same medicine may be available under a generic name and several brand names. The generic medications are usually less expensive than the brand name ones. The generic medications have the same chemical formula, but they may or may not be exactly the same strength as the brand-name medications. Also, some brands of pills contain dye or other things that can cause allergic reactions. It is a good idea to talk to the doctor and the pharmacist about whether it is important to use a specific brand of medicine.

Any medicine can cause an allergic reaction. Examples are hives, itching, rashes, swelling, and trouble breathing. Even a tiny amount of a medicine can cause a reaction in patients who are allergic to that medicine. Be *sure* to talk to the doctor before restarting a medicine that has caused an allergic reaction and tell the doctor about any reactions to medicine that your child has had before.

Taking more than one medicine at the same time may cause more side effects or cause one of the medicines to not work as well. Always ask the doctor, nurse, or pharmacist before adding another

medicine, either prescription or bought without a prescription in a store or on the Internet. Be sure that each doctor knows about *all* of the medicines your child is taking. Also tell the doctor about any vitamins, herbal medicines, or supplements your child may be taking. Some of these may have side effects alone or when taken with this medication. It is a very good idea to keep a list with you of the names and doses of all medicines that your child is taking.

Everyone taking medicine should have a physical examination at least once a year.

If you think that your child may be using drugs or alcohol, please tell the doctor right away.

Pregnancy requires special care in the use of medicine. Some medicines can cause birth defects if taken by a pregnant mother. **Please tell the doctor immediately if you suspect the teenager is at risk of becoming pregnant.** The doctor may wish to discuss sexual behavior and/or birth control with your daughter.

Printed information like this applies to children and adolescents in general. If you have questions about the medicine, or if you notice changes or anything unusual, please ask the doctor or nurse. As scientific research advances, knowledge increases and advice changes. Even experts do not always agree. Many medicines have not been "approved" by the U.S. Food and Drug Administration (FDA) for use in children or use for particular problems. For this reason, use of the medicine for a problem or age group often is not listed in the *Physicians' Desk Reference*. This does not necessarily mean that the medicine is dangerous or does not work, only that the company that makes the medicine has not received permission to advertise the medicine for use in children. Companies often do not apply for this permission because it is expensive to do the tests needed to apply for approval for use in children. Once a medication is approved by the FDA for any purpose, a doctor is allowed to prescribe it according to research and clinical experience.

Note to Teachers

It is a good idea to talk with the parent(s) about the reason(s) that a medication is being used. If the parent(s) sign consent to release information, it is often helpful for you to talk with the doctor. If the parent(s) give permission, the doctor may ask you to fill out rating forms about your experience with the student's behavior, feelings, academic performance, and medication side effects. This information is very useful in selecting and monitoring medication treatment. If you have observations that you think are important, do not hesitate to share these with the student's parent(s) and treating clinicians (with parental consent).

It is very important that the medicine be taken exactly as the doctor instructs. However, everyone forgets to give a medicine on time once in a while. It is a good idea to ask the parent(s) in advance what to do if this happens. Do not stop or change the time you are giving a medicine at school without parental permission. If a medication is to be taken with food, but lunchtime or snack time changes, be sure to notify the parent(s) so appropriate adjustments can be made.

All medicines should be kept in a secure place and should be supervised by an adult. If someone takes too much of a medicine, follow your school procedure for an urgent medical problem.

Taking medicine is a private matter and is best managed discreetly and confidentially. It is important to be sensitive to the student's feelings about taking medicine.

If you suspect that the student is using drugs or alcohol, please tell the parent(s) or a school counselor right away.

Please tell the parent(s) or school nurse if you suspect medication side effects.

Modifications of the classroom environment or assignments may be useful in addition to medication. The student may need to be evaluated for additional help or a 504 plan or an Individualized Education Plan for learning problems or emotional or behavioral issues.

Any expression of suicidal thoughts or feelings or self-harm by a child or adolescent is a signal of distress and should be taken seriously. These behaviors should not be dismissed as "attention seeking." School procedures for safety issues should be followed.

What Is Risperidone (Risperdal)?

This medicine is called an *atypical* or *second-generation antipsychotic*. It is sometimes called an *atypical psychotropic agent* or simply an *atypical*. It comes in brand name Risperdal and generic tablets and liquid, Risperdal M-Tab and generic dispersible (rapid disintegrating) tablets, and Risperdal Consta long-acting injection (shot). The dispersible tablets melt fast in the mouth.

How Can This Medicine Help?

Risperidone is used to treat psychosis, such as in schizophrenia, mania, or very severe depression. It can reduce *positive symptoms* such as hallucinations (hearing voices or seeing things that are not there); delusions (troubling beliefs that other people do not share); agitation; and very unusual thinking, speech, and behavior. It is also used to lessen the *negative symptoms* of schizophrenia, such as lack of interest in doing things (apathy), lack of motivation, social withdrawal, and lack of energy.

Risperidone may be used as a *mood stabilizer* in patients with bipolar disorder or severe mood swings. It can reduce mania and may be able to help maintain a stable mood over the long term.

Risperidone is used to treat irritability and associated dysfunctional behaviors in people with autism spectrum disorders.

Sometimes risperidone is used to reduce severe aggression or very serious behavioral problems in young people with conduct disorder, autism spectrum disorder, or pervasive developmental disorder or intellectual disability.

Risperidone may be used for behavior problems after a head injury.

It is also used to reduce motor and vocal tics (fast, repeated movements or sounds) and behavioral problems in people with Tourette's disorder.

This medicine is very powerful and is used to treat very serious problems or symptoms that other medicines do not help. Be patient; the positive effects of this medicine may not appear for 2–3 weeks.

How Does This Medicine Work?

Cells in the brain communicate using chemicals called *neurotransmitters*. Too much or too little of these substances in parts of the brain can cause problems. Risperidone works by blocking the action of two of these neurotransmitters, *dopamine* and *serotonin*, in certain areas of the brain.

How Long Does This Medicine Last?

Risperidone is usually taken once or twice a day. Risperdal Consta lasts for 2 weeks, but when it is first started, an oral antipsychotic medicine must be taken also for about 3 weeks, until enough Consta builds up in the blood to work.

How Will the Doctor Monitor This Medicine?

The doctor will review your child's medical history and physical examination before starting risperidone. The doctor may order some blood or urine tests to be sure your child does not have a hidden medical condition that would make it unsafe to use this medicine. The doctor or nurse will measure your child's height, weight, pulse, and blood pressure before starting risperidone. The doctor may order other tests, such as baseline tests for blood sugar and cholesterol or an ECG (electrocardiogram or heart rhythm test).

Be sure to tell the doctor if anyone in the family has diabetes, high blood pressure, high cholesterol, or heart disease.

Before your child starts taking risperidone and every so often afterward, a test such as the Abnormal Involuntary Movement Scale (AIMS) may be used to check your child's tongue, legs, and arms for unusual movements that could be caused by the medicine.

After the medicine is started, the doctor will want to have regular appointments with you and your child to see how the medicine is working, to see if a dose change is needed, to watch for side effects, to see if risperidone is still needed, and to see if any other treatment is needed. The doctor or nurse will check your child's height, weight, pulse, and blood pressure, and watch for abnormal movements. Sometimes blood tests are needed to watch for diabetes or increased cholesterol.

What Side Effects Can This Medicine Have?

Any medicine can have side effects, including an allergy to the medicine. Because each patient is different, the doctor will monitor the youth closely, especially when the medicine is started. The doctor will work with you to increase the positive effects and decrease the negative effects of the medicine. Please tell the doctor if any of the listed side effects appear or if you think that the medicine is causing any other problems. Not all of the rare or unusual side effects are listed.

Side effects are most common after starting the medicine or after a dose increase. Many side effects can be avoided or lessened by starting with a very low dose and increasing it slowly—ask the doctor.

Allergic Reaction

Tell the doctor in a day or two (if possible, before the next dose of medicine):

- Hives
- Itching
- Rash

Stop the medicine and get *immediate* medical care:

- Trouble breathing or chest tightness
- Swelling of lips, tongue, or throat

Common, but Not Usually Serious, Side Effects

Discuss the following side effects with your child's doctor when convenient. These side effects often can be helped by lowering the dose of medicine, changing the times medicine is taken, or adding another medicine.

- Daytime sleepiness or tiredness—Do not allow your child to drive, ride a bicycle or motorcycle, or operate machinery if this happens. This problem may be lessened by taking the medicine at bedtime.
- Dry mouth—Have your child try using sugar-free gum or candy.
- Constipation—Encourage your child to drink more fluids and eat high-fiber foods; if necessary, the doctor may recommend a fiber medicine such as Benefiber or a stool softener such as Colace or mineral oil.
- Dizziness—This side effect is worse when the child stands up quickly, especially when getting out of bed in the morning; try having the child stand up slowly.
- Increased appetite
- Weight gain—Seek nutritional counseling; provide your child with low-calorie snacks and encourage regular exercise.
- Increased risk of sunburn—Have your child wear sunscreen or protective clothing or stay out of the sun.
- Nausea
- Vomiting
- Insomnia (trouble sleeping)

Less Common, but Not Usually Serious, Side Effects

Discuss the following side effects with your child's doctor when convenient. These side effects often can be helped by lowering the dose of medicine, changing the times medicine is taken, or adding another medicine.

- Drooling
- Increased restlessness or inability to sit still
- Shaking of hands and fingers
- Decreased or slowed movement and decreased facial expressions
- Decreased sexual interest or ability
- Changes in menstrual cycle
- Increase in breast size or discharge from the breasts (in both boys and girls)

Less Common, but Potentially Serious, Side Effects

Call the doctor *immediately:*

- Stiffness of the tongue, jaw, neck, back, or legs
- Seizure (fit, convulsion)—This is more common in people with a history of seizures or head injury.
- Increased thirst, frequent urination (having to go to the bathroom often), lethargy, tiredness, dizziness, and blurred vision—These could be signs of diabetes, especially if your child is overweight or there is a family history of diabetes. **Talk to a doctor within a day.**

Very Rare, but Serious, Side Effects

- Extreme stiffness or lack of movement, very high fever, mental confusion, irregular pulse rate, or eye pain—**This is a medical emergency. Go to an emergency room right away.**
- Sudden stiffness and inability to breathe or swallow—**Go to an emergency room or call 911.** Tell the paramedics, nurses, and doctors that the patient is taking risperidone. Other medicines can be used to treat this problem fast.

What Else Should I Know About Side Effects?

Most side effects lessen over time. If they are troublesome, talk with your child's doctor. Some side effects can be decreased by taking a smaller dose of medicine, by stopping the medicine, by changing to another medicine, or by adding another medicine.

Many young people who take risperidone gain weight. The weight gain may be from increased appetite and from ways that the medicine changes how the body processes food. Risperidone may also change the way that the body handles glucose (sugar) and cause high blood sugar levels (*hyperglycemia*). People who take risperidone, especially those who gain a lot of weight, are at increased risk of developing *diabetes* and of having increased fats (*lipids—cholesterol and triglycerides*) in their blood. Over time, both diabetes and increased fats in the blood may lead to heart disease, stroke, and other complications. The FDA has put warnings on all atypical agents about the increased risks of hyperglycemia, diabetes, and increased blood cholesterol and triglycerides when taking one of these medicines. It is much easier to prevent weight gain than to lose weight later. When your child first starts taking risperidone, it is a good idea to be sure that he or she eats a well-balanced diet without "junk food" and with healthy snacks like fruits and vegetables, not sweets or fried foods. He or she should drink water or skim milk, not pop, sodas, soft drinks, or sugary juices. Regular exercise is important for maintaining a healthy weight (and may also help with sleep).

The medicine may increase the level of *prolactin*, a natural hormone made in the part of the brain called the *pituitary*. This may cause side effects such as breast tenderness or swelling or production of milk in both boys and girls. It also may interfere with sexual functioning in teenage boys and with regular menstrual cycles (periods) in teenage girls. A blood test can measure the level of prolactin. If these side effects do not go away and are troublesome, talk with your child's doctor about substituting another medicine for risperidone.

One very rare side effect that may not go away is *tardive dyskinesia* (or TD). Patients with tardive dyskinesia have involuntary movements (movements that they cannot help making) of the body, especially the mouth and tongue. The patient may look as though he or she is making faces over and over again. Jerky movements of the arms, legs, or body may occur. There may be fine, wormlike, or sudden repeated movements of the tongue, or the person may appear to be chewing something or smacking or puckering his or her lips. The fingers may look as though they are rolling something. If you notice any unusual movements, be sure to tell the doctor. The doctor may use the AIMS test to look for these movements.

Neuroleptic malignant syndrome is a very rare side effect that can lead to death. The symptoms are severe muscle stiffness, high fever, increased heart rate and blood pressure, irregular heartbeat (pulse), and sweating. It may lead to unconsciousness. If you suspect this, **call 911 or go to an emergency room right away.**

Sometimes this medicine can cause a *dystonic reaction*. This is a sudden stiffening of the muscles, most often in the jaw, neck, tongue, face, or shoulders. If this happens, and your child is not having trouble breathing, you may give a dose of diphenhydramine (Benadryl). Follow the dose instructions on the package for your child's age. This should relax the muscles in a few minutes. Then call your doctor to tell him or her what happened. If the muscles do not relax, take your child to the emergency department.

Some Interactions With Other Medicines or Food

Please note that the following are only the most likely interactions with other medicines or food.

Risperidone may be taken with or without food.

Risperidone liquid should *not* be taken with tea or cola. It may be taken with water, orange juice, coffee, or low-fat milk.

Paroxetine (Paxil), fluoxetine (Prozac), and other selective serotonin reuptake inhibitor (SSRI) antidepressants can increase the levels of risperidone and increase the risk of side effects.

Carbamazepine (Tegretol) can decrease the levels of risperidone so that it does not work as well.

Heart problems are more common if other medicines that affect the heart are being taken as well. Be sure to tell all your child's doctors and your pharmacist about all medications your child is taking.

It is better to limit drinks with caffeine (coffee, tea, soft drinks) because caffeine works in the opposite way from this medicine, and the positive effects might be decreased.

What Could Happen if This Medicine Is Stopped Suddenly?

Involuntary movements, or *withdrawal dyskinesias*, may appear within 1–4 weeks of lowering the dose or stopping the medicine. Usually these go away, but they can last for days to months. If this medicine is stopped suddenly, emotional disturbance (such as irritability, nervousness, moodiness, or oppositional behavior) or physical problems (such as stomachache, loss of appetite, nausea, vomiting, diarrhea, sweating, indigestion, trouble sleeping, trembling, or shaking) may appear. These problems usually last only a few days to a few weeks. If they happen, you should tell your child's doctor. The medicine dose may need to be lowered more slowly (tapered). Always check with the doctor before stopping a medicine.

How Long Will This Medicine Be Needed?

How long your child will need to take this medicine depends partly on the reason that it was prescribed. Some problems last for only a few months, whereas others last much longer. It is important to ask the doctor whether medicine is still needed, especially with medicines as powerful as this one. Every few months, you should discuss with your child's doctor the reasons for using the medicine and whether the medicine may be stopped or the dose lowered.

What Else Should I Know About This Medicine?

There are other medicines that are used for the same kinds of problems. If your child is having bad side effects or the medicine does not seem to be working, ask the doctor if another medicine might work as well or better and have fewer side effects for your child. Each person reacts differently to medicines.

Taking this medicine could make overheating or heatstroke more likely. Have your child decrease activity in hot weather, stay out of the sun, and drink water to prevent this.

Notes

Use this space to take notes or to write down questions you want to ask the doctor.

_____

_____

_____

_____

_____

_____

_____

_____

_____

_____

_____

Medication Information for Parents and Teachers

Sertraline—Zoloft

General Information About Medication

Each child and adolescent is different. No one has exactly the same combination of medical and psychological problems. It is a good idea to talk with the doctor or nurse about the reasons a medicine is being used. It is very important to keep all appointments and to be in touch by telephone if you have concerns. It is important to communicate with the doctor, nurse, or therapist. An *advanced practice nurse* (APN) has additional education and training after becoming a registered nurse (RN). Your child's medication may be prescribed by a medical doctor (MD or DO) or an APN. In addition, a *physician assistant* (PA) working with a physician may prescribe certain medications. In this information sheet, "doctor" includes medical doctors as well as APNs and PAs who prescribe medication. Often a nurse (RN) will be part of the team and answer questions and give information.

It is very important that the medicine be taken exactly as the doctor instructs. However, once in a while, everyone forgets to give a medicine on time. It is a good idea to ask the doctor or nurse what to do if this happens. Do not stop or change a medicine without asking the doctor or nurse first.

If the medicine seems to stop working, it may be because it is not being taken regularly. The youth may be "cheeking" or hiding the medicine or forgetting to take it (especially at school). The doses may be too far apart or a different dose or medicine may be needed. Something at school, at home, or in the neighborhood may be upsetting the youth, or he or she may need special help for learning disabilities or tutoring. Please discuss your concerns with the doctor. **Do not just increase the dose.** It is also very important not to decrease the dose or stop the medicine without talking to the doctor first. The problem being treated may come back, or there could be uncomfortable or even dangerous results.

All medicines should be kept in a safe place, out of the reach of children, and should be supervised by an adult. If someone takes too much of a medicine, call the doctor, the poison control center, or a hospital emergency room.

Each medicine has a "generic" or chemical name. Just like laundry detergents or paper towels, some medicines are sold by more than one company under different brand names. The same medicine may be available under a generic name and several brand names. The generic medications are usually less expensive than the brand name ones. The generic medications have the same chemical formula, but they may or may not be exactly the same strength as the brand-name medications. Also, some brands of pills contain dye or other things that can cause allergic reactions. It is a good idea to talk to the doctor and the pharmacist about whether it is important to use a specific brand of medicine.

Any medicine can cause an allergic reaction. Examples are hives, itching, rashes, swelling, and trouble breathing. Even a tiny amount of a medicine can cause a reaction in patients who are allergic to that medicine. Be *sure* to talk to the doctor before restarting a medicine that has caused an allergic reaction and tell the doctor about any reactions to medicine that your child has had before.

Taking more than one medicine at the same time may cause more side effects or cause one of the medicines to not work as well. Always ask the doctor, nurse, or pharmacist before adding another

475

medicine, either prescription or bought without a prescription in a store or on the Internet. **Be sure that each doctor knows about *all* of the medicines your child is taking. Also tell the doctor about any vitamins, herbal medicines, or supplements your child may be taking.** Some of these may have side effects alone or when taken with this medication. It is a very good idea to keep a list with you of the names and doses of all medicines that your child is taking.

Everyone taking medicine should have a physical examination at least once a year.

If you think that your child may be using drugs or alcohol, please tell the doctor right away.

Pregnancy requires special care in the use of medicine. Some medicines can cause birth defects if taken by a pregnant mother. **Please tell the doctor immediately if you suspect the teenager is at risk of becoming pregnant.** The doctor may wish to discuss sexual behavior and/or birth control with your daughter.

Printed information like this applies to children and adolescents in general. If you have questions about the medicine, or if you notice changes or anything unusual, please ask the doctor or nurse. As scientific research advances, knowledge increases and advice changes. Even experts do not always agree. Many medicines have not been "approved" by the U.S. Food and Drug Administration (FDA) for use in children or use for particular problems. For this reason, use of the medicine for a problem or age group often is not listed in the *Physicians' Desk Reference*. This does not necessarily mean that the medicine is dangerous or does not work, only that the company that makes the medicine has not received permission to advertise the medicine for use in children. Companies often do not apply for this permission because it is expensive to do the tests needed to apply for approval for use in children. Once a medication is approved by the FDA for any purpose, a doctor is allowed to prescribe it according to research and clinical experience.

Note to Teachers

It is a good idea to talk with the parent(s) about the reason(s) that a medication is being used. If the parent(s) sign consent to release information, it is often helpful for you to talk with the doctor. If the parent(s) give permission, the doctor may ask you to fill out rating forms about your experience with the student's behavior, feelings, academic performance, and medication side effects. This information is very useful in selecting and monitoring medication treatment. If you have observations that you think are important, do not hesitate to share these with the student's parent(s) and treating clinicians (with parental consent).

It is very important that the medicine be taken exactly as the doctor instructs. However, everyone forgets to give a medicine on time once in a while. It is a good idea to ask the parent(s) in advance what to do if this happens. Do not stop or change the time you are giving a medicine at school without parental permission. If a medication is to be taken with food, but lunchtime or snack time changes, be sure to notify the parent(s) so appropriate adjustments can be made.

All medicines should be kept in a secure place and should be supervised by an adult. If someone takes too much of a medicine, follow your school procedure for an urgent medical problem.

Taking medicine is a private matter and is best managed discreetly and confidentially. It is important to be sensitive to the student's feelings about taking medicine.

If you suspect that the student is using drugs or alcohol, please tell the parent(s) or a school counselor right away.

Please tell the parent(s) or school nurse if you suspect medication side effects.

Modifications of the classroom environment or assignments may be useful in addition to medication. The student may need to be evaluated for additional help or a 504 plan or an Individualized Education Plan for learning problems or emotional or behavioral issues.

Any expression of suicidal thoughts or feelings or self-harm by a child or adolescent is a signal of distress and should be taken seriously. These behaviors should not be dismissed as "attention seeking." School procedures for safety issues should be followed.

What Is Sertraline (Zoloft)?

Sertraline (brand name Zoloft) is an antidepressant known as a *selective serotonin reuptake inhibitor* (SSRI). It comes in generic and brand name tablets and generic and brand name liquid form.

How Can This Medicine Help?

Sertraline is used to treat depression and anxiety disorders such as obsessive-compulsive disorder (OCD), posttraumatic stress disorder (PTSD), panic disorder, separation anxiety disorder, selective mutism, social anxiety disorder, generalized anxiety disorder, and premenstrual dysphoric disorder.

How Does This Medicine Work?

Sertraline increases the amount of a *neurotransmitter* called *serotonin* in certain parts of the brain. People with emotional and behavioral problems, such as depression and anxiety, may have low levels of serotonin in certain parts of the brain. SSRIs such as sertraline help by increasing the action of brain serotonin to more normal levels.

How Long Does This Medicine Last?

Sertraline can be taken only once a day for most people.

How Will the Doctor Monitor This Medicine?

The doctor will review your child's medical history and physical examination before starting sertraline. The doctor may order some blood or urine tests to be sure your child does not have a hidden medical condition that would make it unsafe to use this medicine. Extra care is needed when using SSRIs in youth with seizures (epilepsy); heart, liver, or kidney problems; or diabetes. The doctor or nurse may measure your child's pulse, blood pressure, and weight before starting the medicine.

Be sure to tell the doctor if your child or anyone in the family has bipolar disorder or has tried to kill himself or herself.

After the medicine is started, the doctor will want to have regular appointments with you and your child to see how the medicine is working, to see if a dose change is needed, to watch for side effects, to see if sertraline is still needed, and to see if any other treatment is needed. The doctor or nurse may check your child's height, weight, pulse, and blood pressure.

Before using medicine and at times afterward, the doctor may ask your child to fill out a rating scale about depression or anxiety to help see how your child is doing.

What Side Effects Can This Medicine Have?

Any medicine can have side effects, including an allergy to the medicine. Because each patient is different, the doctor will monitor the youth closely, especially when the medicine is started. The doctor will work with you to increase the positive effects and decrease the negative effects of the medicine. Please tell the doctor if any of the listed side effects appear or if you think that the medicine is causing any other problems. Not all of the rare or unusual side effects are listed.

Side effects are most common after starting the medicine or after a dose increase. Many side effects can be avoided or lessened by starting with a very low dose and increasing it slowly—ask the doctor.

Allergic Reaction

Tell the doctor in a day or two (if possible, before the next dose of medicine):

- Hives
- Itching
- Rash

Stop the medicine and get *immediate* medical care:

- Trouble breathing or chest tightness
- Swelling of lips, tongue, or throat

Common Side Effects

Tell the doctor within a week or two, or sooner if the problems are getting worse:

- Nausea, upset stomach, vomiting
- Diarrhea or excessive gas
- Dry mouth—Have your child try using sugar-free gum or candy.
- Constipation—Encourage your child to drink more fluids and eat high-fiber foods; if necessary, the doctor may recommend a fiber medicine such as Benefiber or a stool softener such as Colace or mineral oil.
- Headache
- Anxiety or nervousness
- Insomnia (trouble sleeping)
- Restlessness, increased activity level
- Daytime sleepiness or tiredness—Do not allow your child to drive, ride a bicycle or motorcycle, or operate machinery if this side effect is present.
- Dizziness—This side effect is worse when the child stands up quickly, especially when getting out of bed in the morning; try having the child stand up slowly.
- Tremor (shakiness)
- Excessive sweating
- Apathy, lack of interest in school or friends—This may happen after an initial good response to treatment.
- Decreased sexual interest, trouble with sexual functioning
- Weight gain
- Weight loss

Less Common, but More Serious, Side Effects

Call the doctor within a day or two:

- Significant suicidal thoughts or self-injurious behavior
- Increased activity, rapid speech, feeling "speeded up," decreased need for sleep, being very excited or irritable (cranky), agitation, acting out of character
- Bleeding, such as bruising or nosebleeds, or bleeding with surgery

Serious Side Effects

Call the doctor *immediately* or go to the nearest emergency room:

- Seizure (fit, convulsion)
- Stiffness, high fever, confusion, tremors (shaking)
- Overheating or heatstroke—Prevent by decreasing activity in hot weather, staying out of the sun, and drinking water.

Serotonin Syndrome

A very serious side effect called *serotonin syndrome* can happen when certain kinds of medicines (including SSRI antidepressants, clomipramine, and other medicines, such as triptans for migraine headaches, buspirone, linezolid, tramadol, or St. John's wort) are taken by the same person. Very rarely, serotonin syndrome can happen at high doses of just one medicine. The early signs are restlessness, confusion, shaking, skin turning red, sweating, muscle stiffness, sweating, and jerking of muscles. If you see these symptoms, stop the medicine and send or take the youth to an emergency room right away.

Some Interactions With Other Medicines or Food

Please note that the following are only the most likely interactions with other medicines or food.

Sertraline interacts with many other prescription and over-the-counter medicines, including some antibiotics and other psychiatric medicines. It is especially important to tell the doctor and pharmacist about all of the medicines your child is taking or has taken in the past few months, including over-the-counter and herbal medicines. Sometimes one medicine can increase or decrease the blood level of another medicine, so that different doses are needed. Erythromycin and similar antibiotics, as well as antifungal agents such as ketoconazole, may increase levels of sertraline and increase side effects. Sertraline may increase the heart side effects of pimozide (Orap), so those two medicines should not be taken by the same person. Tryptophan or the herbal medicine St. John's Wort also increases serotonin and can cause serious side effects if taken with sertraline. Taking sertraline with aspirin, nonsteroidal anti-inflammatory drugs (NSAIDs) (medications including ibuprofen or naproxen), or anticoagulant medications (including warfarin) increases risk of abnormal bleeding.

It can be *very dangerous* to take an SSRI at the same time as or even within a month of taking another type of medicine called a *monoamine oxidase inhibitor* (MAOI), such as selegiline (Eldepryl), phenelzine (Nardil), tranylcypromine (Parnate), or isocarboxazid (Marplan).

Sertraline can be taken with or without food but should not be taken with grapefruit juice.

Caffeine may increase side effects.

What Could Happen if This Medicine Is Stopped Suddenly?

No known serious medical effects occur if sertraline is stopped suddenly, but there may be uncomfortable feelings, which should be avoided if possible. Your child might have trouble sleeping, nervousness, irritability, dizziness, and flu-like symptoms. Ask the doctor before stopping sertraline or if these symptoms happen while the dose is being decreased.

How Long Will This Medicine Be Needed?

Sertraline may take up to 1–2 months to reach its full effect. If your child has a good response to sertraline, it is a good idea to continue the medicine for at least 6–12 months. It is important to review this with your doctor.

What Else Should I Know About This Medicine?

In youth who have bipolar disorder or who may be at risk for bipolar disorder, any antidepressant medicine may increase the risk of hypomania or mania (excitement, agitation, increased activity, decreased sleep).

In hot weather, make sure your child drinks enough water or other liquids and does not get overheated.

Sometimes, after a person has improved while taking sertraline, he or she loses interest in school or friends or just stops trying. Please tell your child's doctor if this happens—it may be a side effect of the medicine. A lower dose or a different medicine may be needed.

Store the medicine away from sunlight, heat, moisture, and humidity.

Black Box Antidepressant Warning

In 2004, an advisory committee to the FDA decided that there might be an increased risk of suicidal behavior for some youth taking medicines called *antidepressants*. In the research studies that the committee reviewed, about 3%–4% of youth with depression who took an antidepressant medicine—and 1%–2% of youth with depression who took a placebo (pill without active medicine)—talked about suicidal thoughts (thinking about killing themselves or wishing they were dead) or did something to harm themselves. This means that almost twice as many youth who were taking an antidepressant to treat their depression talked about suicide or had suicidal behavior compared with youth with depression who were taking inactive medicine. There were *no* completed suicides in any of these research studies, which included more than 4,000 children and adolescents. For youth being treated for anxiety, there was no difference in suicidal talking or behavior between those taking antidepressant medication and those taking placebo.

The FDA told drug companies to add a *black box warning* label to all antidepressant medicines. Because of this label, a doctor (or advanced practice nurse) prescribing one of these medicines has to warn youth and their families that there might be more suicidal thoughts and actions in youth taking these medicines.

On the other hand, in places where more youth are taking the newer antidepressant medicines, the number of adolescents who commit suicide has gotten smaller. Also, thinking about or attempting suicide is more common in surveys of teenagers in the community than it is in depressed youth treated in research studies with antidepressant medicine.

If a youth is being treated with this medicine and is doing well, then no changes are needed as a result of this warning. Increased suicidal talk or action is most likely to happen in the first few months of treatment with a medicine. If your child has recently started this medicine or is about to start, then you and your doctor (or advanced practice nurse) should watch for any changes in behavior. People who are depressed often have suicidal thoughts or actions. It is hard to know whether suicidal thoughts or actions in depressed people are caused by the depression itself or by the medicine. Also, as their depression is getting better, some people talk more about the suicidal thoughts that they had before but did not talk about. As young people get better from depression, they might be at higher risk of doing something about suicidal thoughts that they have had for some time, because they have more energy.

What Should a Parent Do?

1. Be honest with your child about possible risks and benefits of medicine.
2. Talk to your child about whether he or she is having any suicidal thoughts, and tell your child to come to you if he or she is having such thoughts.
3. You, your child, and your child's doctor or nurse should develop a safety plan. Pick adults whom your child can tell if he or she is thinking about suicide.
4. Be sure to tell your child's doctor, nurse, or therapist if you suspect that your child is using alcohol or drugs or if something has happened that might make your child feel worse, such as a family separation, breaking up with a boyfriend or girlfriend, someone close dying or attempting suicide, physical or sexual abuse, or failure in school.
5. Be sure that there are no guns in the home and that all medicines (including over-the-counter medicines like Tylenol) are closely supervised by an adult and kept in a safe place.
6. Watch for new or worse thoughts of suicide, self-harm, depression, anxiety (nerves), feeling very agitated or restless, being angry or aggressive, having more trouble sleeping, or anything else that you see for the first time, seems worse, or worries your child or you. If these appear, contact a mental health professional **right away.** Do not just stop or change the dose of the medicine on your own. If the problems are serious, and you cannot reach one of your clinicians, call a 24-hour psychiatry emergency telephone number or take your child to an emergency room.

Youth taking antidepressant medicine should be watched carefully by their parent(s), clinician(s) (doctor, advanced practice nurse, nurse, therapist), and other concerned adults for the first weeks of treatment. It is a good idea to have regular contact with the doctor, APN, nurse, or therapist for the first months to check for feelings of depression or sadness, thoughts of killing or harming himself or herself, and any problems with the medication. If you have questions, be sure to ask the doctor, APN, nurse, or therapist.

For more information, see http://www.parentsmedguide.org/.

Notes

Use this space to take notes or to write down questions you want to ask the doctor.

_____

_____

_____

_____

_____

_____

_____

_____

_____

_____

_____

_____

_____

From Dulcan MK, Ballard R (editors): _Helping Parents and Teachers Understand Medications for Behavioral and Emotional Problems: A Resource Book of Medication Information Handouts,_ Fourth Edition. Washington, DC, American Psychiatric Publishing, 2015

Medication Information for Parents and Teachers

Thiothixene

General Information About Medication

Each child and adolescent is different. No one has exactly the same combination of medical and psychological problems. It is a good idea to talk with the doctor or nurse about the reasons a medicine is being used. It is very important to keep all appointments and to be in touch by telephone if you have concerns. It is important to communicate with the doctor, nurse, or therapist. An *advanced practice nurse* (APN) has additional education and training after becoming a registered nurse (RN). Your child's medication may be prescribed by a medical doctor (MD or DO) or an APN. In addition, a *physician assistant* (PA) working with a physician may prescribe certain medications. In this information sheet, "doctor" includes medical doctors as well as APNs and PAs who prescribe medication. Often a nurse (RN) will be part of the team and answer questions and give information.

It is very important that the medicine be taken exactly as the doctor instructs. However, once in a while, everyone forgets to give a medicine on time. It is a good idea to ask the doctor or nurse what to do if this happens. Do not stop or change a medicine without asking the doctor or nurse first.

If the medicine seems to stop working, it may be because it is not being taken regularly. The youth may be "cheeking" or hiding the medicine or forgetting to take it (especially at school). The doses may be too far apart or a different dose or medicine may be needed. Something at school, at home, or in the neighborhood may be upsetting the youth, or he or she may need special help for learning disabilities or tutoring. Please discuss your concerns with the doctor. **Do not just increase the dose.** It is also very important not to decrease the dose or stop the medicine without talking to the doctor first. The problem being treated may come back, or there could be uncomfortable or even dangerous results.

All medicines should be kept in a safe place, out of the reach of children, and should be supervised by an adult. If someone takes too much of a medicine, call the doctor, the poison control center, or a hospital emergency room.

Each medicine has a "generic" or chemical name. Just like laundry detergents or paper towels, some medicines are sold by more than one company under different brand names. The same medicine may be available under a generic name and several brand names. The generic medications are usually less expensive than the brand name ones. The generic medications have the same chemical formula, but they may or may not be exactly the same strength as the brand-name medications. Also, some brands of pills contain dye or other things that can cause allergic reactions. It is a good idea to talk to the doctor and the pharmacist about whether it is important to use a specific brand of medicine.

Any medicine can cause an allergic reaction. Examples are hives, itching, rashes, swelling, and trouble breathing. Even a tiny amount of a medicine can cause a reaction in patients who are allergic to that medicine. Be *sure* to talk to the doctor before restarting a medicine that has caused an allergic reaction and tell the doctor about any reactions to medicine that your child has had before.

Taking more than one medicine at the same time may cause more side effects or cause one of the medicines to not work as well. Always ask the doctor, nurse, or pharmacist before adding another

483

medicine, either prescription or bought without a prescription in a store or on the Internet. **Be sure that each doctor knows about** *all* **of the medicines your child is taking. Also tell the doctor about any vitamins, herbal medicines, or supplements your child may be taking.** Some of these may have side effects alone or when taken with this medication. It is a very good idea to keep a list with you of the names and doses of all medicines that your child is taking.

Everyone taking medicine should have a physical examination at least once a year.

If you think that your child may be using drugs or alcohol, please tell the doctor right away.

Pregnancy requires special care in the use of medicine. Some medicines can cause birth defects if taken by a pregnant mother. **Please tell the doctor immediately if you suspect the teenager is at risk of becoming pregnant.** The doctor may wish to discuss sexual behavior and/or birth control with your daughter.

Printed information like this applies to children and adolescents in general. If you have questions about the medicine, or if you notice changes or anything unusual, please ask the doctor or nurse. As scientific research advances, knowledge increases and advice changes. Even experts do not always agree. Many medicines have not been "approved" by the U.S. Food and Drug Administration (FDA) for use in children or use for particular problems. For this reason, use of the medicine for a problem or age group often is not listed in the *Physicians' Desk Reference*. This does not necessarily mean that the medicine is dangerous or does not work, only that the company that makes the medicine has not received permission to advertise the medicine for use in children. Companies often do not apply for this permission because it is expensive to do the tests needed to apply for approval for use in children. Once a medication is approved by the FDA for any purpose, a doctor is allowed to prescribe it according to research and clinical experience.

Note to Teachers

It is a good idea to talk with the parent(s) about the reason(s) that a medication is being used. If the parent(s) sign consent to release information, it is often helpful for you to talk with the doctor. If the parent(s) give permission, the doctor may ask you to fill out rating forms about your experience with the student's behavior, feelings, academic performance, and medication side effects. This information is very useful in selecting and monitoring medication treatment. If you have observations that you think are important, do not hesitate to share these with the student's parent(s) and treating clinicians (with parental consent).

It is very important that the medicine be taken exactly as the doctor instructs. However, everyone forgets to give a medicine on time once in a while. It is a good idea to ask the parent(s) in advance what to do if this happens. Do not stop or change the time you are giving a medicine at school without parental permission. If a medication is to be taken with food, but lunchtime or snack time changes, be sure to notify the parent(s) so appropriate adjustments can be made.

All medicines should be kept in a secure place and should be supervised by an adult. If someone takes too much of a medicine, follow your school procedure for an urgent medical problem.

Taking medicine is a private matter and is best managed discreetly and confidentially. It is important to be sensitive to the student's feelings about taking medicine.

If you suspect that the student is using drugs or alcohol, please tell the parent(s) or a school counselor right away.

Please tell the parent(s) or school nurse if you suspect medication side effects.

Modifications of the classroom environment or assignments may be useful in addition to medication. The student may need to be evaluated for additional help or a 504 plan or an Individualized Education Plan for learning problems or emotional or behavioral issues.

Any expression of suicidal thoughts or feelings or self-harm by a child or adolescent is a signal of distress and should be taken seriously. These behaviors should not be dismissed as "attention seeking." School procedures for safety issues should be followed.

What Is Thiothixene?

Thiothixene is sometimes called a *typical*, *conventional*, or *first-generation antipsychotic* medicine. It is also called a *neuroleptic*. It used to be called a *major tranquilizer*. It comes in generic capsules. It used to come in brand name Navane, so sometimes it is still called that.

How Can This Medicine Help?

Thiothixene is used to treat psychosis, such as in schizophrenia, mania, or very severe depression. It can reduce hallucinations (hearing voices or seeing things that are not there) and delusions (troubling beliefs that other people do not share). It can help the patient be less upset and agitated. It can improve the patient's ability to think clearly.

Sometimes thiothixene is used to decrease severe aggression or very serious behavioral problems in young people with conduct disorder, intellectual disability, or autism spectrum disorder.

This medicine is very powerful and should be used to treat very serious problems or symptoms that other medicines do not help. Be patient; the positive effects of this medicine may not appear for 2–3 weeks.

How Does This Medicine Work?

Cells in the brain (neurons) communicate using chemicals called *neurotransmitters*. Too much or too little of these substances in certain parts of the brain can cause problems. Thiothixene reduces the activity of one of these neurotransmitters, *dopamine*. Blocking the effect of dopamine in certain parts of the brain reduces what have been called *positive symptoms* of psychosis: delusions; hallucinations; disorganized and unusual thinking, speaking, and behavior; excessive activity (agitation); and lack of activity (catatonia). Blocking dopamine can also reduce tics. Reducing dopamine action in other parts of the brain may lead to the side effects of this medicine.

How Long Does This Medicine Last?

Thiothixene is usually taken twice a day.

How Will the Doctor Monitor This Medicine?

The doctor will review your child's medical history and physical examination before starting thiothixene. The doctor may order some blood or urine tests to be sure your child does not have a hidden medical condition. The doctor or nurse may measure your child's pulse and blood pressure before starting thiothixene.

Before starting thiothixene and every so often afterward, a test such as the AIMS (Abnormal Involuntary Movement Scale) may be used to check your child's tongue, legs, and arms for unusual movements that could be caused by the medicine.

After the medicine is started, the doctor will want to have regular appointments with you and your child to see how the medicine is working, to see if a dose change is needed, to watch for side effects, to see if thiothixene is still needed, and to see if any other treatment is needed. The doctor or nurse may check your child's height, weight, pulse, and blood pressure and watch for abnormal movements.

What Side Effects Can This Medicine Have?

Any medicine can have side effects, including an allergy to the medicine. Because each patient is different, the doctor will monitor the youth closely, especially when the medicine is started. The doctor will work with you to increase the positive effects and decrease the negative effects of the medicine. Please tell the doctor if any of the listed side effects appear or if you think that the medicine is causing any other problems. Not all of the rare or unusual side effects are listed.

Side effects are most common after starting the medicine or after a dose increase. Many side effects can be avoided or lessened by starting with a very low dose and increasing it slowly—ask the doctor.

Allergic Reaction

Tell the doctor in a day or two (if possible, before the next dose of medicine):

- Hives
- Itching
- Rash

Stop the medicine and get *immediate* medical care:

- Trouble breathing or chest tightness
- Swelling of lips, tongue, or throat

Common, but Not Usually Serious, Side Effects

Discuss the following side effects with your child's doctor within a week or two. They often can be helped by lowering the dose of medicine, changing the times medicine is taken, or adding another medicine.

- Dry mouth—Have your child try using sugar-free gum or candy.
- Constipation—Encourage your child to drink more fluids and eat high-fiber foods; if necessary, the doctor may recommend a fiber medicine such as Benefiber or a stool softener such as Colace or mineral oil.
- Increased risk of sunburn—Have your child wear sunscreen or protective clothing or stay out of the sun.
- Mild trouble urinating
- Blurred vision
- Weight gain—Seek nutritional counseling; provide your child with low-calorie snacks and encourage regular exercise.
- Sadness, irritability, nervousness, clinginess, not wanting to go to school
- Restlessness or inability to sit still
- Shaking of hands and fingers

Less Common, but Not Usually Serious, Side Effects

Discuss the following side effects with your child's doctor within a week or two. They often can be helped by lowering the dose of medicine, changing the times medicine is taken, or adding another medicine.

- Daytime sleepiness or tiredness—Do not allow your child to drive, ride a bicycle or motorcycle, or operate machinery if this happens. This problem may be lessened by taking the medicine at bedtime.
- Dizziness—This side effect is worse when the child stands up quickly, especially when getting out of bed in the morning; try having the child stand up slowly.
- Decreased or slowed movement and decreased facial expressions
- Drooling
- Decreased sexual interest or ability
- Changes in menstrual cycle
- Increase in breast size or discharge from the breasts (in both boys and girls)—This may go away with time.

Less Common, but Potentially Serious, Side Effects

Call the doctor or go to an emergency room *right away*:

- Stiffness of the tongue, jaw, neck, back, or legs
- Overheating or heatstroke—Prevent by decreasing activity in hot weather, staying out of the sun, and drinking water.
- Seizure (fit, convulsion)—This is more likely in people with a history of seizures or head injury.
- Severe confusion

Rare, but Serious, Side Effects

- Extreme stiffness or lack of movement, very high fever, mental confusion, irregular pulse rate, or eye pain—**This is a medical emergency. Go to an emergency room right away.**
- Sudden stiffness and inability to breathe or swallow—**Go to an emergency room or call 911.** Tell the paramedics, nurses, and doctors that the patient is taking thiothixene. Other medicines can be used to treat this problem fast.

What Else Should I Know About Side Effects?

Most side effects lessen over time. If they are troublesome, talk with your child's doctor. Some side effects can be decreased by taking a smaller dose of medicine, by stopping the medicine, by changing to another medicine, or by adding another medicine (see the table).

One side effect that may not go away is *tardive dyskinesia* (or TD). Patients with tardive dyskinesia have involuntary movements of the body, especially the mouth and tongue. The patient may look as though he or she is making faces over and over again. Jerky movements of the arms, legs, or body may occur. There may be fine, wormlike, or sudden repeated movements of the tongue, or the person may appear to be chewing something or smacking or puckering his or her lips. The fingers may look as though they are rolling something. If you notice any unusual movements, be sure to tell the doctor. The doctor may use the AIMS test to look for these movements.

The medicine may increase the level of *prolactin*, a natural hormone made in the part of the brain called the *pituitary*. This may cause side effects such as breast tenderness or swelling or production of milk, in both boys and girls. It also may interfere with sexual functioning in teenage boys and with regular menstrual cycles (periods) in teenage girls. A blood test can measure the level of prolactin. If these side effects do not go away and are troublesome, talk with your child's doctor about substituting another medicine for thiothixene.

Heart problems are more common if other medicines are being taken also. Be sure to tell all your child's doctors and your pharmacist about all medications your child is taking.

Neuroleptic malignant syndrome is a very rare side effect that can lead to death. The symptoms are severe muscle stiffness, high fever, increased heart rate and blood pressure, irregular heartbeat (pulse), and sweating. It may lead to unconsciousness. If you suspect this, **call 911 or go to an emergency room right away.**

Sometimes this medicine can cause a *dystonic reaction*. This is a sudden stiffening of the muscles, most often in the jaw, neck, tongue, face, or shoulders. If this happens, and your child is not having trouble breathing, you may give a dose of diphenhydramine (Benadryl). Follow the dose instructions on the package for your child's age. This should relax the muscles in a few minutes. Then call your doctor to tell him or her what happened. If the muscles do not relax, take your child to the emergency department.

Some Interactions With Other Medicines or Food

Please note that the following are only the most likely interactions with other medicines or food.

Thiothixene may be taken with or without food. If the medicine causes stomach upset, taking it with food may help.

It is better to limit drinks with caffeine (coffee, tea, soft drinks) because caffeine works in the opposite way from this medicine, and the positive effects might be decreased.

What Could Happen if This Medicine Is Stopped Suddenly?

Involuntary movements, or *withdrawal dyskinesias*, may appear within 1–4 weeks of lowering the dose or stopping the medicine. Usually these go away, but they can last for days to months. If thiothixene is stopped suddenly, emotional problems such as irritability, nervousness, moodiness; behavior problems; or physical problems such as stomachache, loss of appetite, nausea, vomiting, diarrhea, sweating, indigestion, trouble sleeping, trembling, or shaking may appear. These problems usually last only a few days to a few weeks. If they happen, tell your child's doctor. The medicine dose may need to be lowered more slowly (tapered). Always check with the doctor before stopping a medicine.

How Long Will This Medicine Be Needed?

How long your child will need to be on thiothixene depends partly on the reason that it was prescribed. Some problems last for only a few months, whereas others last much longer. Sometimes thiothixene is used for only a short time until other medicines or behavioral treatments start to work. Some people need to take thiothixene for years. It is especially important with medicines as powerful as this one to ask the doctor whether it is still needed. Every few months, you should discuss with your child's doctor the reasons for using thiothixene and whether it is time for a trial of lowering the dose.

What Else Should I Know About This Medicine?

There are many other medicines that are used for the same kinds of problems. If your child is having bad side effects or the medicine does not seem to be working, ask the doctor if another medicine in this group might work as well or better and have fewer side effects for your child.

Be sure to tell the doctor if there is anyone in your family who died suddenly or had a heart problem.

Notes

Use this space to take notes or to write down questions you want to ask the doctor.

_____

_____

_____

_____

_____

_____

_____

_____

_____

_____

Medication Information for Parents and Teachers

Topiramate—Topamax, Topiragen, Trokendi XR, Qudexy SR

General Information About Medication

Each child and adolescent is different. No one has exactly the same combination of medical and psychological problems. It is a good idea to talk with the doctor or nurse about the reasons a medicine is being used. It is very important to keep all appointments and to be in touch by telephone if you have concerns. It is important to communicate with the doctor, nurse, or therapist. An *advanced practice nurse* (APN) has additional education and training after becoming a registered nurse (RN). Your child's medication may be prescribed by a medical doctor (MD or DO) or an APN. In addition, a *physician assistant* (PA) working with a physician may prescribe certain medications. In this information sheet, "doctor" includes medical doctors as well as APNs and PAs who prescribe medication. Often a nurse (RN) will be part of the team and answer questions and give information.

It is very important that the medicine be taken exactly as the doctor instructs. However, once in a while, everyone forgets to give a medicine on time. It is a good idea to ask the doctor or nurse what to do if this happens. Do not stop or change a medicine without asking the doctor or nurse first.

If the medicine seems to stop working, it may be because it is not being taken regularly. The youth may be "cheeking" or hiding the medicine or forgetting to take it (especially at school). The doses may be too far apart or a different dose or medicine may be needed. Something at school, at home, or in the neighborhood may be upsetting the youth, or he or she may need special help for learning disabilities or tutoring. Please discuss your concerns with the doctor. **Do not just increase the dose.** It is also very important not to decrease the dose or stop the medicine without talking to the doctor first. The problem being treated may come back, or there could be uncomfortable or even dangerous results.

All medicines should be kept in a safe place, out of the reach of children, and should be supervised by an adult. If someone takes too much of a medicine, call the doctor, the poison control center, or a hospital emergency room.

Each medicine has a "generic" or chemical name. Just like laundry detergents or paper towels, some medicines are sold by more than one company under different brand names. The same medicine may be available under a generic name and several brand names. The generic medications are usually less expensive than the brand name ones. The generic medications have the same chemical formula, but they may or may not be exactly the same strength as the brand-name medications. Also, some brands of pills contain dye or other things that can cause allergic reactions. It is a good idea to talk to the doctor and the pharmacist about whether it is important to use a specific brand of medicine.

Any medicine can cause an allergic reaction. Examples are hives, itching, rashes, swelling, and trouble breathing. Even a tiny amount of a medicine can cause a reaction in patients who are allergic to that medicine. Be *sure* to talk to the doctor before restarting a medicine that has caused an allergic reaction and tell the doctor about any reactions to medicine that your child has had before.

491

Taking more than one medicine at the same time may cause more side effects or cause one of the medicines to not work as well. Always ask the doctor, nurse, or pharmacist before adding another medicine, either prescription or bought without a prescription in a store or on the Internet. Be sure that each doctor knows about *all* of the medicines your child is taking. Also tell the doctor about any vitamins, herbal medicines, or supplements your child may be taking. Some of these may have side effects alone or when taken with this medication. It is a very good idea to keep a list with you of the names and doses of all medicines that your child is taking.

Everyone taking medicine should have a physical examination at least once a year.

If you think that your child may be using drugs or alcohol, please tell the doctor right away.

Pregnancy requires special care in the use of medicine. Some medicines can cause birth defects if taken by a pregnant mother. **Please tell the doctor immediately if you suspect the teenager is at risk of becoming pregnant.** The doctor may wish to discuss sexual behavior and/or birth control with your daughter.

Printed information like this applies to children and adolescents in general. If you have questions about the medicine, or if you notice changes or anything unusual, please ask the doctor or nurse. As scientific research advances, knowledge increases and advice changes. Even experts do not always agree. Many medicines have not been "approved" by the U.S. Food and Drug Administration (FDA) for use in children or use for particular problems. For this reason, use of the medicine for a problem or age group often is not listed in the *Physicians' Desk Reference*. This does not necessarily mean that the medicine is dangerous or does not work, only that the company that makes the medicine has not received permission to advertise the medicine for use in children. Companies often do not apply for this permission because it is expensive to do the tests needed to apply for approval for use in children. Once a medication is approved by the FDA for any purpose, a doctor is allowed to prescribe it according to research and clinical experience.

Note to Teachers

It is a good idea to talk with the parent(s) about the reason(s) that a medication is being used. If the parent(s) sign consent to release information, it is often helpful for you to talk with the doctor. If the parent(s) give permission, the doctor may ask you to fill out rating forms about your experience with the student's behavior, feelings, academic performance, and medication side effects. This information is very useful in selecting and monitoring medication treatment. If you have observations that you think are important, do not hesitate to share these with the student's parent(s) and treating clinicians (with parental consent).

It is very important that the medicine be taken exactly as the doctor instructs. However, everyone forgets to give a medicine on time once in a while. It is a good idea to ask the parent(s) in advance what to do if this happens. Do not stop or change the time you are giving a medicine at school without parental permission. If a medication is to be taken with food, but lunchtime or snack time changes, be sure to notify the parent(s) so appropriate adjustments can be made.

All medicines should be kept in a secure place and should be supervised by an adult. If someone takes too much of a medicine, follow your school procedure for an urgent medical problem.

Taking medicine is a private matter and is best managed discreetly and confidentially. It is important to be sensitive to the student's feelings about taking medicine.

If you suspect that the student is using drugs or alcohol, please tell the parent(s) or a school counselor right away.

Please tell the parent(s) or school nurse if you suspect medication side effects.

Modifications of the classroom environment or assignments may be useful in addition to medication. The student may need to be evaluated for additional help or a 504 plan or an Individualized Education Plan for learning problems or emotional or behavioral issues.

Any expression of suicidal thoughts or feelings or self-harm by a child or adolescent is a signal of distress and should be taken seriously. These behaviors should not be dismissed as "attention seeking." School procedures for safety issues should be followed.

What Is Topiramate (Topamax, Topiragen, Trokendi XR, Qudexy SR)?

Topiramate was first used to treat seizures (fits, convulsions), so it is sometimes called an *anticonvulsant*. Now it is also used for behavioral problems or bipolar disorder regardless of whether the patient has seizures. It also may be used when the patient has a history of severe mood changes, sometimes called *mood swings*. When used in psychiatry, this medicine is more commonly called a *mood stabilizer*. Topiramate is now also used to prevent migraine headaches in teenagers as well as adults. It is sometimes used to treat bulimia nervosa, binge-eating disorder, and weight gain in people taking antipsychotic medicines.

Topiramate comes in brand name Topamax and Topiragen and generic tablets, brand name Topamax and generic sprinkle capsules, and brand name Qudexy SR and Trokendi XR and generic extended-release forms.

How Can This Medicine Help?

Topiramate can reduce aggression, anger, and severe mood swings. It can treat mania or prevent relapse (mania coming back).

How Does This Medicine Work?

Topiramate is thought to work by stabilizing a part of the brain cell (the cell membrane or envelope) and by changing the concentrations of certain *neurotransmitters* (chemicals in the brain) such as *GABA* and *glutamate*.

How Long Does This Medicine Last?

Topiramate needs to be taken twice a day. The extended-release forms can be taken once a day.

How Will the Doctor Monitor This Medicine?

The doctor will review your child's medical history and physical examination before starting topiramate. The doctor or nurse may measure your child's pulse and blood pressure before starting this medicine. The doctor may order a baseline blood test of liver and kidney functions.

After the medicine is started, the doctor will want to have regular appointments with you and your child to see how the medicine is working, to see if a dose change is needed, to watch for side effects, to see if topiramate is still needed, and to see if any other treatment is needed. The doctor or nurse may check your child's height, weight, pulse, and blood pressure and may order a blood test to monitor bicarbonate.

What Side Effects Can This Medicine Have?

Any medicine can have side effects, including an allergy to the medicine. Because each patient is different, the doctor will monitor the youth closely, especially when the medicine is started. The doctor will work with you to increase the positive effects and decrease the negative effects of the medicine. Please tell the doctor if any of the listed side effects appear or if you think that the medicine is causing any other problems. Not all of the rare or unusual side effects are listed.

Side effects are most common after starting the medicine or after a dose increase. Many side effects can be avoided or lessened by starting with a very low dose and increasing it slowly—ask the doctor.

Allergic Reaction

Tell the doctor in a day or two (if possible, before the next dose of medicine):

- Hives
- Itching
- Rash

Stop the medicine and get *immediate* medical care:

- Trouble breathing or chest tightness
- Swelling of lips, tongue, or throat

Allergic reaction to topiramate may be more common in people who are allergic to sulfa drugs.

General Side Effects

These side effects are more common when first starting the medicine. Tell the doctor within a week or two:

- Daytime sleepiness—Do not allow your child to drive, ride a bicycle or motorcycle, or operate machinery if this happens.
- Dizziness
- Vision problems
- Unsteadiness when walking
- Speech problems
- Slowed movements
- Skin feeling like "pins and needles"
- Decreased sweating
- Fever
- Decreased appetite, weight loss
- Nausea, vomiting
- Stomach cramps
- Tremor (shakiness)
- Decreased concentration or attention

Behavior and Emotional Side Effects

Call the doctor right away:

- New or increased suicidal thoughts or behaviors

Call the doctor within a day or two:

- New or increased anxiety (nervousness) or depression (sadness)
- Irritability
- Memory problems
- Confusion

Possibly Dangerous Side Effects

Call the doctor *immediately*:

- Clumsiness or poor coordination
- Bloody or cloudy urine (could be from a kidney stone)
- Unexplained fever or chills
- Sharp back pain (could be a kidney stone)
- Blurred vision or eye pain
- Unexplained fast breathing, very fast heartbeat, extreme fatigue

Some Interactions With Other Medicines or Food

Please note that the following are only the most likely interactions with other medicines or food.

Caffeine may increase side effects.

Topiramate interacts with many other medicines. Taking it with another medicine may make one or both not work as well or may cause more side effects. Be sure that each doctor knows about *all* of the medicines being taken.

Topiramate may decrease the blood levels of birth control pills (oral contraceptives) so that they do not work as well—this may lead to accidental pregnancy. An additional method of birth control may be needed.

Taking topiramate together with valproate (Depakote) may increase ammonia in the blood. If your child seems tired and confused please be sure to talk with the doctor right away.

What Could Happen if This Medicine Is Stopped Suddenly?

Stopping topiramate suddenly could cause an increase in very dangerous seizures (convulsions) if your child is being treated for epilepsy (seizures).

How Long Will This Medicine Be Needed?

The length of time a person needs to take topiramate depends on what problem is being treated. For example, someone with an impulse control disorder usually takes the medicine only until behavioral therapy begins to work. Someone with bipolar disorder may need to take the medicine for many years. Please ask the doctor about the length of treatment needed.

What Else Should I Know About This Medicine?

Taking topiramate with food may decrease stomach upset.

While taking topiramate, diets low in carbohydrates (such as Atkins, South Beach, or ketogenic diet [to treat severe epilepsy]) should be avoided to prevent kidney stones. It is also important to drink plenty of liquids to decrease the risk of kidney stones.

Be sure that your child drinks plenty of water and avoids very vigorous physical activities, dehydration, and exposure to very hot temperatures because rarely children who take topiramate may develop decreased sweating and dangerously increased body temperature.

Keep the medicine in a safe place under close supervision. Keep the pill container tightly closed and in a dry place, away from bathrooms, showers, and humidifiers.

Notes

Use this space to take notes or to write down questions you want to ask the doctor.

_____

_____

_____

_____

_____

_____

_____

_____

_____

_____

_____

_____

Medication Information for Parents and Teachers

Trazodone—Oleptro

General Information About Medication

Each child and adolescent is different. No one has exactly the same combination of medical and psychological problems. It is a good idea to talk with the doctor or nurse about the reasons a medicine is being used. It is very important to keep all appointments and to be in touch by telephone if you have concerns. It is important to communicate with the doctor, nurse, or therapist. An *advanced practice nurse* (APN) has additional education and training after becoming a registered nurse (RN). Your child's medication may be prescribed by a medical doctor (MD or DO) or an APN. In addition, a *physician assistant* (PA) working with a physician may prescribe certain medications. In this information sheet, "doctor" includes medical doctors as well as APNs and PAs who prescribe medication. Often a nurse (RN) will be part of the team and answer questions and give information.

It is very important that the medicine be taken exactly as the doctor instructs. However, once in a while, everyone forgets to give a medicine on time. It is a good idea to ask the doctor or nurse what to do if this happens. Do not stop or change a medicine without asking the doctor or nurse first.

If the medicine seems to stop working, it may be because it is not being taken regularly. The youth may be "cheeking" or hiding the medicine or forgetting to take it (especially at school). The doses may be too far apart or a different dose or medicine may be needed. Something at school, at home, or in the neighborhood may be upsetting the youth, or he or she may need special help for learning disabilities or tutoring. Please discuss your concerns with the doctor. **Do not just increase the dose.** It is also very important not to decrease the dose or stop the medicine without talking to the doctor first. The problem being treated may come back, or there could be uncomfortable or even dangerous results.

All medicines should be kept in a safe place, out of the reach of children, and should be supervised by an adult. If someone takes too much of a medicine, call the doctor, the poison control center, or a hospital emergency room.

Each medicine has a "generic" or chemical name. Just like laundry detergents or paper towels, some medicines are sold by more than one company under different brand names. The same medicine may be available under a generic name and several brand names. The generic medications are usually less expensive than the brand name ones. The generic medications have the same chemical formula, but they may or may not be exactly the same strength as the brand-name medications. Also, some brands of pills contain dye or other things that can cause allergic reactions. It is a good idea to talk to the doctor and the pharmacist about whether it is important to use a specific brand of medicine.

Any medicine can cause an allergic reaction. Examples are hives, itching, rashes, swelling, and trouble breathing. Even a tiny amount of a medicine can cause a reaction in patients who are allergic to that medicine. Be *sure* to talk to the doctor before restarting a medicine that has caused an allergic reaction and tell the doctor about any reactions to medicine that your child has had before.

Taking more than one medicine at the same time may cause more side effects or cause one of the medicines to not work as well. Always ask the doctor, nurse, or pharmacist before adding another

medicine, either prescription or bought without a prescription in a store or on the Internet. Be sure that each doctor knows about *all* of the medicines your child is taking. Also tell the doctor about any vitamins, herbal medicines, or supplements your child may be taking. Some of these may have side effects alone or when taken with this medication. It is a very good idea to keep a list with you of the names and doses of all medicines that your child is taking.

Everyone taking medicine should have a physical examination at least once a year.

If you think that your child may be using drugs or alcohol, please tell the doctor right away.

Pregnancy requires special care in the use of medicine. Some medicines can cause birth defects if taken by a pregnant mother. **Please tell the doctor immediately if you suspect the teenager is at risk of becoming pregnant.** The doctor may wish to discuss sexual behavior and/or birth control with your daughter.

Printed information like this applies to children and adolescents in general. If you have questions about the medicine, or if you notice changes or anything unusual, please ask the doctor or nurse. As scientific research advances, knowledge increases and advice changes. Even experts do not always agree. Many medicines have not been "approved" by the U.S. Food and Drug Administration (FDA) for use in children or use for particular problems. For this reason, use of the medicine for a problem or age group often is not listed in the *Physicians' Desk Reference*. This does not necessarily mean that the medicine is dangerous or does not work, only that the company that makes the medicine has not received permission to advertise the medicine for use in children. Companies often do not apply for this permission because it is expensive to do the tests needed to apply for approval for use in children. Once a medication is approved by the FDA for any purpose, a doctor is allowed to prescribe it according to research and clinical experience.

Note to Teachers

It is a good idea to talk with the parent(s) about the reason(s) that a medication is being used. If the parent(s) sign consent to release information, it is often helpful for you to talk with the doctor. If the parent(s) give permission, the doctor may ask you to fill out rating forms about your experience with the student's behavior, feelings, academic performance, and medication side effects. This information is very useful in selecting and monitoring medication treatment. If you have observations that you think are important, do not hesitate to share these with the student's parent(s) and treating clinicians (with parental consent).

It is very important that the medicine be taken exactly as the doctor instructs. However, everyone forgets to give a medicine on time once in a while. It is a good idea to ask the parent(s) in advance what to do if this happens. Do not stop or change the time you are giving a medicine at school without parental permission. If a medication is to be taken with food, but lunchtime or snack time changes, be sure to notify the parent(s) so appropriate adjustments can be made.

All medicines should be kept in a secure place and should be supervised by an adult. If someone takes too much of a medicine, follow your school procedure for an urgent medical problem.

Taking medicine is a private matter and is best managed discreetly and confidentially. It is important to be sensitive to the student's feelings about taking medicine.

If you suspect that the student is using drugs or alcohol, please tell the parent(s) or a school counselor right away.

Please tell the parent(s) or school nurse if you suspect medication side effects.

Modifications of the classroom environment or assignments may be useful in addition to medication. The student may need to be evaluated for additional help or a 504 plan or an Individualized Education Plan for learning problems or emotional or behavioral issues.

Any expression of suicidal thoughts or feelings or self-harm by a child or adolescent is a signal of distress and should be taken seriously. These behaviors should not be dismissed as "attention seeking." School procedures for safety issues should be followed.

What Is Trazodone (Oleptro)?

Trazodone is called an *antidepressant*. In young people, it is most often used for insomnia (trouble falling asleep) together with other medicines for emotional or behavioral problems. It comes in generic tablets. An extended-release tablet called Oleptro has been developed for use in adults.

How Can This Medicine Help?

Trazodone can help people fall asleep at night. It may also decrease depression, anxiety (nervousness), irritability (crankiness), and aggression. It is sometimes used to help chronic migraine headaches.

How Does This Medicine Work?

People with emotional and behavior problems may have low levels of a brain chemical (*neurotransmitter*) called *serotonin*. Trazodone is believed to help by increasing brain serotonin to more normal activity.

How Long Does This Medicine Last?

The medicine lasts about a day for most people, but the sleepiness effect should be gone by morning if the medicine is taken at bedtime. If your child is still sleepy in the morning, talk with the doctor. Oleptro is designed to be taken once a day.

How Will the Doctor Monitor This Medicine?

The doctor will review your child's medical history and physical examination before starting trazodone. The doctor or nurse may measure your child's pulse and blood pressure.

Be sure to tell the doctor if your child or anyone in the family has bipolar illness or has tried to kill himself or herself.

After the medicine is started, the doctor will want to have regular appointments with you and your child to see how the medicine is working, to see if a dose change is needed, to watch for side effects, to see if trazodone is still needed, and to see if any other treatment is needed. The doctor or nurse may check your child's height, weight, pulse, and blood pressure.

Before using medicine and at times afterward, the doctor may ask your child to fill out a rating scale about depression, to help see how your child is doing. The doctor may ask you and your child to keep a log of sleep and awake times.

What Side Effects Can This Medicine Have?

Any medicine can have side effects, including an allergy to the medicine. Because each patient is different, the doctor will monitor the youth closely, especially when the medicine is started. The doctor will work with you to increase the positive effects and decrease the negative effects of the medicine. Please tell the doctor if any of the listed side effects appear or if you think that the medicine is causing any other problems. Not all of the rare or unusual side effects are listed.

Side effects are most common after starting the medicine or after a dose increase. Many side effects can be avoided or lessened by starting with a very low dose and increasing it slowly—ask the doctor.

Allergic Reaction

Tell the doctor in a day or two (if possible, before the next dose of medicine):

- Hives
- Itching
- Rash

Stop the medicine and get *immediate* medical care:

- Trouble breathing or chest tightness
- Swelling of lips, tongue, or throat

Common Side Effects

Tell the doctor within a week or two, or sooner if the problems are getting worse over time:

- Daytime drowsiness or sleepiness—Do not allow your child to drive, ride a bicycle or motorcycle, or operate machinery if this happens.
- Dry mouth—Have your child try using sugar-free gum or candy.
- Dizziness or light-headedness, especially when standing or sitting up fast
- Headache
- Blurred vision
- Nausea
- Constipation
- Decreased appetite
- Seeing trails or shadows that are not there
- Tremors (shaking)
- More frequent erections (in boys)

Rare, but Serious, Side Effects

Go to an emergency room *right away*:

- Erection of the penis lasting more than 1 hour (called *priapism*)—This may be painful and could cause permanent damage.

502

- Yellowing of skin or eyes, dark urine, pale bowel movements, abdominal pain or fullness, unexplained flu-like symptoms, itchy skin—These side effects are extremely rare but could be signs of liver damage.

Serotonin Syndrome

A very serious side effect called *serotonin syndrome* can happen when certain kinds of medicines (including SSRI antidepressants, clomipramine, and other medicines, such as triptans for migraine headaches, buspirone, linezolid, tramadol, or St. John's wort) are taken by the same person. Very rarely, serotonin syndrome can happen at high doses of just one medicine. The early signs are restlessness, confusion, shaking, skin turning red, sweating, muscle stiffness, sweating, and jerking of muscles. If you see these symptoms, stop the medicine and send or take the youth to an emergency room right away.

Some Interactions With Other Medicines or Food

Please note that the following are only the most likely interactions with other medicines or food.

Trazodone works more quickly if taken on an empty stomach.

It is better to limit drinks with caffeine (coffee, tea, soft drinks) because caffeine works in the opposite way from trazodone, may increase the side effects of the medicine, and might decrease the positive effects.

Other antidepressant medicines and some medicines used to fight infections may increase the levels of trazodone, increasing side effects.

When carbamazepine (Tegretol) is combined with trazodone, Tegretol levels and side effects may increase, and trazodone levels may decrease, causing it to not work as well.

Trazodone should not be used with linezolid, methylene blue, or pimozide (Orap).

It can be *very dangerous* to take trazodone at the same time as, or even within several weeks of, taking another type of medicine called a *monoamine oxidase inhibitor* (MAOI), such as selegiline (Eldepryl), phenelzine (Nardil), tranylcypromine (Parnate), or isocarboxazid (Marplan).

What Could Happen if This Medicine Is Stopped Suddenly?

There are no known medical problems from stopping this medicine, although there may be uncomfortable feelings, or the original problems may come back. Always talk to the doctor before stopping a medication.

How Long Will This Medicine Be Needed?

Trazodone may not reach its full effect for several weeks. Your child may need to keep taking the medicine for at least several months.

When trazodone is used to improve sleep, a behavioral program, such as regular soothing routines at bedtime and increased exercise in the daytime, should be used in combination with the medicine. Finding developmentally appropriate bed- and wake-times and sticking to them is very important. These strategies should be continued after the medicine is stopped or when the medicine is used only occasionally.

What Else Should I Know About This Medicine?

In youth who have bipolar disorder or may be at risk for bipolar disorder, any antidepressant medicine may increase the risk of hypomania or mania (excitement, agitation, increased activity, decreased sleep).

Priapism, or erection of the penis lasting for a very long time, is a very rare but serious side effect that may require surgery. If there is any sign of this, **the boy should go to an emergency room right away.**

It is very dangerous to drink alcohol or take illegal drugs while taking trazodone.

Black Box Antidepressant Warning

In 2004, an advisory committee to the FDA decided that there might be an increased risk of suicidal behavior for some youth taking medicines called *antidepressants*. In the research studies that the committee reviewed, about 3%–4% of youth with depression who took an antidepressant medicine—and 1%–2% of youth with depression who took a placebo (pill without active medicine)—talked about suicidal thoughts (thinking about killing themselves or wishing they were dead) or did something to harm themselves. This means that almost twice as many youth who were taking an antidepressant to treat their depression talked about suicide or had suicidal behavior compared with youth with depression who were taking inactive medicine. There were *no* completed suicides in any of these research studies, which included more than 4,000 children and adolescents. For youth being treated for anxiety, there was no difference in suicidal talking or behavior between those taking antidepressant medication and those taking placebo.

The FDA told drug companies to add a *black box warning* label to all antidepressant medicines. Because of this label, a doctor prescribing one of these medicines has to warn youth and their families that there might be more suicidal thoughts and actions in youth taking these medicines.

On the other hand, in places where more youth are taking the newer antidepressant medicines, the number of adolescents who commit suicide has gotten smaller. Also, thinking about or attempting suicide is more common in surveys of teenagers in the community than it is in depressed youth treated in research studies with antidepressant medicine.

If a youth is being treated with this medicine and is doing well, then no changes are needed as a result of this warning. Increased suicidal talk or action is most likely to happen in the first few months of treatment with a medicine. If your child has recently started this medicine or is about to start, then you and your doctor (or advanced practice nurse) should watch for any changes in behavior. People who are depressed often have suicidal thoughts or actions. It is hard to know whether suicidal thoughts or actions in depressed people are caused by the depression itself or by the medicine. Also, as their depression is getting better, some people talk more about the suicidal thoughts that they had before but did not talk about. As young people get better from depression, they might be at higher risk of doing something about suicidal thoughts that they have had for some time, because they have more energy.

What Should a Parent Do?

1. Be honest with your child about possible risks and benefits of medicine.

2. Talk to your child about whether he or she is having any suicidal thoughts, and tell your child to come to you if he or she is having such thoughts.

3. You, your child, and your child's doctor or nurse should develop a safety plan. Pick adults whom your child can tell if he or she is thinking about suicide.

4. Be sure to tell your child's doctor, nurse, or therapist if you suspect that your child is using alcohol or drugs or if something has happened that might make your child feel worse, such as a family separation, breaking up with a boyfriend or girlfriend, someone close dying or attempting suicide, physical or sexual abuse, or failure in school.

5. Be sure that there are no guns in the home and that all medicines (including over-the-counter medicines like Tylenol) are closely supervised by an adult and kept in a safe place.

6. Watch for new or worse thoughts of suicide, self-harm, depression, anxiety (nerves), feeling very agitated or restless, being angry or aggressive, having more trouble sleeping, or anything else that you see for the first time, seems worse, or worries your child or you. If these appear, contact a mental health professional **right away.** Do not just stop or change the dose of the medicine on your own. If the problems are serious, and you cannot reach one of your clinicians, call a 24-hour psychiatry emergency telephone number or take your child to an emergency room.

Youth taking antidepressant medicine should be watched carefully by their parent(s), clinician(s) (doctor, advanced practice nurse, nurse, therapist), and other concerned adults for the first weeks of treatment. It is a good idea to have regular contact with the doctor, APN, nurse, or therapist for the first months to check for feelings of depression or sadness, thoughts of killing or harming himself or herself, and any problems with the medication. If you have questions, be sure to ask the doctor, APN, nurse, or therapist.

For more information, see http://www.parentsmedguide.org/.

Notes

Use this space to take notes or to write down questions you want to ask the doctor.

From Dulcan MK, Ballard R (editors): *Helping Parents and Teachers Understand Medications for Behavioral and Emotional Problems: A Resource Book of Medication Information Handouts*, Fourth Edition. Washington, DC, American Psychiatric Publishing, 2015

Trifluoperazine

General Information About Medication

Each child and adolescent is different. No one has exactly the same combination of medical and psychological problems. It is a good idea to talk with the doctor or nurse about the reasons a medicine is being used. It is very important to keep all appointments and to be in touch by telephone if you have concerns. It is important to communicate with the doctor, nurse, or therapist. An *advanced practice nurse* (APN) has additional education and training after becoming a registered nurse (RN). Your child's medication may be prescribed by a medical doctor (MD or DO) or an APN. In addition, a *physician assistant* (PA) working with a physician may prescribe certain medications. In this information sheet, "doctor" includes medical doctors as well as APNs and PAs who prescribe medication. Often a nurse (RN) will be part of the team and answer questions and give information.

It is very important that the medicine be taken exactly as the doctor instructs. However, once in a while, everyone forgets to give a medicine on time. It is a good idea to ask the doctor or nurse what to do if this happens. Do not stop or change a medicine without asking the doctor or nurse first.

If the medicine seems to stop working, it may be because it is not being taken regularly. The youth may be "cheeking" or hiding the medicine or forgetting to take it (especially at school). The doses may be too far apart or a different dose or medicine may be needed. Something at school, at home, or in the neighborhood may be upsetting the youth, or he or she may need special help for learning disabilities or tutoring. Please discuss your concerns with the doctor. **Do not just increase the dose.** It is also very important not to decrease the dose or stop the medicine without talking to the doctor first. The problem being treated may come back, or there could be uncomfortable or even dangerous results.

All medicines should be kept in a safe place, out of the reach of children, and should be supervised by an adult. If someone takes too much of a medicine, call the doctor, the poison control center, or a hospital emergency room.

Each medicine has a "generic" or chemical name. Just like laundry detergents or paper towels, some medicines are sold by more than one company under different brand names. The same medicine may be available under a generic name and several brand names. The generic medications are usually less expensive than the brand name ones. The generic medications have the same chemical formula, but they may or may not be exactly the same strength as the brand-name medications. Also, some brands of pills contain dye or other things that can cause allergic reactions. It is a good idea to talk to the doctor and the pharmacist about whether it is important to use a specific brand of medicine.

Any medicine can cause an allergic reaction. Examples are hives, itching, rashes, swelling, and trouble breathing. Even a tiny amount of a medicine can cause a reaction in patients who are allergic to that medicine. Be *sure* to talk to the doctor before restarting a medicine that has caused an allergic reaction and tell the doctor about any reactions to medicine that your child has had before.

Taking more than one medicine at the same time may cause more side effects or cause one of the medicines to not work as well. Always ask the doctor, nurse, or pharmacist before adding another

medicine, either prescription or bought without a prescription in a store or on the Internet. Be sure that each doctor knows about *all* of the medicines your child is taking. Also tell the doctor about any vitamins, herbal medicines, or supplements your child may be taking. Some of these may have side effects alone or when taken with this medication. It is a very good idea to keep a list with you of the names and doses of all medicines that your child is taking.

Everyone taking medicine should have a physical examination at least once a year.

If you think that your child may be using drugs or alcohol, please tell the doctor right away.

Pregnancy requires special care in the use of medicine. Some medicines can cause birth defects if taken by a pregnant mother. **Please tell the doctor immediately if you suspect the teenager is at risk of becoming pregnant.** The doctor may wish to discuss sexual behavior and/or birth control with your daughter.

Printed information like this applies to children and adolescents in general. If you have questions about the medicine, or if you notice changes or anything unusual, please ask the doctor or nurse. As scientific research advances, knowledge increases and advice changes. Even experts do not always agree. Many medicines have not been "approved" by the U.S. Food and Drug Administration (FDA) for use in children or use for particular problems. For this reason, use of the medicine for a problem or age group often is not listed in the *Physicians' Desk Reference*. This does not necessarily mean that the medicine is dangerous or does not work, only that the company that makes the medicine has not received permission to advertise the medicine for use in children. Companies often do not apply for this permission because it is expensive to do the tests needed to apply for approval for use in children. Once a medication is approved by the FDA for any purpose, a doctor is allowed to prescribe it according to research and clinical experience.

Note to Teachers

It is a good idea to talk with the parent(s) about the reason(s) that a medication is being used. If the parent(s) sign consent to release information, it is often helpful for you to talk with the doctor. If the parent(s) give permission, the doctor may ask you to fill out rating forms about your experience with the student's behavior, feelings, academic performance, and medication side effects. This information is very useful in selecting and monitoring medication treatment. If you have observations that you think are important, do not hesitate to share these with the student's parent(s) and treating clinicians (with parental consent).

It is very important that the medicine be taken exactly as the doctor instructs. However, everyone forgets to give a medicine on time once in a while. It is a good idea to ask the parent(s) in advance what to do if this happens. Do not stop or change the time you are giving a medicine at school without parental permission. If a medication is to be taken with food, but lunchtime or snack time changes, be sure to notify the parent(s) so appropriate adjustments can be made.

All medicines should be kept in a secure place and should be supervised by an adult. If someone takes too much of a medicine, follow your school procedure for an urgent medical problem.

Taking medicine is a private matter and is best managed discreetly and confidentially. It is important to be sensitive to the student's feelings about taking medicine.

If you suspect that the student is using drugs or alcohol, please tell the parent(s) or a school counselor right away.

Please tell the parent(s) or school nurse if you suspect medication side effects.

Modifications of the classroom environment or assignments may be useful in addition to medication. The student may need to be evaluated for additional help or a 504 plan or an Individualized Education Plan for learning problems or emotional or behavioral issues.

Any expression of suicidal thoughts or feelings or self-harm by a child or adolescent is a signal of distress and should be taken seriously. These behaviors should not be dismissed as "attention seeking." School procedures for safety issues should be followed.

What Is Trifluoperazine?

Trifluoperazine is sometimes called a *typical* or *first-generation antipsychotic* medicine. It is also called a *neuroleptic* or *phenothiazine*. It used to be called a *major tranquilizer*. It comes in generic tablets. It used to come in brand name Stelazine, so it is sometimes still called that.

How Can This Medicine Help?

Trifluoperazine is used to treat psychosis, such as in schizophrenia, mania, or very severe depression. It can reduce hallucinations (hearing voices or seeing things that are not there) and delusions (troubling beliefs that other people do not share). It can help the patient be less upset and agitated. It can improve the patient's ability to think clearly.

Sometimes trifluoperazine is used to decrease severe aggression or very serious behavioral problems in young people with conduct disorder, intellectual disability, or autism spectrum disorder.

This medicine is very powerful and should be used to treat very serious problems or symptoms that other medicines do not help. Be patient; the positive effects of this medicine may not appear for 2–3 weeks.

How Does This Medicine Work?

Cells in the brain (neurons) communicate using chemicals called *neurotransmitters*. Too much or too little of these substances in certain parts of the brain can cause problems. Trifluoperazine reduces the activity of one of these neurotransmitters, *dopamine*. Blocking the effect of dopamine in certain parts of the brain reduces what have been called *positive symptoms* of psychosis: delusions; hallucinations; disorganized and unusual thinking, speaking, and behavior; excessive activity (agitation); and lack of activity (catatonia). Blocking dopamine can also reduce tics. Reducing dopamine action in other parts of the brain may lead to the side effects of this medicine.

How Long Does This Medicine Last?

Trifluoperazine usually may be taken only once a day, unless divided doses are used to lessen side effects.

How Will the Doctor Monitor This Medicine?

The doctor will review your child's medical history and physical examination before starting trifluoperazine. The doctor may order some blood or urine tests to be sure your child does not have a hidden medical condition. The doctor or nurse may measure your child's pulse and blood pressure before starting trifluoperazine.

Before starting trifluoperazine and every so often afterward, a test such as the AIMS (Abnormal Involuntary Movement Scale) may be used to check your child's tongue, legs, and arms for unusual movements that could be caused by the medicine.

After the medicine is started, the doctor will want to have regular appointments with you and your child to see how the medicine is working, to see if a dose change is needed, to watch for side effects, to see if trifluoperazine is still needed, and to see if any other treatment is needed. The doctor or nurse may check your child's height, weight, pulse, and blood pressure and watch for abnormal movements.

What Side Effects Can This Medicine Have?

Any medicine can have side effects, including an allergy to the medicine. Because each patient is different, the doctor will monitor the youth closely, especially when the medicine is started. The doctor will work with you to increase the positive effects and decrease the negative effects of the medicine. Please tell the doctor if any of the listed side effects appear or if you think that the medicine is causing any other problems. Not all of the rare or unusual side effects are listed.

Side effects are most common after starting the medicine or after a dose increase. Many side effects can be avoided or lessened by starting with a very low dose and increasing it slowly—ask the doctor.

Allergic Reaction

Tell the doctor in a day or two (if possible, before the next dose of medicine):

- Hives
- Itching
- Rash

Stop the medicine and get *immediate* medical care:

- Trouble breathing or chest tightness
- Swelling of lips, tongue, or throat

Common, but Not Usually Serious, Side Effects

Discuss the following side effects with your child's doctor within a week or two. They often can be helped by lowering the dose of medicine, changing the times medicine is taken, or adding another medicine.

- Dry mouth—Have your child try using sugar-free gum or candy.
- Constipation—Encourage your child to drink more fluids and eat high-fiber foods; if necessary, the doctor may recommend a fiber medicine such as Benefiber or a stool softener such as Colace or mineral oil.
- Increased risk of sunburn—Have your child wear sunscreen or protective clothing or stay out of the sun.
- Mild trouble urinating
- Blurred vision
- Weight gain—Seek nutritional counseling; provide your child with low-calorie snacks and encourage regular exercise.
- Sadness, irritability, nervousness, clinginess, not wanting to go to school
- Restlessness or inability to sit still
- Shaking of hands and fingers

Less Common, but Not Usually Serious, Side Effects

Discuss the following side effects with your child's doctor within a week or two. They often can be helped by lowering the dose of medicine, changing the times medicine is taken, or adding another medicine.

- Daytime sleepiness or tiredness—Do not allow your child to drive, ride a bicycle or motorcycle, or operate machinery if this happens. This problem may be lessened by taking the medicine at bedtime.
- Dizziness—This side effect is worse when the child stands up quickly, especially when getting out of bed in the morning; try having the child stand up slowly.
- Decreased or slowed movement and decreased facial expressions
- Drooling
- Decreased sexual interest or ability
- Changes in menstrual cycle
- Increase in breast size or discharge from the breasts (in both boys and girls)—This may go away with time.

Less Common, but Potentially Serious, Side Effects

Call the doctor or go to an emergency room *right away*:

- Stiffness of the tongue, jaw, neck, back, or legs
- Overheating or heatstroke—Prevent by decreasing activity in hot weather, staying out of the sun, and drinking water.
- Seizure (fit, convulsion)—This is more likely in people with a history of seizures or head injury.
- Severe confusion

Rare, but Serious, Side Effects

- Extreme stiffness or lack of movement, very high fever, mental confusion, irregular pulse rate, or eye pain—**This is a medical emergency. Go to an emergency room right away.**
- Sudden stiffness and inability to breathe or swallow—**Go to an emergency room or call 911.** Tell the paramedics, nurses, and doctors that the patient is taking trifluoperazine. Other medicines can be used to treat this problem fast.
- Increased thirst, frequent urination, lethargy, tiredness, dizziness—These could be signs of diabetes, especially if your child is overweight or there is a family history of diabetes. **Talk to a doctor within a day.**

What Else Should I Know About Side Effects?

Most side effects lessen over time. If they are troublesome, talk with your child's doctor. Some side effects can be decreased by taking a smaller dose of medicine, by stopping the medicine, by changing to another medicine, or by adding another medicine (see the table).

One side effect that may not go away is *tardive dyskinesia* (or TD). Patients with tardive dyskinesia have involuntary movements of the body, especially the mouth and tongue. The patient may look as though he or she is making faces over and over again. Jerky movements of the arms, legs, or body may occur. There may be fine, wormlike, or sudden repeated movements of the tongue, or the person may appear to be chewing something or smacking or puckering his or her lips. The fingers may look as though they are rolling something. If you notice any unusual movements, be sure to tell the doctor. The doctor may use the AIMS test to look for these movements.

The medicine may increase the level of *prolactin*, a natural hormone made in the part of the brain called the *pituitary*. This may cause side effects such as breast tenderness or swelling or production of milk, in both boys and girls. It also may interfere with sexual functioning in teenage boys and with regular menstrual cycles (periods) in teenage girls. A blood test can measure the level of prolactin. If these side effects do not go away and are troublesome, talk with your child's doctor about substituting another medicine for trifluoperazine.

Heart problems are more common if other medicines are being taken as well. Be sure to tell all your child's doctors and your pharmacist about all medications your child is taking.

Neuroleptic malignant syndrome is a very rare side effect that can lead to death. The symptoms are severe muscle stiffness, high fever, increased heart rate and blood pressure, irregular heartbeat (pulse), and sweating. It may lead to unconsciousness. If you suspect this, **call 911 or go to an emergency room right away.**

Sometimes this medicine can cause a *dystonic reaction*. This is a sudden stiffening of the muscles, most often in the jaw, neck, tongue, face, or shoulders. If this happens, and your child is not having trouble breathing, you may give a dose of diphenhydramine (Benadryl). Follow the dose instructions on the package for your child's age. This should relax the muscles in a few minutes. Then call your doctor to tell him or her what happened. If the muscles do not relax, take your child to the emergency department.

Some Interactions With Other Medicines or Food

Please note that the following are only the most likely interactions with other medicines or food.

Trifluoperazine may be taken with or without food. If the medicine causes stomach upset, taking it with food may help.

It is better to limit drinks with caffeine (coffee, tea, soft drinks) because caffeine works in the opposite way from this medicine, and the positive effects might be decreased.

Trifluoperazine can interact with other medications including antibiotics and other psychiatric medications in ways that may cause serious side effects. Be sure to tell your child's doctor about all medications that your child is taking.

What Could Happen if This Medicine Is Stopped Suddenly?

Involuntary movements, or *withdrawal dyskinesias*, may appear within 1–4 weeks of lowering the dose or stopping the medicine. Usually these go away, but they can last for days to months. If trifluoperazine is stopped suddenly, emotional problems such as irritability, nervousness, moodiness; behavior problems; or physical problems such as stomachache, loss of appetite, nausea, vomiting, diarrhea, sweating, indigestion, trouble sleeping, trembling, or shaking may appear. These problems usually last only a few days to a few weeks. If they happen, tell your child's doctor. The medicine dose may need to be lowered more slowly (tapered). Always check with the doctor before stopping a medicine.

How Long Will This Medicine Be Needed?

How long your child will need to be on trifluoperazine depends partly on the reason that it was prescribed. Some problems last for only a few months, whereas others last much longer. Sometimes trifluoperazine is used for only a short time until other medicines or behavioral treatments start to work. Some people need to take trifluoperazine for years. It is especially important with medicines as powerful as this one to ask the doctor whether it is still needed. Every few months, you should discuss with your child's doctor the reasons for using trifluoperazine and whether it is time for a trial of lowering the dose.

What Else Should I Know About This Medicine?

There are many other medicines that are used for the same kinds of problems. If your child is having bad side effects or the medicine does not seem to be working, ask the doctor if another medicine in this group might work as well or better and have fewer side effects for your child.

   Be sure to tell the doctor if there is anyone in your family who died suddenly or had a heart problem.

Notes

Use this space to take notes or to write down questions you want to ask the doctor.

_____

_____

_____

_____

_____

_____

_____

_____

_____

_____

_____

_____

_____

_____

From Dulcan MK, Ballard R (editors): *Helping Parents and Teachers Understand Medications for Behavioral and Emotional Problems: A Resource Book of Medication Information Handouts*, Fourth Edition. Washington, DC, American Psychiatric Publishing, 2015

Medication Information for Parents and Teachers

Valproic Acid—Depakene, Stavzor Divalproex—Depakote, Depakote ER, Depakote Sprinkles

General Information About Medication

Each child and adolescent is different. No one has exactly the same combination of medical and psychological problems. It is a good idea to talk with the doctor or nurse about the reasons a medicine is being used. It is very important to keep all appointments and to be in touch by telephone if you have concerns. It is important to communicate with the doctor, nurse, or therapist. An *advanced practice nurse* (APN) has additional education and training after becoming a registered nurse (RN). Your child's medication may be prescribed by a medical doctor (MD or DO) or an APN. In addition, a *physician assistant* (PA) working with a physician may prescribe certain medications. In this information sheet, "doctor" includes medical doctors as well as APNs and PAs who prescribe medication. Often a nurse (RN) will be part of the team and answer questions and give information.

It is very important that the medicine be taken exactly as the doctor instructs. However, once in a while, everyone forgets to give a medicine on time. It is a good idea to ask the doctor or nurse what to do if this happens. Do not stop or change a medicine without asking the doctor or nurse first.

If the medicine seems to stop working, it may be because it is not being taken regularly. The youth may be "cheeking" or hiding the medicine or forgetting to take it (especially at school). The doses may be too far apart or a different dose or medicine may be needed. Something at school, at home, or in the neighborhood may be upsetting the youth, or he or she may need special help for learning disabilities or tutoring. Please discuss your concerns with the doctor. **Do not just increase the dose.** It is also very important not to decrease the dose or stop the medicine without talking to the doctor first. The problem being treated may come back, or there could be uncomfortable or even dangerous results.

All medicines should be kept in a safe place, out of the reach of children, and should be supervised by an adult. If someone takes too much of a medicine, call the doctor, the poison control center, or a hospital emergency room.

Each medicine has a "generic" or chemical name. Just like laundry detergents or paper towels, some medicines are sold by more than one company under different brand names. The same medicine may be available under a generic name and several brand names. The generic medications are usually less expensive than the brand name ones. The generic medications have the same chemical formula, but they may or may not be exactly the same strength as the brand-name medications. Also, some brands of pills contain dye or other things that can cause allergic reactions. It is a good idea to talk to the doctor and the pharmacist about whether it is important to use a specific brand of medicine.

Any medicine can cause an allergic reaction. Examples are hives, itching, rashes, swelling, and trouble breathing. Even a tiny amount of a medicine can cause a reaction in patients who are allergic to that medicine. Be *sure* to talk to the doctor before restarting a medicine that has caused an allergic reaction and tell the doctor about any reactions to medicine that your child has had before.

515

Taking more than one medicine at the same time may cause more side effects or cause one of the medicines to not work as well. Always ask the doctor, nurse, or pharmacist before adding another medicine, either prescription or bought without a prescription in a store or on the Internet. Be sure that each doctor knows about *all* of the medicines your child is taking. Also tell the doctor about any vitamins, herbal medicines, or supplements your child may be taking. Some of these may have side effects alone or when taken with this medication. It is a very good idea to keep a list with you of the names and doses of all medicines that your child is taking.

Everyone taking medicine should have a physical examination at least once a year.

If you think that your child may be using drugs or alcohol, please tell the doctor right away.

Pregnancy requires special care in the use of medicine. Some medicines can cause birth defects if taken by a pregnant mother. **Please tell the doctor immediately if you suspect the teenager is at risk of becoming pregnant.** The doctor may wish to discuss sexual behavior and/or birth control with your daughter.

Printed information like this applies to children and adolescents in general. If you have questions about the medicine, or if you notice changes or anything unusual, please ask the doctor or nurse. As scientific research advances, knowledge increases and advice changes. Even experts do not always agree. Many medicines have not been "approved" by the U.S. Food and Drug Administration (FDA) for use in children or use for particular problems. For this reason, use of the medicine for a problem or age group often is not listed in the *Physicians' Desk Reference*. This does not necessarily mean that the medicine is dangerous or does not work, only that the company that makes the medicine has not received permission to advertise the medicine for use in children. Companies often do not apply for this permission because it is expensive to do the tests needed to apply for approval for use in children. Once a medication is approved by the FDA for any purpose, a doctor is allowed to prescribe it according to research and clinical experience.

Note to Teachers

It is a good idea to talk with the parent(s) about the reason(s) that a medication is being used. If the parent(s) sign consent to release information, it is often helpful for you to talk with the doctor. If the parent(s) give permission, the doctor may ask you to fill out rating forms about your experience with the student's behavior, feelings, academic performance, and medication side effects. This information is very useful in selecting and monitoring medication treatment. If you have observations that you think are important, do not hesitate to share these with the student's parent(s) and treating clinicians (with parental consent).

It is very important that the medicine be taken exactly as the doctor instructs. However, everyone forgets to give a medicine on time once in a while. It is a good idea to ask the parent(s) in advance what to do if this happens. Do not stop or change the time you are giving a medicine at school without parental permission. If a medication is to be taken with food, but lunchtime or snack time changes, be sure to notify the parent(s) so appropriate adjustments can be made.

All medicines should be kept in a secure place and should be supervised by an adult. If someone takes too much of a medicine, follow your school procedure for an urgent medical problem.

Taking medicine is a private matter and is best managed discreetly and confidentially. It is important to be sensitive to the student's feelings about taking medicine.

If you suspect that the student is using drugs or alcohol, please tell the parent(s) or a school counselor right away.

Please tell the parent(s) or school nurse if you suspect medication side effects.

Modifications of the classroom environment or assignments may be useful in addition to medication. The student may need to be evaluated for additional help or a 504 plan or an Individualized Education Plan for learning problems or emotional or behavioral issues.

Any expression of suicidal thoughts or feelings or self-harm by a child or adolescent is a signal of distress and should be taken seriously. These behaviors should not be dismissed as "attention seeking." School procedures for safety issues should be followed.

What Are Valproic Acid (Depakene) and Divalproex (Depakote)?

Valproic acid and divalproex come in many forms, but the active ingredient in all of them is valproic acid. All of the forms can be referred to as *valproate*. It was first used to treat seizures (fits, convulsions), so it is sometimes called an *anticonvulsant* or an *antiepileptic drug (AED)*. Now it is also used for behavioral problems, such as aggression or bipolar disorder, whether or not the patient has seizures. It also may be used when the patient has a history of severe mood changes, sometimes called *mood swings*. When used for emotional or behavioral symptoms, this medicine is more commonly called a *mood stabilizer*.

Valproate comes in tablets (Depakote), gel capsules, liquid syrup, sprinkle capsules, and extended-release tablets (Depakote-ER). Depakote and Depakote-ER tablets have a coating that decreases stomach irritation. A generic valproate capsule (not sprinkle) and liquid are also available. Valproic acid comes in brand name Depakene and generic capsules and brand name Stavzor delayed-release capsules.

How Can This Medicine Help?

Valproate can reduce aggression, anger, and severe mood swings. It can treat mania or prevent relapse (mania coming back).

How Does This Medicine Work?

Valproate is thought to work by stabilizing a part of the brain cell (the cell membrane or envelope) and by changing the concentrations of certain *neurotransmitters* (chemicals in the brain) such as *GABA*.

How Long Does This Medicine Last?

Most forms of valproate are taken two to four times a day. Depakote may be taken twice a day. Depakote-ER can be taken only once a day.

How Will the Doctor Monitor This Medicine?

The doctor will review your child's medical history and physical examination before starting valproate. The doctor may order some blood tests to be sure your child does not have a hidden medical condition that would make it unsafe to use this medicine. The doctor or nurse will measure your child's height, weight, pulse, and blood pressure before starting valproate. The doctor may order a baseline blood test of liver functions.

After the medicine is started, the doctor will want to have regular appointments with you and your child to see how the medicine is working, to see if a dose change is needed, to watch for side effects, to see if valproate is still needed, and to see if any other treatment is needed. The doctor or nurse will check your child's height, weight, pulse, and blood pressure. The doctor will need to order blood tests to make sure that the medicine is at the right dose as well as to look for any side effects in the liver or blood. To see if the medicine is at the right dose, blood should be drawn first thing in the morning, 10–12 hours after the last dose and before the morning dose.

What Side Effects Can This Medicine Have?

Any medicine can have side effects, including an allergy to the medicine. Because each patient is different, the doctor will monitor the youth closely, especially when the medicine is started. The doctor will work with you to increase the positive effects and decrease the negative effects of the medicine. Please tell the doctor if any of the listed side effects appear or if you think that the medicine is causing any other problems. Not all of the rare or unusual side effects are listed.

Side effects are most common after starting the medicine or after a dose increase. Many side effects can be avoided or lessened by starting with a very low dose and increasing it slowly—ask the doctor.

Allergic Reaction

Tell the doctor in a day or two (if possible, before the next dose of medicine):

- Hives
- Itching
- Rash

Stop the medicine and get *immediate* medical care:

- Trouble breathing or chest tightness
- Swelling of lips, tongue, or throat

General Side Effects

Tell the doctor within a week or two:

- Upset stomach—This can be helped by taking medicine with food, or ask the doctor about a different form of the medicine.
- Stomach cramps
- Increased appetite
- Weight gain
- Hand tremor (shakiness)
- Clumsiness and difficulty walking
- Daytime drowsiness, sleepiness, or tiredness—Do not allow your child to drive, ride a bicycle or motorcycle, or operate machinery if this happens.
- Hair loss from the scalp (thinning hair)
- Increased facial or body hair
- Irregular menstrual periods
- Severe acne

Behavioral and Emotional Side Effects

Tell the doctor right away:

- Increased suicidal thoughts or behaviors or new or worse depression or anxiety

Call the doctor within a day or two:

- Increased aggression
- Increased irritability

Possibly Dangerous Side Effects

Call the doctor *immediately*:

- Weakness or feeling sick or unusually tired (for no reason)
- Loss of appetite (for more than a few hours)
- Yellowing of skin or eyes
- Dark urine or pale bowel movements
- Swelling of the legs, feet, or face
- Greatly increased or decreased urination
- Unusual bruising or bleeding
- Sore throat or fever
- Mouth ulcers
- Vomiting (for more than a few hours)
- Persistent stomachache (more than 20 minutes)
- Skin rash
- Seizure (fit, convulsion)
- Blurry vision
- Mental confusion

Some Interactions With Other Medicines or Food

Please note that the following are only the most likely interactions with other medicines or food.

Caffeine may increase side effects.

Valproate interacts with many other medicines. Taking it with another medicine may make one or both not work as well or may cause more side effects. Be sure that each doctor knows about *all* of the medicines being taken.

These medicines (and many others) increase the levels of valproate and increase the risk of serious side effects:

- Cimetidine (Tagamet)
- Fluoxetine (Prozac)
- Fluvoxamine (Luvox)

- Ibuprofen (Motrin) or aspirin
- Erythromycin and similar antibiotics
- Ketoconazole and similar antifungal agents
- Guanfacine (Intuniv)

Taking valproate with lamotrigine (Lamictal) increases the risk of dangerous skin rash. Taking valproate together with another antiepileptic medication—topiramate (Topamax)—may result in a high blood ammonia level that can cause vomiting, tiredness, or confusion.

What Could Happen if This Medicine Is Stopped Suddenly?

Stopping valproate suddenly causes uncomfortable withdrawal symptoms. If the person is taking valproate for epilepsy (seizures), stopping the medicine suddenly could lead to an increase in very dangerous seizures (convulsions).

How Long Will This Medicine Be Needed?

The length of time a person needs to take valproate depends on what problem is being treated. For example, someone with an impulse control disorder usually takes the medicine only until behavioral therapy begins to work. Someone with bipolar disorder may need to take the medicine for many years. Please ask the doctor about the length of treatment needed.

What Else Should I Know About This Medicine?

Taking valproate with food may decrease stomach upset. The liquid may be mixed with another liquid or with food.

Your child should not chew the Depakene capsules or the Depakote tablets; chewing these medicines will irritate the mouth, throat, and stomach. Do not crush or chew Depakote-ER tablets; doing so will destroy the protective coating of the tablet.

Some people taking valproate want to eat a lot more than usual and gain too much weight. It is very important to be sure that your child has a healthy diet without too many sweets or fast food and that your child has regular exercise.

Valproate may cause thinning of hair on the head. Taking a daily multivitamin with minerals may stop this. The hair usually grows back when the valproate is stopped.

When taken during pregnancy, valproate may cause birth defects or lower intelligence in the baby. Your doctor may consider doing a pregnancy test before your daughter starts this medication. If your daughter is sexually active or decides to start sexual activity while taking this medication, she should talk with her doctor about birth control and other health issues related to sex. Call the doctor immediately if your daughter becomes pregnant while taking valproate.

Young women taking valproate may develop *polycystic ovary syndrome*. This very rare condition shows itself as a combination of obesity, acne, excess facial and body hair, and infertility.

People with certain genetic metabolic diseases should not take Depakene or Depakote because of an increased risk of dangerous liver problems. Please ask your doctor about this if your child has a genetic disorder.

Liver failure and inflammation of the pancreas may occur with valproate, but this almost never happens except in children younger than 6 years old who are taking more than one medicine.

Valproate can increase bleeding and decrease blood clotting. Your doctor may want to stop it and change it to another medicine before any surgery or procedure, including dental work.

Valproate is very dangerous in overdose. Keep the medicine in a safe place, under close supervision.

Keep the pill container tightly closed and in a dry place, away from bathrooms, showers, and humidifiers.

The names of the different forms can be confusing. When you get the medicine from the pharmacy, check to be sure you got the right medicine.

Notes

Use this space to take notes or to write down questions you want to ask the doctor.

_____

_____

_____

_____

_____

_____

_____

_____

_____

_____

_____

_____

lication and consistent with standards set by the U.S. Food and Drug Administration and the general medical community and accepted child psychiatric practice. The information on this medication sheet does not cover all the possible uses, precautions, side effects, or interactions of this drug. For a complete listing of side effects, see the manufacturer's package insert, which can be obtained from your physician or pharmacist. As medical research and practice advance, therapeutic standards may change. For this reason and because human and mechanical errors sometimes occur, we recommend that readers follow the advice of a physician who is directly involved in their care or the care of a member of their family.

From Dulcan MK, Ballard R (editors): *Helping Parents and Teachers Understand Medications for Behavioral and Emotional Problems: A Resource Book of Medication Information Handouts*, Fourth Edition. Washington, DC, American Psychiatric Publishing, 2015

Medication Information for Parents and Teachers

Venlafaxine—Effexor
Desvenlafaxine—Pristiq, Khedezla

General Information About Medication

Each child and adolescent is different. No one has exactly the same combination of medical and psychological problems. It is a good idea to talk with the doctor or nurse about the reasons a medicine is being used. It is very important to keep all appointments and to be in touch by telephone if you have concerns. It is important to communicate with the doctor, nurse, or therapist. An *advanced practice nurse* (APN) has additional education and training after becoming a registered nurse (RN). Your child's medication may be prescribed by a medical doctor (MD or DO) or an APN. In addition, a *physician assistant* (PA) working with a physician may prescribe certain medications. In this information sheet, "doctor" includes medical doctors as well as APNs and PAs who prescribe medication. Often a nurse (RN) will be part of the team and answer questions and give information.

It is very important that the medicine be taken exactly as the doctor instructs. However, once in a while, everyone forgets to give a medicine on time. It is a good idea to ask the doctor or nurse what to do if this happens. Do not stop or change a medicine without asking the doctor or nurse first.

If the medicine seems to stop working, it may be because it is not being taken regularly. The youth may be "cheeking" or hiding the medicine or forgetting to take it (especially at school). The doses may be too far apart or a different dose or medicine may be needed. Something at school, at home, or in the neighborhood may be upsetting the youth, or he or she may need special help for learning disabilities or tutoring. Please discuss your concerns with the doctor. **Do not just increase the dose.** It is also very important not to decrease the dose or stop the medicine without talking to the doctor first. The problem being treated may come back, or there could be uncomfortable or even dangerous results.

All medicines should be kept in a safe place, out of the reach of children, and should be supervised by an adult. If someone takes too much of a medicine, call the doctor, the poison control center, or a hospital emergency room.

Each medicine has a "generic" or chemical name. Just like laundry detergents or paper towels, some medicines are sold by more than one company under different brand names. The same medicine may be available under a generic name and several brand names. The generic medications are usually less expensive than the brand name ones. The generic medications have the same chemical formula, but they may or may not be exactly the same strength as the brand-name medications. Also, some brands of pills contain dye or other things that can cause allergic reactions. It is a good idea to talk to the doctor and the pharmacist about whether it is important to use a specific brand of medicine.

Any medicine can cause an allergic reaction. Examples are hives, itching, rashes, swelling, and trouble breathing. Even a tiny amount of a medicine can cause a reaction in patients who are allergic to that medicine. Be *sure* to talk to the doctor before restarting a medicine that has caused an allergic reaction and tell the doctor about any reactions to medicine that your child has had before.

Taking more than one medicine at the same time may cause more side effects or cause one of the medicines to not work as well. **Always ask the doctor, nurse, or pharmacist before adding another medicine, either prescription or bought without a prescription in a store or on the Internet. Be sure that each doctor knows about *all* of the medicines your child is taking. Also tell the doctor about any vitamins, herbal medicines, or supplements your child may be taking.** Some of these may have side effects alone or when taken with this medication. It is a very good idea to keep a list with you of the names and doses of all medicines that your child is taking.

Everyone taking medicine should have a physical examination at least once a year.

If you think that your child may be using drugs or alcohol, please tell the doctor right away.

Pregnancy requires special care in the use of medicine. Some medicines can cause birth defects if taken by a pregnant mother. **Please tell the doctor immediately if you suspect the teenager is at risk of becoming pregnant.** The doctor may wish to discuss sexual behavior and/or birth control with your daughter.

Printed information like this applies to children and adolescents in general. If you have questions about the medicine, or if you notice changes or anything unusual, please ask the doctor or nurse. As scientific research advances, knowledge increases and advice changes. Even experts do not always agree. Many medicines have not been "approved" by the U.S. Food and Drug Administration (FDA) for use in children or use for particular problems. For this reason, use of the medicine for a problem or age group often is not listed in the *Physicians' Desk Reference*. This does not necessarily mean that the medicine is dangerous or does not work, only that the company that makes the medicine has not received permission to advertise the medicine for use in children. Companies often do not apply for this permission because it is expensive to do the tests needed to apply for approval for use in children. Once a medication is approved by the FDA for any purpose, a doctor is allowed to prescribe it according to research and clinical experience.

Note to Teachers

It is a good idea to talk with the parent(s) about the reason(s) that a medication is being used. If the parent(s) sign consent to release information, it is often helpful for you to talk with the doctor. If the parent(s) give permission, the doctor may ask you to fill out rating forms about your experience with the student's behavior, feelings, academic performance, and medication side effects. This information is very useful in selecting and monitoring medication treatment. If you have observations that you think are important, do not hesitate to share these with the student's parent(s) and treating clinicians (with parental consent).

It is very important that the medicine be taken exactly as the doctor instructs. However, everyone forgets to give a medicine on time once in a while. It is a good idea to ask the parent(s) in advance what to do if this happens. Do not stop or change the time you are giving a medicine at school without parental permission. If a medication is to be taken with food, but lunchtime or snack time changes, be sure to notify the parent(s) so appropriate adjustments can be made.

All medicines should be kept in a secure place and should be supervised by an adult. If someone takes too much of a medicine, follow your school procedure for an urgent medical problem.

Taking medicine is a private matter and is best managed discreetly and confidentially. It is important to be sensitive to the student's feelings about taking medicine.

If you suspect that the student is using drugs or alcohol, please tell the parent(s) or a school counselor right away.

Please tell the parent(s) or school nurse if you suspect medication side effects.

Modifications of the classroom environment or assignments may be useful in addition to medication. The student may need to be evaluated for additional help or a 504 plan or an Individualized Education Plan for learning problems or emotional or behavioral issues.

Any expression of suicidal thoughts or feelings or self-harm by a child or adolescent is a signal of distress and should be taken seriously. These behaviors should not be dismissed as "attention seeking." School procedures for safety issues should be followed.

What Are Venlafaxine (Effexor) and Desvenlafaxine (Pristiq, Khedezla)?

Venlafaxine is called an *antidepressant*. It is sometimes called a *serotonin-norepinephrine reuptake inhibitor* (SNRI). It comes in generic immediate-release and extended-release tablets and brand name Effexor-XR and generic controlled-release capsules. The body makes desvenlafaxine when it breaks down venlafaxine. It is available as brand name Pristiq or Khedezla or generic extended-release tablets.

How Can These Medicines Help?

Venlafaxine has been used successfully to treat depression and anxiety (nervousness) in adults. Now it is also used to treat emotional and behavioral problems, including anxiety and depression, in children and adolescents. Desvenlafaxine is a newer form of the medicine that is used for the same problems. Venlafaxine or desvenlafaxine may take as long as 4–8 weeks to reach the full effect.

How Do These Medicines Work?

Venlafaxine and desvenlafaxine work by increasing the brain chemicals *serotonin* and *norepinephrine (neurotransmitters)* to more normal activity levels in certain parts of the brain. They have a somewhat different way of working than the antidepressants that are called *selective serotonin reuptake inhibitors* (or SSRIs).

How Long Do These Medicines Last?

The immediate-release (short-acting) tablets must be taken two or three times a day. The extended-release forms last the whole day when taken only once a day.

How Will the Doctor Monitor These Medicines?

The doctor will review your child's medical history and physical examination before starting venlafaxine or desvenlafaxine. The doctor may order some blood or urine tests to be sure your child does not have a hidden medical condition that would make it unsafe to use this medicine. The doctor or nurse may measure your child's height, weight, pulse, and blood pressure before starting venlafaxine or desvenlafaxine.

Be sure to tell the doctor if your child or anyone in the family has bipolar disorder or has tried to kill himself or herself.

After the medicine is started, the doctor will want to have regular appointments with you and your child to see how the medicine is working, to see if a dose change is needed, to watch for side effects, to see if venlafaxine or desvenlafaxine is still needed, and to see if any other treatment is needed. The doctor or nurse may check your child's height, weight, pulse, and blood pressure. No blood tests are usually required when taking these medicines.

Before using medicine and at times afterward, the doctor may ask your child to fill out a rating scale about depression and anxiety, to help see how your child is doing.

What Side Effects Can These Medicines Have?

Any medicine can have side effects, including an allergy to the medicine. Because each patient is different, the doctor will monitor the youth closely, especially when the medicine is started. The doctor will work with you to increase the positive effects and decrease the negative effects of the medicine. Please tell the doctor if any of the listed side effects appear or if you think that the medicine is causing any other problems. Not all of the rare or unusual side effects are listed.

Side effects are most common after starting the medicine or after a dose increase. Many side effects can be avoided or lessened by starting with a very low dose and increasing it slowly—ask the doctor.

Allergic Reaction

Tell the doctor in a day or two (if possible, before the next dose of medicine):

- Hives
- Itching
- Rash

Stop the medicine and get *immediate* medical care:

- Trouble breathing or chest tightness
- Swelling of lips, tongue, or throat

Common Side Effects

Tell the doctor within a week or two:

- Anxiety and nervousness
- Nausea
- Daytime sleepiness—Do not allow your child to drive, ride a bicycle or motorcycle, or operate machinery if this happens.
- Insomnia (trouble sleeping)
- Decreased appetite
- Weight loss
- Dry mouth—Have your child try using sugar-free gum or candy.
- Dizziness

Occasional Side Effects

Tell the doctor within a week or two:

- Yawning
- Blurred vision or double vision
- Constipation—Encourage your child to drink more fluids and eat high-fiber foods; if necessary, the doctor may recommend a fiber medicine such as Benefiber or a stool softener such as Colace or mineral oil.
- Lack of energy, tiredness
- Excessive sweating
- Trouble with sexual functioning
- Bleeding, such as bruising or nosebleeds
- Increased blood pressure

Less Common, but More Serious, Side Effects

Call the doctor *immediately*:

- Increased activity, rapid speech, feeling "speeded up," decreased need for sleep, being very excited or irritable (cranky)
- Seizure (fit, convulsion)

Serotonin Syndrome

A very serious side effect called *serotonin syndrome* can happen when certain kinds of medicines (including SSRI antidepressants, clomipramine, and other medicines, such as triptans for migraine headaches, buspirone, linezolid, tramadol, or St. John's wort) are taken by the same person. Very rarely, serotonin syndrome can happen at high doses of just one medicine. The early signs are restlessness, confusion, shaking, skin turning red, sweating, muscle stiffness, sweating, and jerking of muscles. If you see these symptoms, stop the medicine and send or take the youth to an emergency room right away.

Some Interactions With Other Medicines or Food

Please note that the following are only the most likely interactions with other medicines or food.

Caffeine may increase side effects.

Cimetidine (Tagamet) should not be used with venlafaxine because it increases the levels of these medicines and may increase side effects.

Taking citalopram with aspirin, nonsteroidal anti-inflammatory drugs (NSAIDs; medications including ibuprofen or naproxen), or anticoagulant medications (such as warfarin) increases risk of abnormal bleeding.

If venlafaxine is taken with haloperidol (Haldol), the levels of haloperidol and its side effects may increase.

It can be *very dangerous* to take venlafaxine at the same time as, or even within several weeks of, taking another type of medicine called a *monoamine oxidase inhibitor* (MAOI), such as selegiline (Eldepryl), phenelzine (Nardil), tranylcypromine (Parnate), or isocarboxazid (Marplan).

What Could Happen if These Medicines Are Stopped Suddenly?

No known serious medical withdrawal effects occur if venlafaxine is stopped suddenly, but there may be uncomfortable feelings such as dizziness, insomnia, nausea, or nervousness, or the problem being treated may come back. These discontinuation symptoms may be more severe with the immediate-release form of venlafaxine, and it is usually recommended that this medication be tapered gradually. Ask the doctor before stopping the medicine.

How Long Will This Medicine Be Needed?

Your child may need to keep taking the medicine for at least 6–12 months so that the emotional or behavioral problem does not come back.

What Else Should I Know About This Medicine?

In youth who have bipolar disorder or who are at risk for bipolar disorder, any antidepressant medicine may increase the risk of hypomania or mania (excitement, agitation, increased activity, decreased sleep).

Black Box Antidepressant Warning

In 2004, an advisory committee to the FDA decided that there might be an increased risk of suicidal behavior for some youth taking medicines called *antidepressants*. In the research studies that the committee reviewed, about 3%–4% of youth with depression who took an antidepressant medicine—and 1%–2% of youth with depression who took a placebo (pill without active medicine)—talked about suicidal thoughts (thinking about killing themselves or wishing they were dead) or did something to harm themselves. This means that almost twice as many youth who were taking an antidepressant to treat their depression talked about suicide or had suicidal behavior compared with youth with depression who were taking inactive medicine. There were *no* completed suicides in any of these research studies, which included more than 4,000 children and adolescents. For youth being treated for anxiety, there was no difference in suicidal talking or behavior between those taking antidepressant medication and those taking placebo.

The FDA told drug companies to add a *black box warning* label to all antidepressant medicines. Because of this label, a doctor (or advanced practice nurse) prescribing one of these medicines has to warn youth and their families that there might be more suicidal thoughts and actions in youth taking these medicines.

On the other hand, in places where more youth are taking the newer antidepressant medicines, the number of adolescents who commit suicide has gotten smaller. Also, thinking about or attempting suicide is more common in surveys of teenagers in the community than it is in depressed youth treated in research studies with antidepressant medicine.

If a youth is being treated with this medicine and is doing well, then no changes are needed as a result of this warning. Increased suicidal talk or action is most likely to happen in the first few months of treatment with a medicine. If your child has recently started this medicine or is about to start, then you and your doctor (or advanced practice nurse) should watch for any changes in behavior. People who are depressed often have suicidal thoughts or actions. It is hard to know whether suicidal thoughts or actions in depressed people are caused by the depression itself or by the medicine. Also, as their depression is getting better, some people talk more about the suicidal thoughts that they had before but did not talk about. As young people get better from depression, they might be at higher risk of doing something about suicidal thoughts that they have had for some time, because they have more energy.

What Should a Parent Do?

1. Be honest with your child about possible risks and benefits of medicine.

2. Talk to your child about whether he or she is having any suicidal thoughts, and tell your child to come to you if he or she is having such thoughts.

3. You, your child, and your child's doctor or nurse should develop a safety plan. Pick adults whom your child can tell if he or she is thinking about suicide.

4. Be sure to tell your child's doctor, nurse, or therapist if you suspect that your child is using alcohol or drugs or if something has happened that might make your child feel worse, such as a family separation, breaking up with a boyfriend or girlfriend, someone close dying or attempting suicide, physical or sexual abuse, or failure in school.

5. Be sure that there are no guns in the home and that all medicines (including over-the-counter medicines like Tylenol) are closely supervised by an adult and kept in a safe place.

6. Watch for new or worse thoughts of suicide, self-harm, depression, anxiety (nerves), feeling very agitated or restless, being angry or aggressive, having more trouble sleeping, or anything else that you see for the first time, seems worse, or worries your child or you. If these appear, contact a mental health professional **right away.** Do not just stop or change the dose of the medicine on your own. If the problems are serious, and you cannot reach one of your clinicians, call a 24-hour psychiatry emergency telephone number or take your child to an emergency room.

Youth taking antidepressant medicine should be watched carefully by their parent(s), clinician(s) (doctor, advanced practice nurse, nurse, therapist), and other concerned adults for the first weeks of treatment. It is a good idea to have regular contact with the doctor, APN, nurse, or therapist for the first months to check for feelings of depression or sadness, thoughts of killing or harming himself or herself, and any problems with the medication. If you have questions, be sure to ask the doctor, APN, nurse, or therapist.

For more information, see http://www.parentsmedguide.org/.

Notes

Use this space to take notes or to write down questions you want to ask the doctor.

_____

_____

_____

_____

_____

_____

_____

_____

_____

_____

_____

_____

_____

_____

Vilazodone—Viibryd

General Information About Medication

Each child and adolescent is different. No one has exactly the same combination of medical and psychological problems. It is a good idea to talk with the doctor or nurse about the reasons a medicine is being used. It is very important to keep all appointments and to be in touch by telephone if you have concerns. It is important to communicate with the doctor, nurse, or therapist. An *advanced practice nurse* (APN) has additional education and training after becoming a registered nurse (RN). Your child's medication may be prescribed by a medical doctor (MD or DO) or an APN. In addition, a *physician assistant* (PA) working with a physician may prescribe certain medications. In this information sheet, "doctor" includes medical doctors as well as APNs and PAs who prescribe medication. Often a nurse (RN) will be part of the team and answer questions and give information.

It is very important that the medicine be taken exactly as the doctor instructs. However, once in a while, everyone forgets to give a medicine on time. It is a good idea to ask the doctor or nurse what to do if this happens. Do not stop or change a medicine without asking the doctor or nurse first.

If the medicine seems to stop working, it may be because it is not being taken regularly. The youth may be "cheeking" or hiding the medicine or forgetting to take it (especially at school). The doses may be too far apart or a different dose or medicine may be needed. Something at school, at home, or in the neighborhood may be upsetting the youth, or he or she may need special help for learning disabilities or tutoring. Please discuss your concerns with the doctor. **Do not just increase the dose.** It is also very important not to decrease the dose or stop the medicine without talking to the doctor first. The problem being treated may come back, or there could be uncomfortable or even dangerous results.

All medicines should be kept in a safe place, out of the reach of children, and should be supervised by an adult. If someone takes too much of a medicine, call the doctor, the poison control center, or a hospital emergency room.

Each medicine has a "generic" or chemical name. Just like laundry detergents or paper towels, some medicines are sold by more than one company under different brand names. The same medicine may be available under a generic name and several brand names. The generic medications are usually less expensive than the brand name ones. The generic medications have the same chemical formula, but they may or may not be exactly the same strength as the brand-name medications. Also, some brands of pills contain dye or other things that can cause allergic reactions. It is a good idea to talk to the doctor and the pharmacist about whether it is important to use a specific brand of medicine.

Any medicine can cause an allergic reaction. Examples are hives, itching, rashes, swelling, and trouble breathing. Even a tiny amount of a medicine can cause a reaction in patients who are allergic to that medicine. Be *sure* to talk to the doctor before restarting a medicine that has caused an allergic reaction and tell the doctor about any reactions to medicine that your child has had before.

Taking more than one medicine at the same time may cause more side effects or cause one of the medicines to not work as well. Always ask the doctor, nurse, or pharmacist before adding another medicine, either prescription or bought without a prescription in a store or on the Internet. Be sure

that each doctor knows about *all* of the medicines your child is taking. Also tell the doctor about any vitamins, herbal medicines, or supplements your child may be taking. Some of these may have side effects alone or when taken with this medication. It is a very good idea to keep a list with you of the names and doses of all medicines that your child is taking.

Everyone taking medicine should have a physical examination at least once a year.

If you think that your child may be using drugs or alcohol, please tell the doctor right away.

Pregnancy requires special care in the use of medicine. Some medicines can cause birth defects if taken by a pregnant mother. **Please tell the doctor immediately if you suspect the teenager is at risk of becoming pregnant.** The doctor may wish to discuss sexual behavior and/or birth control with your daughter.

Printed information like this applies to children and adolescents in general. If you have questions about the medicine, or if you notice changes or anything unusual, please ask the doctor or nurse. As scientific research advances, knowledge increases and advice changes. Even experts do not always agree. Many medicines have not been "approved" by the U.S. Food and Drug Administration (FDA) for use in children or use for particular problems. For this reason, use of the medicine for a problem or age group often is not listed in the *Physicians' Desk Reference*. This does not necessarily mean that the medicine is dangerous or does not work, only that the company that makes the medicine has not received permission to advertise the medicine for use in children. Companies often do not apply for this permission because it is expensive to do the tests needed to apply for approval for use in children. Once a medication is approved by the FDA for any purpose, a doctor is allowed to prescribe it according to research and clinical experience.

Note to Teachers

It is a good idea to talk with the parent(s) about the reason(s) that a medication is being used. If the parent(s) sign consent to release information, it is often helpful for you to talk with the doctor. If the parent(s) give permission, the doctor may ask you to fill out rating forms about your experience with the student's behavior, feelings, academic performance, and medication side effects. This information is very useful in selecting and monitoring medication treatment. If you have observations that you think are important, do not hesitate to share these with the student's parent(s) and treating clinicians (with parental consent).

It is very important that the medicine be taken exactly as the doctor instructs. However, everyone forgets to give a medicine on time once in a while. It is a good idea to ask the parent(s) in advance what to do if this happens. Do not stop or change the time you are giving a medicine at school without parental permission. If a medication is to be taken with food, but lunchtime or snack time changes, be sure to notify the parent(s) so appropriate adjustments can be made.

All medicines should be kept in a secure place and should be supervised by an adult. If someone takes too much of a medicine, follow your school procedure for an urgent medical problem.

Taking medicine is a private matter and is best managed discreetly and confidentially. It is important to be sensitive to the student's feelings about taking medicine.

If you suspect that the student is using drugs or alcohol, please tell the parent(s) or a school counselor right away.

Please tell the parent(s) or school nurse if you suspect medication side effects.

Modifications of the classroom environment or assignments may be useful in addition to medication. The student may need to be evaluated for additional help or a 504 plan or an Individualized Education Plan for learning problems or emotional or behavioral issues.

Any expression of suicidal thoughts or feelings or self-harm by a child or adolescent is a signal of distress and should be taken seriously. These behaviors should not be dismissed as "attention seeking." School procedures for safety issues should be followed.

What Is Vilazodone (Viibryd)?

Vilazodone is called an *antidepressant*. It comes in brand name Viibryd tablets. Its mechanism of action is not fully understood, but it has been used successfully to treat major depression in adults. There is little information on its use in children or adolescents. Vilazodone may take as long as 4–8 weeks to reach its full effect.

How Does This Medicine Work?

Vilazodone works by increasing the brain chemical *serotonin* to more normal activity levels in certain parts of the brain. It is very similar to the antidepressants that are called *selective serotonin reuptake inhibitors* (SSRIs).

How Long Does This Medicine Last?

Vilazodone is usually taken only once a day. It should be taken with food.

How Will the Doctor Monitor This Medicine?

The doctor will review your child's medical history and physical examination before starting vilazodone. The doctor may order some blood or urine tests to be sure your child does not have a hidden medical condition that would make it unsafe to use this medicine. The doctor or nurse may measure your child's height, weight, pulse, and blood pressure before starting vilazodone.

Be sure to tell the doctor if anyone in the family has bipolar disorder or has tried to kill himself or herself.

After the medicine is started, the doctor will want to have regular appointments with you and your child to see how the medicine is working, to see if a dose change is needed, to watch for side effects, to see if vilazodone is still needed, and to see if any other treatment is needed. The doctor or nurse will check your child's height, weight, pulse, and blood pressure. No blood tests are routinely required while taking vilazodone.

Before using medicine and at times afterward, the doctor may ask your child to fill out a rating scale about depression and anxiety, to help see how your child is doing.

What Side Effects Can This Medicine Have?

Any medicine can have side effects, including an allergy to the medicine. Because each patient is different, the doctor will monitor the youth closely, especially when the medicine is started. The doctor will work with you to increase the positive effects and decrease the negative effects of the medicine. Please tell the doctor if any of the listed side effects appear or if you think that the medicine is causing any other problems. Not all of the rare or unusual side effects are listed.

Side effects are most common after starting the medicine or after a dose increase. Many side effects can be avoided or lessened by starting with a very low dose and increasing it slowly—ask the doctor.

Allergic Reaction

Tell the doctor in a day or two (if possible, before the next dose of medicine):

- Hives
- Itching
- Rash

Stop the medicine and get *immediate* medical care:

- Trouble breathing or chest tightness
- Swelling of lips, tongue, or throat

Common Side Effects

Tell the doctor within a week or two:

- Nausea and vomiting
- Diarrhea
- Insomnia (trouble sleeping)

Occasional Side Effects

Tell the doctor within a week or two:

- Blurred vision
- Weakness and dizziness
- Lack of energy, tiredness
- Excessive sweating
- Trouble with sexual functioning

Less Common, but More Serious, Side Effects

Call the doctor *immediately*:

- Increased activity, rapid speech, feeling "speeded up," decreased need for sleep, being very excited or irritable (cranky)
- Increased blood pressure
- Seizure (fit, convulsion)
- Abnormal bleeding or bruising—This is more common if the child is also taking aspirin or a nonsteroidal anti-inflammatory medication, such as ibuprofen or naproxen.

Serotonin Syndrome

A very serious side effect called *serotonin syndrome* can happen when certain kinds of medicines (including SSRI antidepressants, clomipramine, and other medicines, such as triptans for migraine headaches, buspirone, linezolid, tramadol, or St. John's wort) are taken by the same person. Very rarely, serotonin syndrome can happen at high doses of just one medicine. The early signs are restlessness, confusion, shaking, skin turning red, sweating, muscle stiffness, sweating, and jerking of muscles. If you see these symptoms, stop the medicine and send or take the youth to an emergency room right away.

Some Interactions With Other Medicines

Please note that the following are only the most likely interactions with other medicines.

Many medicines used to fight infections may increase levels of vilazodone and increase side effects. Ask the doctor.

It can be *very dangerous* to take vilazodone at the same time as, or even within several weeks of, taking another type of medicine called a *monoamine oxidase inhibitor* (MAOI), such as selegiline (Eldepryl), phenelzine (Nardil), tranylcypromine (Parnate), or isocarboxazid (Marplan).

What Could Happen if This Medicine Is Stopped Suddenly?

No known serious medical withdrawal effects occur if vilazodone is stopped suddenly, but there may be uncomfortable feelings such as dizziness, insomnia, nausea, or nervousness, or the problem being treated may come back. Ask the doctor before stopping the medicine.

How Long Will This Medicine Be Needed?

Your child may need to keep taking the medicine for at least 6–12 months so that the emotional or behavioral problem does not come back.

What Else Should I Know About This Medicine?

In youth who have bipolar disorder or who may be at risk for bipolar disorder, any antidepressant medicine may increase the risk of hypomania or mania (excitement, agitation, increased activity, decreased sleep).

Black Box Antidepressant Warning

In 2004, an advisory committee to the FDA decided that there might be an increased risk of suicidal behavior for some youth taking medicines called *antidepressants*. In the research studies that the committee reviewed, about 3%–4% of youth with depression who took an antidepressant medicine—and 1%–2% of youth with depression who took a placebo (pill without active medicine)—talked about suicidal thoughts (thinking about killing themselves or wishing they were dead) or did something to harm themselves. This means that almost twice as many youth who were taking an antidepressant to treat their depression talked about suicide or had suicidal behavior compared with youth with depression who were taking inactive medicine. There were *no* completed suicides in any of these research studies, which included more than 4,000 children and adolescents. For youth being treated for anxiety, there was no difference in suicidal talking or behavior between those taking antidepressant medication and those taking placebo.

The FDA told drug companies to add a *black box warning* label to all antidepressant medicines. Because of this label, a doctor (or advanced practice nurse) prescribing one of these medicines has to warn youth and their families that there might be more suicidal thoughts and actions in youth taking these medicines.

On the other hand, in places where more youth are taking the newer antidepressant medicines, the number of adolescents who commit suicide has gotten smaller. Also, thinking about or attempting suicide is more common in surveys of teenagers in the community than it is in depressed youth treated in research studies with antidepressant medicine.

If a youth is being treated with this medicine and is doing well, then no changes are needed as a result of this warning. Increased suicidal talk or action is most likely to happen in the first few months of treatment with a medicine. If your child has recently started this medicine, or is about to start, then you and your doctor (or advanced practice nurse) should watch for any changes in behavior. People who are depressed often have suicidal thoughts or actions. It is hard to know whether suicidal thoughts or actions in depressed people are caused by the depression itself or by the medicine. Also, as their depression is getting better, some people talk more about the suicidal thoughts they had before but did not talk about. As young people get better from depression, they might be at higher risk of doing something about suicidal thoughts that they have had for some time, because they have more energy.

What Should a Parent Do?

1. Be honest with your child about possible risks and benefits of medicine.
2. Talk to your child about whether he or she is having any suicidal thoughts, and tell your child to come to you if he or she is having such thoughts.
3. You, your child, and your child's doctor or nurse should develop a safety plan. Pick adults whom your child can tell if he or she is thinking about suicide.
4. Be sure to tell your child's doctor, nurse, or therapist if you suspect that your child is using alcohol or drugs or if something has happened that might make your child feel worse, such as a family separation, breaking up with a boyfriend or girlfriend, someone close dying or attempting suicide, physical or sexual abuse, or failure in school.
5. Be sure that there are no guns in the home and that all medicines (including over-the-counter medicines like Tylenol) are closely supervised by an adult and kept in a safe place.
6. Watch for new or worse thoughts of suicide, self-harm, depression, anxiety (nerves), feeling very agitated or restless, being angry or aggressive, having more trouble sleeping, or anything else that you see for the first time, seems worse, or worries your child or you. If these appear, contact a mental health professional **right away.** Do not just stop or change the dose of the medicine on your own. If the problems are serious, and you cannot reach one of your clinicians, call a 24-hour psychiatry emergency telephone number or take your child to an emergency room.

Youth taking antidepressant medicine should be watched carefully by their parent(s), clinician(s) (doctor, advanced practice nurse, nurse, therapist), and other concerned adults for the first weeks of treatment. It is a good idea to have regular contact with the doctor, APN, nurse, or therapist for the first months to check for feelings of depression or sadness, thoughts of killing or harming himself or herself, and any problems with the medication. If you have questions, be sure to ask the doctor, APN, nurse, or therapist.

For more information, see http://www.parentsmedguide.org.

Notes

Use this space to take notes or to write down questions you want to ask the doctor.

_____

_____

_____

_____

_____

_____

_____

_____

_____

From Dulcan MK, Ballard R (editors): *Helping Parents and Teachers Understand Medications for Behavioral and Emotional Problems: A Resource Book of Medication Information Handouts*, Fourth Edition. Washington, DC, American Psychiatric Publishing, 2015

Vortioxetine—Brintellix

General Information About Medication

Each child and adolescent is different. No one has exactly the same combination of medical and psychological problems. It is a good idea to talk with the doctor or nurse about the reasons a medicine is being used. It is very important to keep all appointments and to be in touch by telephone if you have concerns. It is important to communicate with the doctor, nurse, or therapist. An *advanced practice nurse* (APN) has additional education and training after becoming a registered nurse (RN). Your child's medication may be prescribed by a medical doctor (MD or DO) or an APN. In addition, a *physician assistant* (PA) working with a physician may prescribe certain medications. In this information sheet, "doctor" includes medical doctors as well as APNs and PAs who prescribe medication. Often a nurse (RN) will be part of the team and answer questions and give information.

It is very important that the medicine be taken exactly as the doctor instructs. However, once in a while, everyone forgets to give a medicine on time. It is a good idea to ask the doctor or nurse what to do if this happens. Do not stop or change a medicine without asking the doctor or nurse first.

If the medicine seems to stop working, it may be because it is not being taken regularly. The youth may be "cheeking" or hiding the medicine or forgetting to take it (especially at school). The doses may be too far apart or a different dose or medicine may be needed. Something at school, at home, or in the neighborhood may be upsetting the youth, or he or she may need special help for learning disabilities or tutoring. Please discuss your concerns with the doctor. **Do not just increase the dose.** It is also very important not to decrease the dose or stop the medicine without talking to the doctor first. The problem being treated may come back, or there could be uncomfortable or even dangerous results.

All medicines should be kept in a safe place, out of the reach of children, and should be supervised by an adult. If someone takes too much of a medicine, call the doctor, the poison control center, or a hospital emergency room.

Each medicine has a "generic" or chemical name. Just like laundry detergents or paper towels, some medicines are sold by more than one company under different brand names. The same medicine may be available under a generic name and several brand names. The generic medications are usually less expensive than the brand name ones. The generic medications have the same chemical formula, but they may or may not be exactly the same strength as the brand-name medications. Also, some brands of pills contain dye or other things that can cause allergic reactions. It is a good idea to talk to the doctor and the pharmacist about whether it is important to use a specific brand of medicine.

Any medicine can cause an allergic reaction. Examples are hives, itching, rashes, swelling, and trouble breathing. Even a tiny amount of a medicine can cause a reaction in patients who are allergic to that medicine. Be *sure* to talk to the doctor before restarting a medicine that has caused an allergic reaction and tell the doctor about any reactions to medicine that your child has had before.

Taking more than one medicine at the same time may cause more side effects or cause one of the medicines to not work as well. Always ask the doctor, nurse, or pharmacist before adding another medicine, either prescription or bought without a prescription in a store or on the Internet. Be sure

that each doctor knows about *all* of the medicines your child is taking. **Also tell the doctor about any vitamins, herbal medicines, or supplements your child may be taking.** Some of these may have side effects alone or when taken with this medication. It is a very good idea to keep a list with you of the names and doses of all medicines that your child is taking.

Everyone taking medicine should have a physical examination at least once a year.

If you think that your child may be using drugs or alcohol, please tell the doctor right away.

Pregnancy requires special care in the use of medicine. Some medicines can cause birth defects if taken by a pregnant mother. **Please tell the doctor immediately if you suspect the teenager is at risk of becoming pregnant.** The doctor may wish to discuss sexual behavior and/or birth control with your daughter.

Printed information like this applies to children and adolescents in general. If you have questions about the medicine, or if you notice changes or anything unusual, please ask the doctor or nurse. As scientific research advances, knowledge increases and advice changes. Even experts do not always agree. Many medicines have not been "approved" by the U.S. Food and Drug Administration (FDA) for use in children or use for particular problems. For this reason, use of the medicine for a problem or age group often is not listed in the *Physicians' Desk Reference*. This does not necessarily mean that the medicine is dangerous or does not work, only that the company that makes the medicine has not received permission to advertise the medicine for use in children. Companies often do not apply for this permission because it is expensive to do the tests needed to apply for approval for use in children. Once a medication is approved by the FDA for any purpose, a doctor is allowed to prescribe it according to research and clinical experience.

Note to Teachers

It is a good idea to talk with the parent(s) about the reason(s) that a medication is being used. If the parent(s) sign consent to release information, it is often helpful for you to talk with the doctor. If the parent(s) give permission, the doctor may ask you to fill out rating forms about your experience with the student's behavior, feelings, academic performance, and medication side effects. This information is very useful in selecting and monitoring medication treatment. If you have observations that you think are important, do not hesitate to share these with the student's parent(s) and treating clinicians (with parental consent).

It is very important that the medicine be taken exactly as the doctor instructs. However, everyone forgets to give a medicine on time once in a while. It is a good idea to ask the parent(s) in advance what to do if this happens. Do not stop or change the time you are giving a medicine at school without parental permission. If a medication is to be taken with food, but lunchtime or snack time changes, be sure to notify the parent(s) so appropriate adjustments can be made.

All medicines should be kept in a secure place and should be supervised by an adult. If someone takes too much of a medicine, follow your school procedure for an urgent medical problem.

Taking medicine is a private matter and is best managed discreetly and confidentially. It is important to be sensitive to the student's feelings about taking medicine.

If you suspect that the student is using drugs or alcohol, please tell the parent(s) or a school counselor right away.

Please tell the parent(s) or school nurse if you suspect medication side effects.

Modifications of the classroom environment or assignments may be useful in addition to medication. The student may need to be evaluated for additional help or a 504 plan or an Individualized Education Plan for learning problems or emotional or behavioral issues.

Any expression of suicidal thoughts or feelings or self-harm by a child or adolescent is a signal of distress and should be taken seriously. These behaviors should not be dismissed as "attention seeking." School procedures for safety issues should be followed.

What Is Vortioxetine (Brintellix)?

Vortioxetine is called an *antidepressant*. It comes in brand name Brintellix tablets.

How Can This Medicine Help?

Vortioxetine has been used successfully to treat major depression in adults. There is little information on its use in children or adolescents. Vortioxetine may take as long as 4–8 weeks to reach its full effect.

How Does This Medicine Work?

Vortioxetine works by increasing the brain chemical *serotonin* to more normal activity levels in certain parts of the brain. It is very similar to the antidepressants that are called *selective serotonin reuptake inhibitors* (SSRIs).

How Long Does This Medicine Last?

Vortioxetine is usually taken only once a day. It may be taken with food.

How Will the Doctor Monitor This Medicine?

The doctor will review your child's medical history and physical examination before starting vortioxetine. The doctor may order some blood or urine tests to be sure your child does not have a hidden medical condition that would make it unsafe to use this medicine. The doctor or nurse may measure your child's height, weight, pulse, and blood pressure before starting vortioxetine.

Be sure to tell the doctor if anyone in the family has bipolar disorder or has tried to kill himself or herself.

After the medicine is started, the doctor will want to have regular appointments with you and your child to see how the medicine is working, to see if a dose change is needed, to watch for side effects, to see if vortioxetine is still needed, and to see if any other treatment is needed. The doctor or nurse will check your child's height, weight, pulse, and blood pressure. No blood tests are routinely required while taking vortioxetine.

Before using medicine and at times afterward, the doctor may ask your child to fill out a rating scale about depression and anxiety, to help see how your child is doing.

What Side Effects Can This Medicine Have?

Any medicine can have side effects, including an allergy to the medicine. Because each patient is different, the doctor will monitor the youth closely, especially when the medicine is started. The doctor will work with you to increase the positive effects and decrease the negative effects of the medicine. Please tell the doctor if any of the listed side effects appear or if you think that the medicine is causing any other problems. Not all of the rare or unusual side effects are listed.

Side effects are most common after starting the medicine or after a dose increase. Many side effects can be avoided or lessened by starting with a very low dose and increasing it slowly—ask the doctor.

Allergic Reaction

Tell the doctor in a day or two (if possible, before the next dose of medicine):

- Hives
- Itching
- Rash

Stop the medicine and get *immediate* medical care:

- Trouble breathing or chest tightness
- Swelling of lips, tongue, or throat

Common Side Effects

Tell the doctor within a week or two:

- Nausea and vomiting
- Diarrhea
- Headache
- Constipation—Encourage your child to drink more fluids and eat high-fiber foods; if necessary, the doctor may recommend a fiber medicine such as Benefiber or a stool softener such as Colace or mineral oil.

Occasional Side Effects

Tell the doctor within a week or two:

- Abnormal bleeding or bruising, or bleeding with surgery
- Blurred vision
- Weakness and dizziness
- Lack of energy, tiredness
- Excessive sweating
- Trouble with sexual functioning

Less Common, but More Serious, Side Effects

Call the doctor *immediately*:

- Increased activity, rapid speech, feeling "speeded up," decreased need for sleep, being very excited or irritable (cranky)
- Seizure (fit, convulsion)

Serotonin Syndrome

A very serious side effect called *serotonin syndrome* can happen when certain kinds of medicines (including SSRI antidepressants, clomipramine, and other medicines, such as triptans for migraine headaches, buspirone, linezolid, tramadol, or St. John's wort) are taken by the same person. Very rarely, serotonin syndrome can happen at high doses of just one medicine. The early signs are restlessness, confusion, shaking, skin turning red, sweating, muscle stiffness, sweating, and jerking of muscles. If you see these symptoms, stop the medicine and send or take the youth to an emergency room right away.

Some Interactions With Other Medicines or Food

Please note that the following are only the most likely interactions with other medicines or food.

Vortioxetine can be taken with or without food.

It can be *very dangerous* to take vortioxetine at the same time as, or even within several weeks of, taking another type of medicine called a *monoamine oxidase inhibitor* (MAOI), such as selegiline (Eldepryl), phenelzine (Nardil), tranylcypromine (Parnate), or isocarboxazid (Marplan).

Taking vortioxetine with aspirin, nonsteroidal anti-inflammatory drugs (NSAIDs) (medications including ibuprofen or naproxen), or anticoagulant medications (including warfarin) increases risk of abnormal bleeding.

If given with the antiseizure medication carbamazepine, a higher dose of vortioxetine may be needed.

A lower dose of vortioxetine should be given if the patient is also taking one of the antidepressants bupropion, fluoxetine, or paroxetine.

What Could Happen if This Medicine Is Stopped Suddenly?

No known serious medical withdrawal effects occur if vortioxetine is stopped suddenly, but there may be uncomfortable feelings such as dizziness, insomnia, nausea, or nervousness, or the problem being treated may come back. Ask the doctor before stopping the medicine.

How Long Will This Medicine Be Needed?

Your child may need to keep taking the medicine for at least 6–12 months so that the emotional or behavioral problem does not come back.

What Else Should I Know About This Medicine?

In youth who have bipolar disorder or who may be at risk for bipolar disorder, any antidepressant medicine may increase the risk of hypomania or mania (excitement, agitation, increased activity, decreased sleep).

Black Box Antidepressant Warning

In 2004, an advisory committee to the FDA decided that there might be an increased risk of suicidal behavior for some youth taking medicines called *antidepressants*. In the research studies that the committee reviewed, about 3%–4% of youth with depression who took an antidepressant medicine—and 1%–2% of youth with depression who took a placebo (pill without active medicine)—talked about suicidal thoughts (thinking about killing themselves or wishing they were dead) or did something to harm themselves. This means that almost twice as many youth who were taking an antidepressant to treat their depression talked about suicide or had suicidal behavior compared with youth with depression who were taking inactive medicine. There were *no* completed suicides in any of these research studies, which included more than 4,000 children and adolescents. For youth being treated for anxiety, there was no difference in suicidal talking or behavior between those taking antidepressant medication and those taking placebo.

The FDA told drug companies to add a *black box warning* label to all antidepressant medicines. Because of this label, a doctor (or advanced practice nurse) prescribing one of these medicines has to warn youth and their families that there might be more suicidal thoughts and actions in youth taking these medicines.

On the other hand, in places where more youth are taking the newer antidepressant medicines, the number of adolescents who commit suicide has gotten smaller. Also, thinking about or attempting suicide is more common in surveys of teenagers in the community than it is in depressed youth treated in research studies with antidepressant medicine.

If a youth is being treated with this medicine and is doing well, then no changes are needed as a result of this warning. Increased suicidal talk or action is most likely to happen in the first few months of treatment with a medicine. If your child has recently started this medicine, or is about to start, then you and your doctor (or advanced practice nurse) should watch for any changes in behavior. People who are depressed often have suicidal thoughts or actions. It is hard to know whether suicidal thoughts or actions in depressed people are caused by the depression itself or by the medicine. Also, as their depression is getting better, some people talk more about the suicidal thoughts they had before but did not talk about. As young people get better from depression, they might be at higher risk of doing something about suicidal thoughts that they have had for some time, because they have more energy.

What Should a Parent Do?

1. Be honest with your child about possible risks and benefits of medicine.
2. Talk to your child about whether he or she is having any suicidal thoughts, and tell your child to come to you if he or she is having such thoughts.
3. You, your child, and your child's doctor or nurse should develop a safety plan. Pick adults whom your child can tell if he or she is thinking about suicide.
4. Be sure to tell your child's doctor, nurse, or therapist if you suspect that your child is using alcohol or drugs or if something has happened that might make your child feel worse, such as a family separation, breaking up with a boyfriend or girlfriend, someone close dying or attempting suicide, physical or sexual abuse, or failure in school.
5. Be sure that there are no guns in the home and that all medicines (including over-the-counter medicines like Tylenol) are closely supervised by an adult and kept in a safe place.
6. Watch for new or worse thoughts of suicide, self-harm, depression, anxiety (nerves), feeling very agitated or restless, being angry or aggressive, having more trouble sleeping, or anything else that you see for the first time, seems worse, or worries your child or you. If these appear, contact a mental health professional **right away.** Do not just stop or change the dose of the medicine on your own. If the problems are serious, and you cannot reach one of your clinicians, call a 24-hour psychiatry emergency telephone number or take your child to an emergency room.

Youth taking antidepressant medicine should be watched carefully by their parent(s), clinician(s) (doctor, advanced practice nurse, nurse, therapist), and other concerned adults for the first weeks of treatment. It is a good idea to have regular contact with the doctor, APN, nurse, or therapist for the first months to check for feelings of depression or sadness, thoughts of killing or harming himself or herself, and any problems with the medication. If you have questions, be sure to ask the doctor, APN, nurse, or therapist.

For more information, see http://www.parentsmedguide.org.

Notes

Use this space to take notes or to write down questions you want to ask the doctor.

_____

_____

_____

_____

_____

_____

_____

_____

_____

_____

_____

_____

From Dulcan MK, Ballard R (editors): *Helping Parents and Teachers Understand Medications for Behavioral and Emotional Problems: A Resource Book of Medication Information Handouts*, Fourth Edition. Washington, DC, American Psychiatric Publishing, 2015

Medication Information for Parents and Teachers

Ziprasidone—Geodon

General Information About Medication

Each child and adolescent is different. No one has exactly the same combination of medical and psychological problems. It is a good idea to talk with the doctor or nurse about the reasons a medicine is being used. It is very important to keep all appointments and to be in touch by telephone if you have concerns. It is important to communicate with the doctor, nurse, or therapist. An *advanced practice nurse* (APN) has additional education and training after becoming a registered nurse (RN). Your child's medication may be prescribed by a medical doctor (MD or DO) or an APN. In addition, a *physician assistant* (PA) working with a physician may prescribe certain medications. In this information sheet, "doctor" includes medical doctors as well as APNs and PAs who prescribe medication. Often a nurse (RN) will be part of the team and answer questions and give information.

It is very important that the medicine be taken exactly as the doctor instructs. However, once in a while, everyone forgets to give a medicine on time. It is a good idea to ask the doctor or nurse what to do if this happens. Do not stop or change a medicine without asking the doctor or nurse first.

If the medicine seems to stop working, it may be because it is not being taken regularly. The youth may be "cheeking" or hiding the medicine or forgetting to take it (especially at school). The doses may be too far apart or a different dose or medicine may be needed. Something at school, at home, or in the neighborhood may be upsetting the youth, or he or she may need special help for learning disabilities or tutoring. Please discuss your concerns with the doctor. **Do not just increase the dose.** It is also very important not to decrease the dose or stop the medicine without talking to the doctor first. The problem being treated may come back, or there could be uncomfortable or even dangerous results.

All medicines should be kept in a safe place, out of the reach of children, and should be supervised by an adult. If someone takes too much of a medicine, call the doctor, the poison control center, or a hospital emergency room.

Each medicine has a "generic" or chemical name. Just like laundry detergents or paper towels, some medicines are sold by more than one company under different brand names. The same medicine may be available under a generic name and several brand names. The generic medications are usually less expensive than the brand name ones. The generic medications have the same chemical formula, but they may or may not be exactly the same strength as the brand-name medications. Also, some brands of pills contain dye or other things that can cause allergic reactions. It is a good idea to talk to the doctor and the pharmacist about whether it is important to use a specific brand of medicine.

Any medicine can cause an allergic reaction. Examples are hives, itching, rashes, swelling, and trouble breathing. Even a tiny amount of a medicine can cause a reaction in patients who are allergic to that medicine. Be *sure* to talk to the doctor before restarting a medicine that has caused an allergic reaction and tell the doctor about any reactions to medicine that your child has had before.

Taking more than one medicine at the same time may cause more side effects or cause one of the medicines to not work as well. Always ask the doctor, nurse, or pharmacist before adding another

547

medicine, either prescription or bought without a prescription in a store or on the Internet. **Be sure that each doctor knows about *all* of the medicines your child is taking. Also tell the doctor about any vitamins, herbal medicines, or supplements your child may be taking.** Some of these may have side effects alone or when taken with this medication. It is a very good idea to keep a list with you of the names and doses of all medicines that your child is taking.

Everyone taking medicine should have a physical examination at least once a year.

If you think that your child may be using drugs or alcohol, please tell the doctor right away.

Pregnancy requires special care in the use of medicine. Some medicines can cause birth defects if taken by a pregnant mother. **Please tell the doctor immediately if you suspect the teenager is at risk of becoming pregnant.** The doctor may wish to discuss sexual behavior and/or birth control with your daughter.

Printed information like this applies to children and adolescents in general. If you have questions about the medicine, or if you notice changes or anything unusual, please ask the doctor or nurse. As scientific research advances, knowledge increases and advice changes. Even experts do not always agree. Many medicines have not been "approved" by the U.S. Food and Drug Administration (FDA) for use in children or use for particular problems. For this reason, use of the medicine for a problem or age group often is not listed in the *Physicians' Desk Reference*. This does not necessarily mean that the medicine is dangerous or does not work, only that the company that makes the medicine has not received permission to advertise the medicine for use in children. Companies often do not apply for this permission because it is expensive to do the tests needed to apply for approval for use in children. Once a medication is approved by the FDA for any purpose, a doctor is allowed to prescribe it according to research and clinical experience.

Note to Teachers

It is a good idea to talk with the parent(s) about the reason(s) that a medication is being used. If the parent(s) sign consent to release information, it is often helpful for you to talk with the doctor. If the parent(s) give permission, the doctor may ask you to fill out rating forms about your experience with the student's behavior, feelings, academic performance, and medication side effects. This information is very useful in selecting and monitoring medication treatment. If you have observations that you think are important, do not hesitate to share these with the student's parent(s) and treating clinicians (with parental consent).

It is very important that the medicine be taken exactly as the doctor instructs. However, everyone forgets to give a medicine on time once in a while. It is a good idea to ask the parent(s) in advance what to do if this happens. Do not stop or change the time you are giving a medicine at school without parental permission. If a medication is to be taken with food, but lunchtime or snack time changes, be sure to notify the parent(s) so appropriate adjustments can be made.

All medicines should be kept in a secure place and should be supervised by an adult. If someone takes too much of a medicine, follow your school procedure for an urgent medical problem.

Taking medicine is a private matter and is best managed discreetly and confidentially. It is important to be sensitive to the student's feelings about taking medicine.

If you suspect that the student is using drugs or alcohol, please tell the parent(s) or a school counselor right away.

Please tell the parent(s) or school nurse if you suspect medication side effects.

Modifications of the classroom environment or assignments may be useful in addition to medication. The student may need to be evaluated for additional help or a 504 plan or an Individualized Education Plan for learning problems or emotional or behavioral issues.

Any expression of suicidal thoughts or feelings or self-harm by a child or adolescent is a signal of distress and should be taken seriously. These behaviors should not be dismissed as "attention seeking." School procedures for safety issues should be followed.

What Is Ziprasidone (Geodon)?

This medicine is called an *atypical* or *second-generation antipsychotic*. It is sometimes called an *atypical psychotropic agent* or simply an *atypical*. It comes in brand name Geodon and generic capsules and a fast-acting injection (shot).

How Can This Medicine Help?

Ziprasidone is used to treat psychosis, such as in schizophrenia, mania, or very severe depression. It can reduce *positive symptoms* such as hallucinations (hearing voices or seeing things that are not there); delusions (troubling beliefs that other people do not share); agitation; and very unusual thinking, speech, and behavior. It is also used to lessen the *negative symptoms* of schizophrenia, such as lack of interest in doing things (apathy), lack of motivation, social withdrawal, and lack of energy.

Ziprasidone may be used as a *mood stabilizer* in patients with bipolar disorder or severe mood swings. It can reduce mania and may be able to help maintain a stable mood over the long term.

Sometimes ziprasidone is used to reduce severe aggression or very serious behavioral problems in young people with conduct disorder, intellectual disability, or autism spectrum disorder.

Ziprasidone may be used for behavior problems after a head injury.

This medicine is very powerful and is used to treat very serious problems or symptoms that other medicines do not help. Be patient; the positive effects of this medicine may not appear for 2–3 weeks.

How Does This Medicine Work?

Cells in the brain communicate using chemicals called *neurotransmitters*. Too much or too little of these substances in parts of the brain can cause problems. Ziprasidone works by blocking the action of two of these neurotransmitters, *dopamine* and *serotonin*, in certain areas of the brain.

How Long Does This Medicine Last?

Ziprasidone is usually taken twice a day, with food.

How Will the Doctor Monitor This Medicine?

The doctor will review your child's medical history and physical examination before starting ziprasidone. The doctor may order some blood or urine tests to be sure your child does not have a hidden medical condition that would make it unsafe to use this medicine. The doctor or nurse may measure your child's height, weight, pulse, and blood pressure before starting ziprasidone. The doctor may order other tests, such as baseline tests for blood sugar and cholesterol. An ECG (electrocardiogram or heart rhythm test) may be done before and after starting the medicine. A blood test for potassium also may be done.

Be sure to tell the doctor if anyone in the family has diabetes, high blood pressure, high cholesterol, or heart disease or if a family member died suddenly.

Before starting ziprasidone and every so often afterward, a test such as the AIMS (Abnormal Involuntary Movement Scale) may be used to check your child's tongue, legs, and arms for unusual movements that could be caused by the medicine.

After the medicine is started, the doctor will want to have regular appointments with you and your child to see how the medicine is working, to see if a dose change is needed, to watch for side effects, to see if ziprasidone is still needed, and to see if any other treatment is needed. The doctor or nurse may check your child's height, weight, pulse, and blood pressure, and watch for abnormal movements. Sometimes blood tests are needed to watch for diabetes or increased cholesterol.

What Side Effects Can This Medicine Have?

Any medicine can have side effects, including an allergy to the medicine. Because each patient is different, the doctor will monitor the youth closely, especially when the medicine is started. The doctor will work with you to increase the positive effects and decrease the negative effects of the medicine. Please tell the doctor if any of the listed side effects appear or if you think that the medicine is causing any other problems. Not all of the rare or unusual side effects are listed.

Side effects are most common after starting the medicine or after a dose increase. Many side effects can be avoided or lessened by starting with a very low dose and increasing it slowly—ask the doctor.

Allergic Reaction

Tell the doctor in a day or two (if possible, before the next dose of medicine):

- Hives
- Itching
- Rash

Stop the medicine and get *immediate* medical care:

- Trouble breathing or chest tightness
- Swelling of lips, tongue, or throat

Common, but Not Usually Serious, Side Effects

Discuss the following side effects with your child's doctor when convenient. These side effects often can be helped by lowering the dose of medicine, changing the times medicine is taken, or adding another medicine.

- Daytime sleepiness or tiredness—Do not allow your child to drive, ride a bicycle or motorcycle, or operate machinery if this happens. This problem may be lessened by taking the medicine at bedtime.
- Dry mouth—Have your child try using sugar-free gum or candy.
- Constipation—Encourage your child to drink more fluids and eat high-fiber foods; if necessary, the doctor may recommend a fiber medicine such as Benefiber or a stool softener such as Colace or mineral oil.
- Upset stomach
- Increased appetite
- Weight gain—Seek nutritional counseling; provide your child with low-calorie snacks and encourage regular exercise.

Rare, but Not Usually Serious, Side Effects

Discuss the following side effects with your child's doctor when convenient. These side effects often can be helped by lowering the dose of medicine, changing the times medicine is taken, or adding another medicine.

- Dizziness—This side effect is worse when the child stands up quickly, especially when getting out of bed in the morning; try having the child stand up slowly.
- Increased restlessness or inability to sit still
- Shaking of hands and fingers
- Decreased or slowed movement and decreased facial expressions

Less Common, but Potentially Serious, Side Effects

Call the doctor *immediately*:

- Stiffness of the tongue, jaw, neck, back, or legs
- Seizure (fit, convulsion)—This is more common in people with a history of seizures or head injury.
- Irregular heartbeat (pulse), palpitations, or fainting
- Increased thirst, frequent urination (having to go to the bathroom often), lethargy, tiredness, dizziness, and blurred vision—These could be signs of diabetes, especially if your child is overweight or there is a family history of diabetes. **Talk to a doctor within a day.**

Very Rare, but Serious, Side Effects

Go to an emergency room right away or call 911:

- Extreme stiffness or lack of movement, very high fever, mental confusion, irregular pulse rate, or eye pain
- Sudden stiffness and inability to breathe or swallow. Tell the paramedics, nurses, and doctors that the patient is taking ziprasidone. Other medicines can be used to treat this problem fast.
- Fever, skin rash, swollen lymph nodes (glands)—This can be a sign of a *very* serious drug reaction called DRESS (drug rash with eosinophilia and systemic symptoms) syndrome.

What Else Should I Know About Side Effects?

Most side effects lessen over time. If they are troublesome, talk with your child's doctor. Some side effects can be decreased by taking a smaller dose of medicine, by stopping the medicine, by changing to another medicine, or by adding another medicine.

Sometimes people who take ziprasidone gain weight. Children seem to have more problems with this than adults. This is less a problem with ziprasidone than with other atypical antipsychotics. The weight gain may be from increased appetite and from ways that the medicine changes how the body processes food. Ziprasidone may also change the way that the body handles glucose (sugar) and cause high blood sugar levels (*hyperglycemia*). People who take ziprasidone, especially those who gain a lot of weight, are at increased risk of developing *diabetes* and of having increased fats (*lipids—cholesterol and triglycerides*) in their blood. Over time, both diabetes and increased fats in the blood may lead to heart disease, stroke, and other complications. The FDA has put warnings on all atypical agents about the increased risks of hyperglycemia, diabetes, and increased blood cholesterol and triglycerides when taking one of these medicines. It is much easier to prevent weight gain than to lose weight later. When your child first starts taking ziprasidone, it is a good idea to be sure that he or she eats a well-balanced diet without "junk food" and with healthy snacks like fruits and vegetables, not sweets or fried foods. He or she should drink water or skim milk, not pop, sodas, soft drinks, or sugary juices. Regular exercise is important for maintaining a healthy weight (and may also help with sleep).

One very rare side effect that may not go away is *tardive dyskinesia* (or TD). Patients with tardive dyskinesia have involuntary movements (movements that they cannot help making) of the body, especially the mouth and tongue. The patient may look as though he or she is making faces over and over again. Jerky movements of the arms, legs, or body may occur. There may be fine, wormlike, or sudden repeated movements of the tongue, or the person may appear to be chewing something or smacking or puckering his or her lips. The fingers may look as though they are rolling something. If you notice any unusual movements, be sure to tell the doctor. The doctor may use the AIMS test to look for these movements.

Neuroleptic malignant syndrome is a very rare side effect that can lead to death. The symptoms are severe muscle stiffness, high fever, increased heart rate and blood pressure, irregular heartbeat (pulse), and sweating. It may lead to unconsciousness. If you suspect this, **call 911 or go to an emergency room right away.**

Sometimes this medicine can cause a *dystonic reaction*. This is a sudden stiffening of the muscles, most often in the jaw, neck, tongue, face, or shoulders. If this happens, and your child is not having trouble breathing, you may give a dose of diphenhydramine (Benadryl). Follow the dose instructions on the package for your child's age. This should relax the muscles in a few minutes. Then call your doctor to tell him or her what happened. If the muscles do not relax, take your child to the emergency department.

Rarely, the medicine may increase the level of *prolactin*, a natural hormone made in the part of the brain called the *pituitary*. This may cause side effects such as breast tenderness or swelling or production of milk in both boys and girls. It also may interfere with sexual functioning in teenage boys and with regular menstrual cycles (periods) in teenage girls. A blood test can measure the level of prolactin. If these side effects do not go away and are troublesome, talk with your child's doctor about substituting another medicine for ziprasidone.

Some Interactions With Other Medicines or Food

Please note that the following are only the most likely interactions other medicines or food.

Heart problems are more common if other medicines that affect the heart or antibiotics such as erythromycin are being taken also. Be sure to tell all your child's doctors and your pharmacist about all medications your child is taking.

Ziprasidone should be taken with food to improve absorption.

Carbamazepine (Tegretol) and phenytoin (Dilantin) may decrease levels of ziprasidone, making it not work as well.

It is better to limit drinks with caffeine (coffee, tea, soft drinks) because caffeine works in the opposite way from this medicine, and the positive effects might be decreased.

What Could Happen if This Medicine Is Stopped Suddenly?

Involuntary movements, or *withdrawal dyskinesias*, may appear within 1–4 weeks of lowering the dose or stopping the medicine. Usually these go away, but they can last for days to months. If ziprasidone is stopped suddenly, emotional disturbance (such as irritability, nervousness, moodiness, or oppositional behavior) or physical problems (such as stomachache, loss of appetite, nausea, vomiting, diarrhea, sweating, indigestion, trouble sleeping, trembling, or shaking) may appear. These problems usually last only a few days to a few weeks. If they happen, you should tell your child's doctor. The medicine dose may need to be lowered more slowly (tapered). Always check with the doctor before stopping a medicine.

How Long Will This Medicine Be Needed?

How long your child will need to take this medicine depends partly on the reason that it was prescribed. Some problems last for only a few months, whereas others last much longer. It is important to ask the doctor whether the medicine is still needed, especially with medicines as powerful as this one. Every few months, you should discuss with your child's doctor the reasons for using ziprasidone and whether the medicine may be stopped or the dose lowered.

What Else Should I Know About This Medicine?

There are other medicines that are used for the same kinds of problems. If your child is having bad side effects or the medicine does not seem to be working, ask the doctor if another medicine might work as well or better and have fewer side effects for your child. Each person reacts differently to medicines.

Notes

Use this space to take notes or to write down questions you want to ask the doctor.

_____

_____

_____

_____

_____

_____

_____

_____

_____

_____

_____

concerning drug dosages, schedules, routes of administration, and side effects is accurate as of the time of publication and consistent with standards set by the U.S. Food and Drug Administration and the general medical community and accepted child psychiatric practice. The information on this medication sheet does not cover all the possible uses, precautions, side effects, or interactions of this drug. For a complete listing of side effects, see the manufacturer's package insert, which can be obtained from your physician or pharmacist. As medical research and practice advance, therapeutic standards may change. For this reason and because human and mechanical errors sometimes occur, we recommend that readers follow the advice of a physician who is directly involved in their care or the care of a member of their family.

From Dulcan MK, Ballard R (editors): *Helping Parents and Teachers Understand Medications for Behavioral and Emotional Problems: A Resource Book of Medication Information Handouts*, Fourth Edition. Washington, DC, American Psychiatric Publishing, 2015

Appendix 1

Medicines With FDA Indication for Attention-Deficit/Hyperactivity Disorder (ADHD)

Stimulant Medications

Methylphenidate

Generic (IR; 3–4 hours)	Tablet Oral solution
Methylin (IR; 3–4 hours)	Tablet Chewable tablet Oral solution (grape)
Ritalin (IR; 3–4 hours)	Tablet
Ritalin SR (6–8 hours)	Wax matrix
Metadate ER (6–8 hours)	Wax matrix
Ritalin LA (8–10 hours)	Capsule with beads (sprinkle)
Metadate CD (6–8 hours)	Capsule Diffucap with beads (sprinkle)
Concerta (10–12 hours)	Oros osmotic controlled-release tablet
Generic XR (10–12 hours)	Oros osmotic controlled-release tablet
Daytrana (10–12 hours, or less if removed early)	Transdermal system (skin patch)
Quillivant XR (10–12 hours)	Oral suspension (banana)

Dexmethylphenidate

Focalin (IR; 3–4 hours)	Tablet
Generic IR (3–4 hours)	Tablet
Focalin XR (8–10 hours)	Capsule with beads (sprinkle)
Generic XR (8–10 hours)	Capsule with beads (sprinkle)

Dextroamphetamine

Dexedrine (IR; 3–5 hours)	Tablet
Generic (IR; 3–5 hours)	Tablet
Dexedrine Spansule (6–8 hours)	Capsule with particles
Dextroamphetamine ER (6–8 hours)	Capsule
ProCenta (dextroamphetamine sulfate) (3–5 hours)	Oral solution
Zenzedi (dextroamphetamine sulfate) (3–5 hours)	Tablet
Generic dextroamphetamine sulfate (3–5 hours)	Tablet
Vyvanse (12 hours)	Capsule

Mixed Salts Amphetamine	
Adderall (IR; 3–5 hours)	Tablet
Generic (IR; 3–5 hours)	Tablet
Adderall XR (10–12 hours)	Capsule with beads (sprinkle)
Generic XR (10–12 hours)	Capsule with beads (sprinkle)
Nonstimulant Medications	
Strattera (atomoxetine) (24 hours)	Capsule
Kapvay (clonidine) (24 hours when taken twice daily)	Extended-release tablets (may not be crushed)
Intuniv (guanfacine) (24 hours)	Extended-release tablets (may not be crushed)

Note. ER=extended-release; IR=immediate-release; LA=long-acting; SR=sustained-release; XR=extended-release

Appendix 2

Medicines Typically Used for Anxiety and Depression

Generic name	Brand name(s)
Alprazolam*	Xanax
Buspirone*	
Citalopram	Celexa
Clomipramine†	Anafranil
Clonazepam*	Klonopin
Desvenlafaxine	Pristiq
Diazepam*	Valium
Duloxetine	Cymbalta
Escitalopram	Lexapro
Fluoxetine	Prozac
Fluvoxamine	Luvox
Levomilnacipran	Fetzima
Lorazepam*	Ativan
Mirtazapine	Remeron
Paroxetine	Paxil, Pexeva
Sertraline	Zoloft
Venlafaxine	Effexor
Vilazodone	Viibryd
Vortioxetine	Brintellex

*Anxiety only
†Obsessive-compulsive disorder only

Appendix 3

Medicines Typically Used for Psychosis

Generic name	Brand name
Aripiprazole	Abilify
Asenapine	Saphris
Chlorpromazine	Thorazine*
Clozapine	Clozaril
Fluphenazine	Prolixin
Haloperidol	Haldol
Iloperidone	Fanapt
Loxapine	Loxitane
Lurasidone	Latuda
Olanzapine	Zyprexa
Paliperidone	Invega
Perphenazine	Trilafon*
Quetiapine	Seroquel
Risperidone	Risperdal
Thiothixene	
Trifluoperazine	
Ziprasidone	Geodon

*The medication is no longer available under this brand name, but the medication is sometimes still referred to by this name.

Appendix 4

Medicines Typically Used for Mood Stabilization or Reducing Aggression

Generic name	Brand name(s)
Aripiprazole	Abilify
Asenapine	Saphris
Carbamazepine	Carbatrol, Tegretol, Carbatrol, Epitol, Equetro, Tegretol XR
Gabapentin	Neurontin
Iloperidone	Fanapt
Lamotrigine	Lamictal
Lithium	Lithobid
Lurasidone	Latuda
Olanzapine	Zyprexa
Oxcarbazepine	Trileptal, Oxtellar XR
Paliperidone	Invega
Quetiapine	Seroquel
Risperidone	Risperdal
Topiramate	Topamax, Topiragen, Trokendi XR, Qudexy SR
Valproic acid, Divalproex sodium	Depakene, Depakote, Stavzor
Ziprasidone	Geodon

Index of Medicines
by Brand Name

*The medication is no longer available under this brand name, but the medication is sometimes still referred to by this name.